THE
BONES & JOINTS

ATLAS *of* TUMOR RADIOLOGY

PHILIP J. HODES, M.D., *Editor-in-Chief*

Sponsored by

THE AMERICAN COLLEGE OF RADIOLOGY

—*with the cooperation of:*
AMERICAN CANCER SOCIETY
AMERICAN ROENTGEN RAY SOCIETY
CANCER CONTROL PROGRAM, USPHS
EASTMAN KODAK COMPANY
JAMES PICKER FOUNDATION
RADIOLOGICAL SOCIETY OF NORTH AMERICA

THE
BONES & JOINTS

by

GWILYM S. LODWICK, M.D.

*Professor and Chairman, Department of Radiology,
University of Missouri, Columbia*

DRAWINGS BY JANE GORDON

YEAR BOOK MEDICAL PUBLISHERS · INC.
35 EAST WACKER DRIVE, CHICAGO

COPYRIGHT © 1971 BY THE AMERICAN COLLEGE OF RADIOLOGY

20 NORTH WACKER DRIVE, CHICAGO, ILLINOIS 60606

Library of Congress Catalog Card Number: 73-138830

International Standard Book Number: 0-8151-5625-1

PRINTED IN U.S.A.

Editor's Preface

IN 1960, the Committee on Radiology of the National Research Council began to consider the preparation of a tumor atlas for radiology similar in concept to the Armed Forces Institute of Pathology's "Atlas of Tumor Pathology." So successfully had the latter filled a need in pathology that it seemed reasonable to establish a similar resource for radiology. Therefore a subcommittee of the Committee on Radiology was appointed to study the concept and make recommendations.

That original committee, made up of Dr. Russell H. Morgan (Chairman), Dr. Marshall H. Brucer and Dr. Eugene P. Pendergrass, reported that a need did indeed exist and recommended that something be done about it. That report was unanimously accepted by the parent committee.

Soon thereafter, there occurred a normal change of the membership of the Committee on Radiology of the Council. This was followed by a change of the "Atlas" subcommittee, which now included Dr. E. Richard King (Chairman), Dr. Leo G. Rigler and Dr. Barton R. Young. To this new subcommittee was assigned the task of finding how the "Atlas" was to be published. Numerous avenues were explored; none seemed wholly satisfactory.

With the passing of time, it became increasingly apparent that the American College of Radiology had to be brought into the picture. It had prime teaching responsibilities; it had a Commission on Education; it seemed the logical responsible agent to launch the "Atlas." Confident of the merits of this approach, the entire Committee on Radiology of the Council became involved in focusing the attention of the American College of Radiology upon the matter.* In 1964, as the result of their persuasiveness, the Board of Chancellors of the American College of Radiology named an ad hoc committee to explore and define the scholarly scope of the "Atlas" and the probable costs. In 1965, the ad hoc committee recommended that the College sponsor and publish the "Atlas." Accordingly, an Editorial Advisory Committee was chosen to work within the Commission on Education with authority to select an Editor-in-Chief. At the same time, the College provided

---

* At that time, the Committee on Radiology included, in addition to the subcommittee, Drs. John A. Campbell, James B. Dealy, Jr., Melvin M. Figley, Hymer L. Friedell, Howard B. Latourette, Alexander Margulis, Ernest A. Mendelsohn, Charles M. Nice, Jr., and Edward W. Webster.

funds for starting the project and began representations for grants-in-aid without which the "Atlas" would never be published.

No history of the "Atlas of Tumor Radiology" would be complete without specific recording of the generous response of the several radiological societies, as well as the private and Federal granting institutions whose names appear on the title page and below among our acknowledgments. It was their tangible evidence of confidence in the project that provided everyone with enthusiasm and eagerness to achieve our goal.

The "Atlas of Tumor Radiology" includes all major organ systems. It is intended to be a systematic body of pictorial and written information dealing with the roentgen manifestations of tumors. No attempt has been made to provide an atlas equivalent of a medical encyclopedia. Nevertheless the "Atlas" is designed to serve as an important reference source and teaching file for all physicians, not radiologists alone.

The thirteen volumes of the "Atlas," to be completed in 1971-72, are: *The Hemopoietic and Lymphatic Systems,* by Gerald D. Dodd and Sidney Wallace; *The Bones and Joints,* by Gwilym S. Lodwick (published); *The Lower Respiratory Tract and Thoracic Contents,* by Roy R. Greening and J. Haynes Heslep; *The Gastrointestinal Tract,* by Arthur K. Finklestein and George N. Stein; *The Upper Urinary Tract,* by John A. Evans and Morton A. Bosniak; *The Lower Urinary Tract,* by John A. Evans and Morton A. Bosniak; *The Breast,* by David M. Witten (published); *The Head and Neck,* by Gilbert H. Fletcher and Bao-Shan Jing (published); *The Nervous System and the Eye,* by Ernest W. Wood, Juan M. Taveras and Michael S. Tenner; *The Female Reproductive System,* by G. Melvin Stevens; *The Endocrines,* by Howard L. Steinbach and Hideyo Minagi (published); *The Accessory Digestive Organs,* by Robert E. Wise; and *The Spine,* by Bernard S. Epstein.

Some overlapping of material in several volumes is inevitable, for example, tumors of the female generative system, tumors of the endocrine glands and tumors of the urinary tract. This is considered to be an asset. It assures the specialist completeness in the volume or volumes that concern him and provides added breadth and depth of knowledge for those interested in the entire series.

The broad scope of the "Atlas of Tumor Radiology" has precluded its preparation by a single or even several authors. To maintain uniformity of format, rather rigid criteria were established early. These included manner of presentation, size of illustrations, as well as style of headings, subheadings and legends. The authors were encouraged to keep the text at a minimum, freeing as much space as possible for large illustrations and meaningful legends. The "Atlas" is to be just that, an "atlas," not a series of "texts." The authors were urged, also, to keep the bibliography brief.

The selection of suitable authors for the "Atlas" was extremely difficult, and to a degree invidious. For the final choice, the Editor-in-Chief accepts full responsibility. It is but fair to record, however, that his Editorial Advisory Committee accepted his recommendations. The format of the "Atlas," too, was the choice of the Editor-in-Chief, again with the concurrence of his advisory group. Should the "Atlas of Tumor Radiology" fall short of its goals, the fault will lie with the Editor-in-Chief alone; his Editorial Advisory Committee was selfless in its dedication to the purposes of the "Atlas," rendering invaluable advice and guidance whenever asked to do so.

As medical knowledge expands, medical concepts change. In medicine, the written word considered true today may not be so tomorrow. The text of the "Atlas," considered true today, therefore may not be true tomorrow. What may not change, what may ever remain true, may be the illustrations of the "Atlas of Tumor Radiology." Their legends may change as our conceptual levels advance. But the validity of the roentgen findings there recorded should endure. Thus, if the fidelity with which the roentgenograms have been reproduced is of superior order, the illustrations in the "Atlas" should long serve as sources for reference no matter what revisions of the text become necessary with advancing medical knowledge.

ACKNOWLEDGMENTS

The American College of Radiology, its Commission on Education, the Editorial Advisory Committee, the authors and the Editor-in-Chief wish to acknowledge their grateful appreciation:

1. For the grants-in-aid so willingly and repeatedly provided by The American Cancer Society, The American Roentgen Ray Society, The Cancer Control Program, National Center for Chronic Disease Control (USPHS Grant No. 59481), The James Picker Foundation, and the Radiological Society of North America.

2. For the superb glossy print reproductions provided by the Radiography Markets Division, Eastman Kodak Company. Special mention must be made of the sustained interest of Mr. George R. Struck, its Assistant Vice-President and General Manager. We applaud particularly Mr. William S. Cornwell, Technical Associate and Editor Emeritus of Kodak's *Medical Radiography and Photography*, as well as his associates, Mr. Charles C. Heckman and Mr. Stanley J. Pietrzkowski and others in the Photo Service Division, whose expertise provided the "Atlas" with its incomparable photographic reproductions.

3. To Year Book Medical Publishers, for their personal involvement with and judicious guidance in the many problems of publication. There were occasions when the publisher questioned the quality of certain illustrations. Almost always the judgment of the authors and the Editor-in-Chief prevailed because of the importance of the original roentgenograms and the singular fidelity of their reproduction.

4. To the Associate Editors, particularly Mrs. Anabel I. Janssen, whose talents lightened the burden of the Editor-in-Chief and helped establish the style of presentation of the material.

5. To the Staff of the American College of Radiology, especially Messrs. William C. Stronach, Otha Linton, Keith Gundlach and William Melton, for continued conceptual and administrative efforts of unusual competence.

Of particular note is the fact that all of the cases contained in this volume come from the Armed Forces Institute of Pathology. As the author has included their respective A.F.I.P. registry numbers, this volume of the "Atlas," to a degree, becomes an extension of that tumor registry.

Dr. Lodwick's interest in computers has long been known. The manner in which he employs this electronic device in the diagnosis of bone tumors will prove a stimulating experience.

Important though these facets may be, of most importance we consider the glossary of descriptive terms developed by Dr. Lodwick. His beautiful drawings and their related parent roentgenograms add a new dimension and new meaning to terms ordinarily used to describe the roentgen changes observed in bone tumors. Indeed, we believe that this volume, with its photographic glossary, may serve as a common verbal bond for all interested in the roentgen manifestation of bone diseases.

The "Atlas of Tumor Radiology" is being published in a time when massive scientific effort is taking place at an unprecedented rate and on an unprecedented scale. We hope that our final product will provide an authoritative summary of our current knowledge of the roentgen manifestations of tumors.

PHILIP J. HODES
Editor-in-Chief

*Jefferson Medical College of
Thomas Jefferson University*

Editorial Advisory Committee

HARRY L. BERMAN   VINCENT P. COLLINS   E. RICHARD KING
            LEO G. RIGLER   PHILIP RUBIN

Author's Preface

THIS VOLUME of the Atlas of Tumor Radiology has at once been fun to prepare, instructive, a chore, a millstone, a challenge, and a professional risk. The tests of its value will be its effectiveness in providing earlier correct diagnosis and better patient care. If these are achieved, the work will have been worth the effort.

Excepting in classic lesions, bone tumors generally are difficult to evaluate. They are rare, few radiologists seeing more than one in a year. Their shifting histologic classification too, has added difficulties and a degree of uncertainty. Indeed, broad differences in opinion exist among pathologists even today. Happily, there will arise few occasions in this volume when genealogy will be questioned. Should such questions arise, the original Armed Forces Institute of Pathology (AFIP) accession numbers will provide easy identification of all parent material for critical review.

Part 1 of this volume illustrates the public model of bone disease and also discusses a system employing computer techniques that has proved effective in predicting the histologic diagnosis of bone tumors. The model includes a glossary of terms with appropriate diagrams and roentgenograms that provide the language used by the radiologist or the computer in establishing a diagnosis. Part 1 also includes the grading principles and the decision tree, which formalizes the logic of bone tumor diagnosis. The decision tree, in effect, contains most of the rules of bone tumor diagnosis.

The key element missing in the presentation will be the probability matrix. It was too voluminous to be included; also it seemed less likely to stand the erosions of time and experience. Those interested in obtaining more information concerning the matrix may do so by contacting me.

Parts 2 to 8 comprise the atlas portion of the volume. Here one will find ample description and application of the principles laid down in Part 1. Extremely important is the fact that the atlas, per se, can stand alone without reference to Part 1. The illustrations are many; the legends self-explanatory. Those willing to master Part 1, however, will find much satisfaction in its applications to Parts 2 to 8. Also, it will heighten one's perception and appreciation of all roentgen findings in all bone lesions irrespective of cause.

In Parts 2 to 8 of the atlas, each major tumor category successively demonstrates first the classic radiologic patterns, then the less typical, and finally patterns seemingly totally unrelated. The presentation is consonant with the wide range of radiologic patterns that may exist for any given type of bone tumor. Having learned well the lessons included in Part 1, one can approach the challenges of less typical tumor patterns with assurance and comfort.

A work as complex as this one cannot be the effort of a single individual, but rather it is that of a team which has been focusing on the problem for many years. Without question the most brilliant, dedicated and informed person in this effort has been Dr. Lent C. Johnson, head of the Orthopedic Registry at the Armed Forces Institute of Pathology in Washington, D.C. Happily do I acknowledge him as my teacher, critic, advisor and confidant since the early 1950s. Indeed, without access to his laboratories and his Orthopedic Registry, this work would have been impossible.

Any effort to improve diagnosis must be based on a sound foundation in gross and microscopic pathology. With his superior competence in radiographic and histologic interpretation, Dr. Johnson has provided this foundation. Equally important has been his uncommon objectivity, an ability to look at a problem from a fresh point of view without the constraint and inhibition of the past. This, Lent Johnson has repeatedly provided me.

Our early efforts in modeling neoplastic disease of bone were closely collaborative. Through time and distance, they have diverged and gotten slightly out of phase. Appropriately, Dr. Johnson is writing his own contribution to this fascinating subject. Though published separately, it will provide a background of support for much that appears in this volume.

Credit is due also to Col. William Thompson, a former director of the Registry of Radiologic Pathology at the Armed Forces Institute. I am particularly grateful to Comdr. Elias Theros, present director of the Registry, whose encouragement and help did much to lighten my burden.

For more than eight years this work has been supported by a grant from the National Cancer Institute of the National Institutes of Health (USPHS Grant No. CA-06263). A special fellowship from the Institute of General Medical Science (USPHS Grant No. 1-F3-GM-35,853-01) for a year abroad was also of inestimable value since it gave me the time to develop the sequential logic of the decision tree, and to formulate the Limited Bayes Concept in computer diagnosis.

In the early and mid-1960s additional intellectual major support was received from Dr. Cosmo Haun, Dr. Arch Templeton, Dr. Daniel Brunk, Dr. Lee Lusted and Dr. James Lehr, now director of Radiology Computer Research. Each in his own way provided knowledge and inspiration without which our efforts at computerization would have foundered. Mr. Arch Turner deserves mention for his effort in systematically organizing the Truth Table approach to grading. To their accomplishments have been added those of Dr. Peter Reichertz, until recently director of Radiology Computer Research.

Special recognition is due the Editor-in-Chief, Dr. Philip J. Hodes, who worked valiantly to bring the volume to fruition. Dr. Hodes always reflected deep personal concern in the progress of this work, invariably was positive and offered excellent advice.

Many others must be mentioned, especially Marjorie C. Tolan, R.T., for her organizational skills; Ann Donaldson of London, England, for her careful and consistent effort in collecting and organizing cases; Merle Wolfmeier for her dedication in manuscript preparation; Mrs. Jane Gordon for her meticulous preparation of illustrative material; Mr. William Cornwell of Eastman Kodak for his magnificent photographs; and last, Dr. Vernon Peterson, NIGMS research trainee in radiology, for his invaluable help in organizing and preparing the final manuscript.

Finally, I would say that the original concept of writing this book resulted from encouragement by my professor of earlier years, Dr. Carl Gillies, whose knowledge of the radiology of bone disease is truly profound.

GWILYM S. LODWICK

Dedicated to TONY

PART 1
Radiologic Concepts, 1

PART 2
Giant Cell and Cystic Tumors, 83

PART 3
Fibrous Tumors, 145

PART 4
Cartilaginous Tumors, 205

PART 5
Osseous Tumors, 257

PART 6
Round Cell Tumors, 337

PART 7
Tumors of the Joints and Soft Tissues, 401

PART 8
Miscellaneous Tumors, 413
Contributors of AFIP Radiographs, 436

Index, 443

PART 1

Radiologic Concepts

A. Logical Diagnosis

WHEN WE SEE a familiar image in the roentgenogram, what is our approach to diagnosis? Do we use a formalized analytic procedure? Very seldom, because identification is usually automatic and so instantaneous that it is difficult later to be objective about the individual components of the image. Diagnosis in medicine depends heavily on automatic recognition. Unfortunately, when a disease is infrequently seen, few individuals will have had sufficient experience to become really skilled, in which instance automatic recognition is no longer possible and a systematized examination and review of findings is necessary. This is especially true with primary neoplasms of bone, whose incidence is about two cases per 100,000 population per year. With this low rate, assuming equal distribution of material, each radiologist should see a single primary bone tumor about every other year. It is impossible to develop proficient automatic recognition with this kind of exposure.

Because bone tumors are difficult to diagnose but more because the contrast in bone is ideal for radiographic research, an effort has been made to automate the recognition of bone lesions through application of decision theory and computer techniques. The long-range goal is totally automated recognition. At the moment, some of the elements of this decision scheme which relate particularly to computer-mediated scanning await further technologic advances, and in the immediate future, completely automatic computer-mediated diagnosis is unlikely. Even more fundamental is the question of how to solve the problem of automated image analysis of radiographic images without learning what and how to scan. Automatic recognition using the radiologist's built-in computer is highly successful, and in the face of success achieved without special techniques, the time and effort to develop the kinds of criteria required for computer diagnosis may not have seemed necessary. However, to solve the problem of what to scan, we have developed an orderly sequence of steps for systematizing the acquisition and management of data derived from the radiographic image (Fig. **1**). These steps include:

1. Development of a model with which it is possible to derive both qualitative and quantitative data from the radiographic image and record them in three dimensions.
2. Application of the model to a large enough series of cases to acquire statistically valid data.
3. Elimination of redundancy in the model through statistical testing of signs and symptoms.

4. Development of decision schemes to compare information from an undiagnosed lesion with stored data acquired from application of the model to known material and from personal experience.

Depending on the kinds of information and the kinds of decision schemes, the result of computer evaluation may be reported either as a single diagnosis, which theoretically may by definition be the only possible one, such as growth rate IA (p. 62), or as a differential diagnosis listed by order of probability, such as Ewing's sarcoma .95, reticulum cell sarcoma .05.

Automatic image analysis carried out in the built-in computer of the radiologist has been programed by heredity and provided a probability matrix by environment. It seems unnecessary for the radiologist to develop a logical decision scheme for instantaneous recognition; it is preprogramed in his computer. However, in developing decision schemes for computer-assisted diagnosis, we have found it necessary to examine concepts carefully and to record them with crystalline clarity. Further, we do not have the resource of logic which was programed by heredity, but must develop our own. The formulation of man-built logical decision schemes, with the frequent

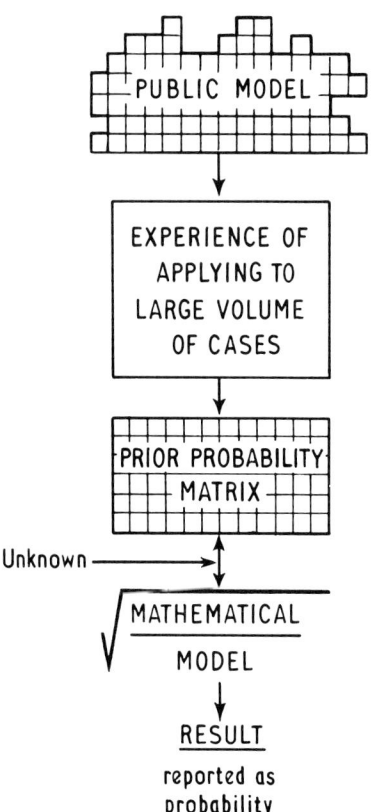

Figure 1.—Elements of the diagnostic system. In image analysis, the "public model" is the language for communicating the features of the image. The frequency of each image feature in the model is obtained by experience and is stored as probability in the matrix. The mathematical model carries out the function of comparing the unknown with the known. In this application the Limited Bayes Concept is employed, which is a sequential decision scheme consisting of decision trees which utilize Boolean logic and Bayesian analysis for those diagnostic elements which have a substantial measure of uncertainty.

testing and retesting required for perfection, results in the development of basically simple decision pathways. When joined with the statistically valid data acquired from large numbers of cases, such man-made decision schemes can be exceedingly useful to the inexperienced radiologist. However, if the data relating to the frequency of the various signs and symptoms of disease are clearly presented and are assimilated by the radiologist, he may soon be able to apply his own hereditary programing to make decisions. This, in a sense, is what this book hopes to offer: What are the components of the radiographic image most useful to diagnosis? What is the frequency rate of these components in the various kinds of bone lesions? What are the best techniques for synthesizing the diagnosis from these components which comprise the image?

This is not to say that hereditary programing accompanied by a matrix of statistically sound information results in the best possible world. True, our minds are capable of effectively dealing with large masses of data, sorting out the important facts and arriving at the correct diagnosis in a surprising number of cases. However, in dealing with three or more kinds of data simultaneously, we often are confused; also, we can overlook or forget important information, to the extent that we may fail even to consider the right diagnosis. The decision schemes programed in the computer are probably cruder than those of the human mind. But the properly programed computer cannot forget, and it also is capable of handling an almost infinite number of variables with mathematical accuracy and, if implemented by a large enough data base, with statistical validity. There is indeed a strong case for symbiotic relationship between man and machine. Each element of this man–machine team has its faults and its virtues which fortunately complement those of the other. For this reason, even though completely automated image analysis will undoubtedly be accomplished in the future, the best possible diagnosis will require that questionable cases be reviewed by the radiologist. Hence, for the forseeable future, there will be a continuing need for this book, or better ones, to assist the human computer in the logic of decision-making.

B. The Public Model of Neoplastic Disease of Bone

TO EXAMINE any concept in detail, particularly if it be a concept of the real world, one good method is to create a model of that concept. To build a model, one must identify all of its components, define them, develop their interrelationships and assess the degree to which a model built from these components resembles the real world. Since the real world is usually a variable and dynamic process, the components of the model must reflect both qualitative and quantitative information of this order. If the model is to be useful to individuals other than its architects, it must be so skillfully defined and designed that its structure and use are understandable by others. What has been a personal model then becomes a public model. Because we have found the modeling concept essential to our study of bone disease, particularly with respect to computer-assisted diagnosis, and feel that the inherent organizational unity of a good model is a proper vehicle for any serious student to understand the concepts of diagnosing bone disease, we have elected to present this analysis of radiographic image information in the form of a model. The success of this concept will depend largely on the extent to which the model is "public."

We have built our model around the concept that it should describe any solitary lesion of bone. We have not attempted to model the generalized and multiple lesions of the skeletal system or to deal in more than a general way with the lesions which exclusively involve the soft tissues external to bone. This particular model is designed to reflect only alterations in structure which are visible to the human eye in the standard high-quality radiographic presentation of the diseased part. Only a single example of tomography and of angiographic analysis is included. Unless otherwise noted, structure is assumed to be within the range of normal expected for the age and sex of the patient in question.

The basic image which we are modeling consists of photographic reflections of a range of densities varying from those of cortical bone at one end of the spectrum to fat at the other. The modeled disease process consists of variations of *expected* density due to alterations in the normal structure caused by the disease. These density variations are affected by (1) the addition to or removal of normal structure which consists of mineral salts that absorb x-rays, (2) the differential replacement of normal tissues by tissues of different density or organization pattern (such as fat invaded by fibrous tissue), or (3) absolute enlargement of the part due directly or indirectly to the presence of new tissue. The pathologic cause of these structural alterations may be classified as (*a*) destruction or removal of bone mediated through osteoclastic activity (regardless of the kind of stimulus), (*b*) replacement of one kind of normal tissue by another, especially the production or addition of reparative new bone mediated through osteoblastic activity (regardless of the kind of stimulus), (*c*) deposition of mineral salts in organic matrices contained in neoplastic tissues (the degree of resemblance between radiographic patterns of reparative and neoplastic bone formation will depend on differences in the structural organization observable in such areas of increased density), (*d*) the exact location of the tumor relative to existing structures, a very important parameter of change, and (*e*) the factor of age. Although not a kind of information directly obtained from the radiographic examination, age can be extremely important in explaining variations in patterns of disease and on occasion has a direct bearing on diagnosis.

For purposes of studying diagnosis and evaluating growth rate, we have assembled a protocol for the collection of pertinent radiographic information. Described below as an illustrated dictionary of terminology, it has been applied to each case in our study. It contains all of the general classes of information which we have found important for evaluation of a solitary tumor. It is sufficiently detailed to record all qualitative information which we use in computer diagnosis of bone lesions, and it can record substantially more quantitative information than we have found possible to use. As of now, the protocol records nearly all of the subtleties which we have observed in many years of clinical practice in analyzing such lesions, but undoubtedly further criteria will be needed particularly as its application is extended to other kinds of disease. The last page of the protocol (p. 67) lists 50 specific histologic diagnoses, including many not pertinent to this Atlas.

There is an additional list of 10 lesions infrequently observed in bone or periosseous soft tissues which are (1) nonneoplastic diseases, (2) neoplasms still under study or so rare as to be incompletely formulated, and (3) a few wastebasket categories.

Early studies of diagnosis and grading of growth rate in relation to computer-assisted diagnosis were limited to nine primary types of lesions, from which the basic radiographic protocol and descriptive terminology for bone tumors were developed. The protocol represents the content and organization of the public model of solitary neoplastic lesions of bone as of December, 1969. A public model seems to be ever-changing as it is modified in the light of experience.

Most of the components of the public model are illustrated in the Dictionary. The description also of each tumor illustrated in this Atlas follows the organization and terminology of the protocol. A careful study of these illustrations and their descriptions should clear up uncertainties relative to the definitions and application of the descriptive elements.

Illustrated Dictionary of Terminology

Above all else is the importance of a uniform code of descriptive terms. Common terms such as "flocculent," "fleck," "solid," "lumpy," "sunburst" and "laminated" must mean absolutely the same to all concerned with bone tumors. This glossary of terms has taken years to develop and is carefully described, and demonstrated in the text for the illustrations. Whereas reference will be made to our computer method of diagnosis, it will be done in such manner as to emphasize the importance and meaning of descriptive terms. The literature contains the details of the manner in which we arrive at a diagnosis using the computer. It is not reproduced here for obvious reasons.

The reader will find the "differential diagnosis" as well as the "probability index" of the diagnoses suggested by the computer for each illustration. The importance of the probability index will become obvious as the text is studied and analyzed.

The subject materials and the order in which they are presented are extracted directly from the radiographic protocol which is used in the research analysis of each case. A copy of the total protocol can be obtained from the author. All data in the protocol can be recorded on four 80-column Hollerith cards, for input into the computer. The card numbers for each section are shown in the heading, and the numbers in parentheses represent the column numbers required to record the illustrated data on that particular card. Where on-line teleprocessing is available through a visual display unit, the data can be entered directly by interactive communication between the user and the computer.

In this volume, in several instances elements present in the research protocol have been omitted because they are not important to explaining the model.

I. Identification
 (1–3)   Source____ ____ ____
 (4–9)   Patient Number
 ____ ____-____ ____-____ ____
 (10)   Examination Number (Circle One)
         1 2 3 4 5 6 7 8 9 0

(11)   Material Used
       1____Original Film
       2____Transparency
       3____Photograph
       4____Drawing

(12–13) Patient's Age ____ ____ Years

(14)   Age is
       1____Known
       2____An Estimate

INFLUENCE OF AGE ON DIAGNOSIS

Age as a factor in diagnosis could be disregarded entirely if each kind of tumor were reflected in such a completely typical radiographic pattern that it could be recognized on sight. Some tumors are indeed that typical. An osteosarcoma tends to look like an osteosarcoma regardless of whether it occurs at age 6 or 60. The same may be said for parosteal sarcoma, although it is unlikely to be seen at age 60. Parenthetically, one wonders what happens to many of the so highly characteristic benign or slowly growing lesions which we see in the younger age group, because certainly many of these are not discovered or treated. In this context we refer not only to the nonossifying fibroma, the fibroxanthoma and the cortical defect but also to some of the mildly aggressive lesions such as chondroblastoma and chondromyxoid fibroma. Almost certainly, with the passage of time, many of these lesions must stop growing and heal spontaneously.

On the other hand, several types of bone tumors have their peak age incidence at about 35 years, such as the primary fibrosarcomas and chondrosarcomas, which are seldom seen in a younger age group. However, the radiographic patterns of fibrosarcoma and chondrosarcoma in bone do not differ appreciably in different age groups, so that the influence of age in the diagnosis of these two specific lesions is not likely to be great.

Age becomes important when histologically distinct tumors have quite similar radiographic patterns. An example is Ewing's sarcoma and reticulum cell sarcoma, particularly as they are found in a spongy bone such as the ilium. In this situation, where the periosteum does not normally react with the vigorous production of periosteal new bone, the principal findings relate to destruction and proliferation within spongy bone which itself is of relatively low density. Where the distinguishing features provided by periosteal response in long bones are not present in flat bone, the radiologist is obliged to depend more heavily on the age of the patient as an additional clue to the probability of a specific diagnosis.

In short, in deciding on a specific diagnosis, the radiologist should depend primarily on the radiographic cues at his disposal. When such cues do not permit a satisfactory differentiation, one reaches for another kind of evidence, such as age of the patient. If an osteosarcoma looks like a osteosarcoma, it should not be called something else because of age; but if one cannot distinguish between two lesions on radiographic grounds, age can be very helpful in making a logical decision.

KINDS OF CHANGE IN THE RADIOGRAPH (LOCATION, SIZE, SHAPE)

LOCATION.—The exact location of a primary tumor in the skeletal system is of great importance for two reasons: (1) location is at times critical in predicting histologic type because of differences of natural incidence, and (2) differences of location may be of great importance in the assessment of growth rate.

II. LOCATION IN BODY
    A. (15–16) Bone Primarily Involved
        01_____Calcaneus
        02_____Carpal
        03_____Clavicle
        04_____Femur
        05_____Fibula
        06_____Humerus
        07_____Ilium
        08_____Ischium
        09_____Mandible
        10_____Maxilla
        11_____Metacarpal
        12_____Metatarsal
        13_____Patella
        14_____Pubis
        15_____Radius
        16_____Rib
        17_____Sacrum
        18_____Scapula
        19_____Skull
        20_____Spine, Cervical
        21_____Spine, Thoracic
        22_____Spine, Lumbar
        23_____Spine, Sacral
        24_____Spine, Coccygeal
        25_____Tarsal (except Calcaneus)
        26_____Tibia

          27____Ulna
          28____Sternum
          29____Phalanx

Kind of bone related to histologic type.—There is a naturally occurring incidence rate for each kind of tumor within any bone. For example, there is a high rate of incidence for osteosarcoma in the femur, particularly the distal segment. In contrast, the incidence rate for this most common of all primary malignant bone tumors in a vertebra is extraordinarily low. A very rare tumor such as adamantinoma occurs in only a few bones, the tibia, fibula, femur, humerus, radius and ulna and, in these, only in the distal shaft and metaphysis. In the rest of the skeleton adamantinoma is unknown. The frequency rates of the many kinds of primary bone lesions discussed here fall somewhere between those of osteosarcoma and adamantinoma, but the predilection of a tumor for a particular bone may vary greatly, and for this reason location of a tumor in a specific bone of the skeletal system may itself be useful in arriving at a diagnosis, or even in predicting behavior. The probability table (which may be obtained from the author) shows the relative frequency of each of the many tumors in the various bones of the skeletal system. It is based on information from several large collections but is provisional, because future experience will inevitably create many changes.

Notation of the status of the growth plate requires no comment here.

    B. (17) Status of Growth Plate in
              Involved Region
              1____Open
              2____Fused
    C. (18) Axial Position of Center
              1____Central
              2____Eccentric
              3____Cortex
              4____Parosteal
              5____Joint

In the long axis of a bone, especially tubular bones, the center of the lesion may be defined as *central* if it lies on the exact central axis of the bone; *eccentric* if the center of the tumor is to one side of the central axis yet lying between the inner surfaces of the cortex; *cortical* if the center of the tumor lies within the substance of the cortex, and *parosteal* if the center of the lesion is in the soft tissues external to bone (Fig. **2**). The location of a tumor defined by these parameters is of great importance for several reasons. First, this kind of classification accomplishes an excellent reduction of data; that is, by sub-

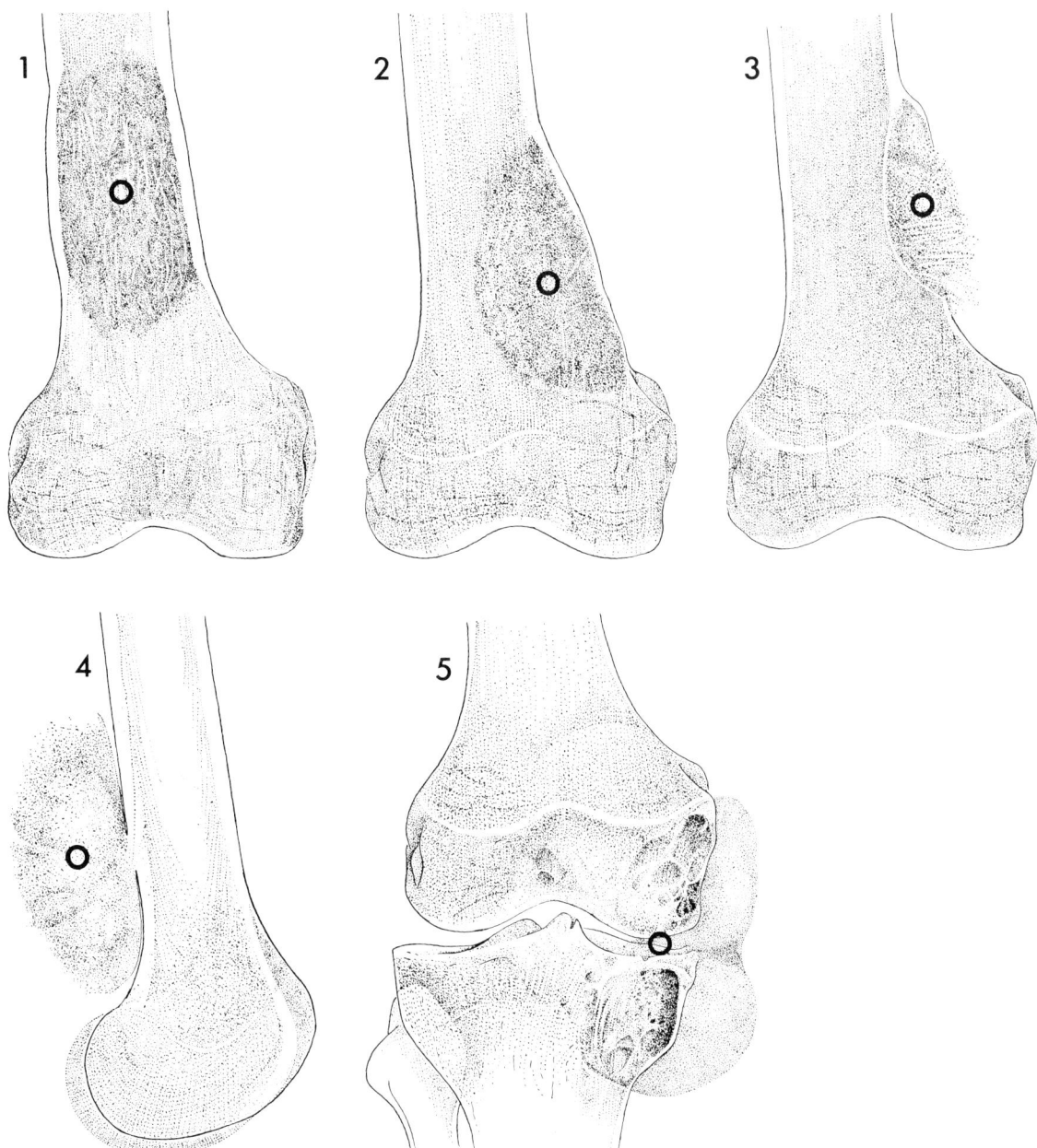

Figure 2.—Axial position of center of the tumor. **1**, central; **2**, eccentric; **3**, cortical; **4**, parosteal; **5**, in joint. The location of the *center* of a tumor is of great importance in estimating histologic type. Diagnosis is a process of data reduction. In the diagnosis of bone disease, substantial data reduction (or elimination of histologic categories) is accomplished by locating the center of the lesion.

dividing tumors into groups, the number of possible diagnoses for any one area is sharply reduced. Second, the techniques for evaluating tumors centered in bone must be managed differently from those for tumors centered in the soft tissues. For example, some tumors invariably fall in the parosteal location, such as myositis ossificans, parosteal chondroma, osteochondroma and parosteal sarcoma; others are invariably found within bone, such as non-ossifying fibroma, bone cysts, chondroblastoma and chondromyxoid fibroma. Yet other kinds of lesions such as chondrosarcoma, fibrosarcoma, osteosarcoma and osteoblastoma may be found in any of the four locations. For assessment of rate of growth, discussed later, it is enough to say here that the rate of growth in the totally parosteal lesion is most difficult to assess radiographically.

    D. (19) Is There Tumor Outside of Bone
                    1_____Yes
                    2_____No
    E. (20) Estimated Fraction (in ninths) of
                  Tumor Outside of Bone (leave blank
                  if not estimable)
                  _____/9
    F. (21) Edge of Extra-Osseous Mass
                  1_____Sharply Defined and/or
                           Encapsulated
                  2_____Ill-Defined

When a tumor is accompanied by moth-eaten or permeated patterns of bone destruction, it is automatically assumed that the cortex is totally penetrated by the tumor, regardless of whether the tumor is centered in the medullary canal, in the cortex or parosteally. With the geographic pattern of bone destruction, judgment as to whether there is tumor outside of bone is based on the presence either of totally penetrated cortex or of a soft tissue mass outside of the cortex, or both. When a tumor within bone has caused expansion of the cortex but apparently has been successfully encapsulated by the expanded shell, the tumor is regarded as being still within bone.

A rough estimation of these relative proportions of a tumor inside and outside of bone is expressed in ninths. In the instance of a parosteal tumor which lies totally in the soft tissues, the estimated fractions would be 9/9ths. In some instances a parosteal tumor will extend inward through the cortex to involve the medullary space.

When the edge of the extraosseous tumor can be clearly seen, an estimation of sharp definition or encapsulation may be made. In many instances, even with a slowly growing lesion, the interface between the tumor front and the normal soft tissues may be difficult to define. The distinction between sharply defined and ill-defined tumor tissue interface has not been found to be of great significance in diagnosis.

    G. (22) Paget's Disease in Involved Bone
          1____Yes
          2____No

  The presence of Paget's disease in a bone involved by neoplasm has considerable impact on the diagnosis of tumor type. For example, the pattern of growth which usually would pass for a fibrosarcoma in normal bone is more likely to represent a rapidly growing osteosarcoma in the presence of Paget's disease.

III. LOCATION IN RELATION TO TUBULAR BONE

A.

	Center of Lesion—Check one (23-24)	Extends into—Check as Many as Applicable	Fraction Within Segment
Adjacent Bone		(25) 1	(26) /9
Joint Space	01	(27) 1	(28) /9
Articular Cortex	02	(29) 1	
Tuberosity or Trochanter	03	(30) 1	(31) /9
Epiphysis	04	(32) 1	(33) /9
Growth Plate	05	(34) 1	
Metaphysis			(35) /9
Peripheral 1/3	06	(36) 1	
Middle 1/3	07	(37) 1	
Central 1/3	08	(38) 1	
Shaft			(39) /9
Distal 1/3	09	(40) 1	
Middle 1/3	10	(41) 1	
Proximal 1/3	11	(42) 1	

B. (43) End of Bone
    1____Proximal
    2____Distal

Location in specific sites within individual bones.—The specific anatomic sites in long bones include the joint and adjacent bone, cortex, the epiphysis, epiphysial plate or line, the metaphysis, and the shaft, both proximally and distally (Fig. 3). The rules for logic in diagnosis employ these anatomic subdivisions to a significant extent. For example, (1) chondroblastoma in a long bone is never diagnosed without involvement of the epiphysis. (2) In contrast, giant cell tumor always involves the metaphysis. When the epiphysial plate is still open, the giant cell tumor involves bone up to the metaphysial side of the plate. When the plate is fused, this tumor almost always involves the epiphysis as well, and often part of the subchondral articular cortex; when the plate is open, giant cell tumor destroys bone up to

The Public Model / 15

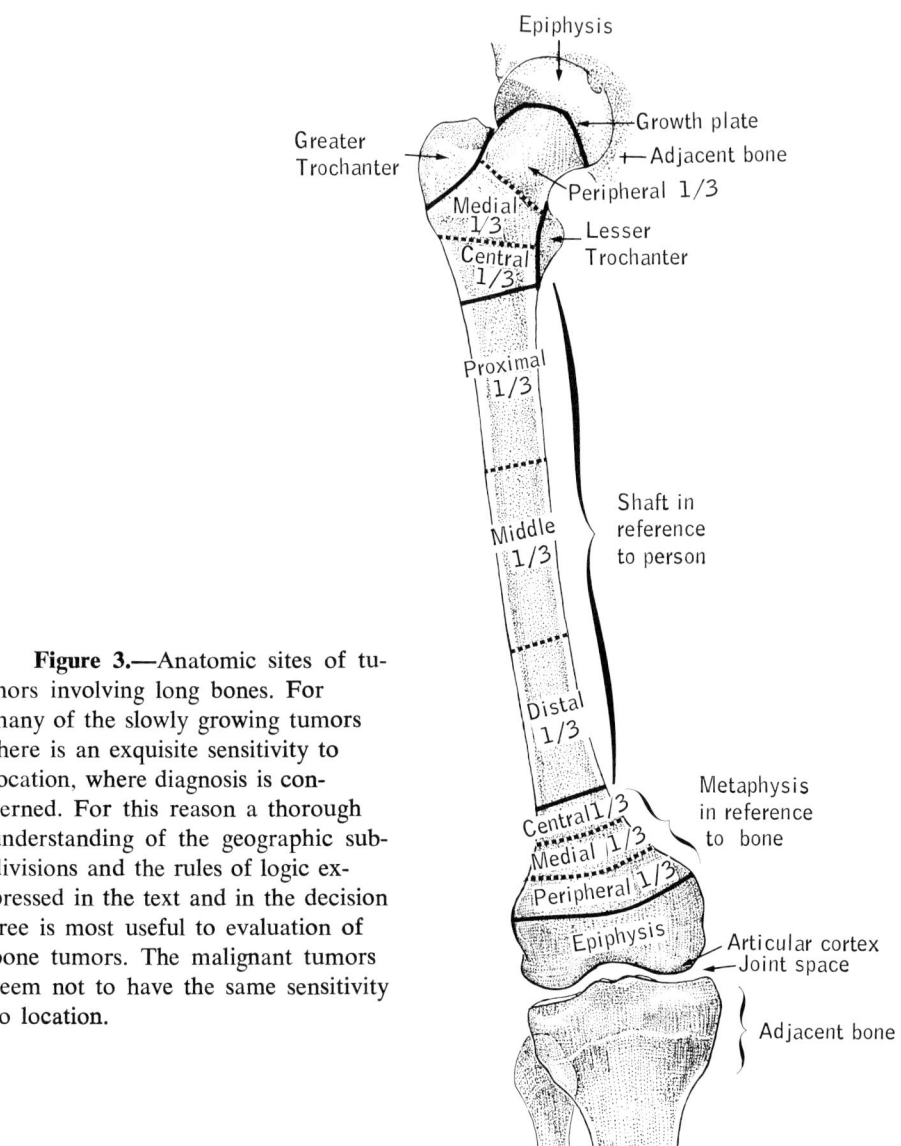

Figure 3.—Anatomic sites of tumors involving long bones. For many of the slowly growing tumors there is an exquisite sensitivity to location, where diagnosis is concerned. For this reason a thorough understanding of the geographic subdivisions and the rules of logic expressed in the text and in the decision tree is most useful to evaluation of bone tumors. The malignant tumors seem not to have the same sensitivity to location.

the plate. (3) The osteochondroma in long bones is invariably found parosteally on the metaphysial side of the plate. (4) Chondromyxoid fibroma nearly always involves the metaphysis of a long bone, although this rule may not hold in some other tubular bones, such as the rib. (5) Certain of the common benign tumors such as benign cortical defect, nonossifying fibroma and fibroxanthoma are found principally in the metaphysis and occasionally in the shaft. Almost invariably a segment of normal bone separates these three from the epiphysial plate or epiphysis. Other rare lesions, such as adamantinoma, are confined to a particular metaphysis and shaft of certain bones. Although most of the remaining primary lesions have favorite locations, they do not follow the rules of diagnosis with the same degree of exactitude as the lesions mentioned.

In the flat bones the anatomic subdivisions are less well observed and defined, and therefore location in these lesions is of less diagnostic significance than in long bones. Certain tumors may be related to specific areas, such as the special dental tumors (ameloblastoma, dentigerous cysts) in the mandible and maxilla.

Certain *special locations* in the skeletal system, particularly in those relating to the reflections and attachments of the joint capsule, have particular diagnostic importance. When erosive or destructive changes are observed at the site of capsular attachment, a disease of synovial origin can be postulated. Similarly, when a primary lesion involves a paranasal sinus a tumor of epithelial origin is of the highest order of precedence.

C. (44) Number of Quadrants of
Circumference Involved
1.____
2.____
3.____
4.____

The *number of quadrants of circumference involved* relates principally

Figure 4.—Quadrants of circumference involved by tumor. Unpublished data have shown a strong correlation between long-term survival and involvement of only one quadrant of a long bone.

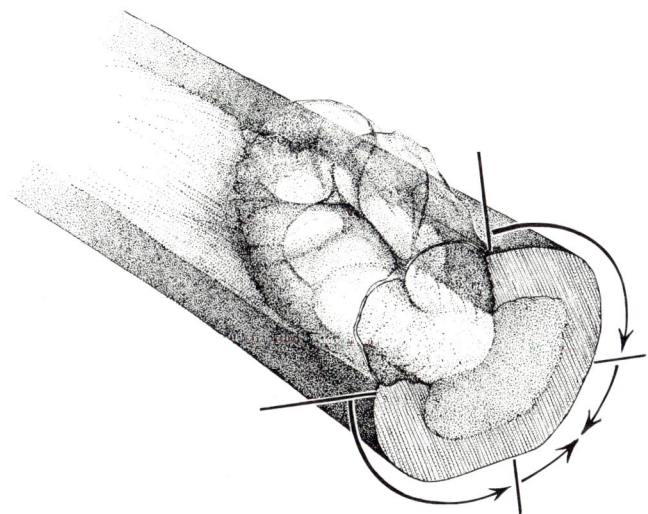

to long bones (Fig. **4**). In a study of material from the Codman Registry carried out many years ago, tumors which involved only one quadrant had a startlingly higher rate of five-year survival than tumors which involved two, three, or four quadrants. This group included not only tumors which arose within bone but a substantial number of parosteal lesions as well.

IV. LOCATION WITHIN SPECIAL BONES

A. Calcaneus
   Pelvis
   Mandible
   Scapula

	Center of Lesion Check One (45)	Extends into- Check as Many as Applicable	Fraction Within Segment
Epiphysis or Apophysis	1 ___	(46) 1 ___	(47) /9
Growth Plate	2 ___	(48) 1 ___	
Metaphysis Analogue	3 ___	(49) 1 ___	(50) /9

Location within Special Bones.—This study is intended to permit accurate evaluation of the significance of locations of the various tumors in specific bones (Fig. **5**). It is commonly thought that giant cell tumor is always found in juxtaposition to a growth plate or involving the metaphysis analogue. In my experience this has been true.

The rules relating histologic type to location in the epiphysis, growth plate and metaphysis in the tubular bones are reliable and very useful in tumor diagnosis. Their reliability in the flat bones is less well known. In the interest of developing further knowledge, the important apophyses and synchondroses are shown in the pelvis and scapula (Fig. **5, A** and **B**).

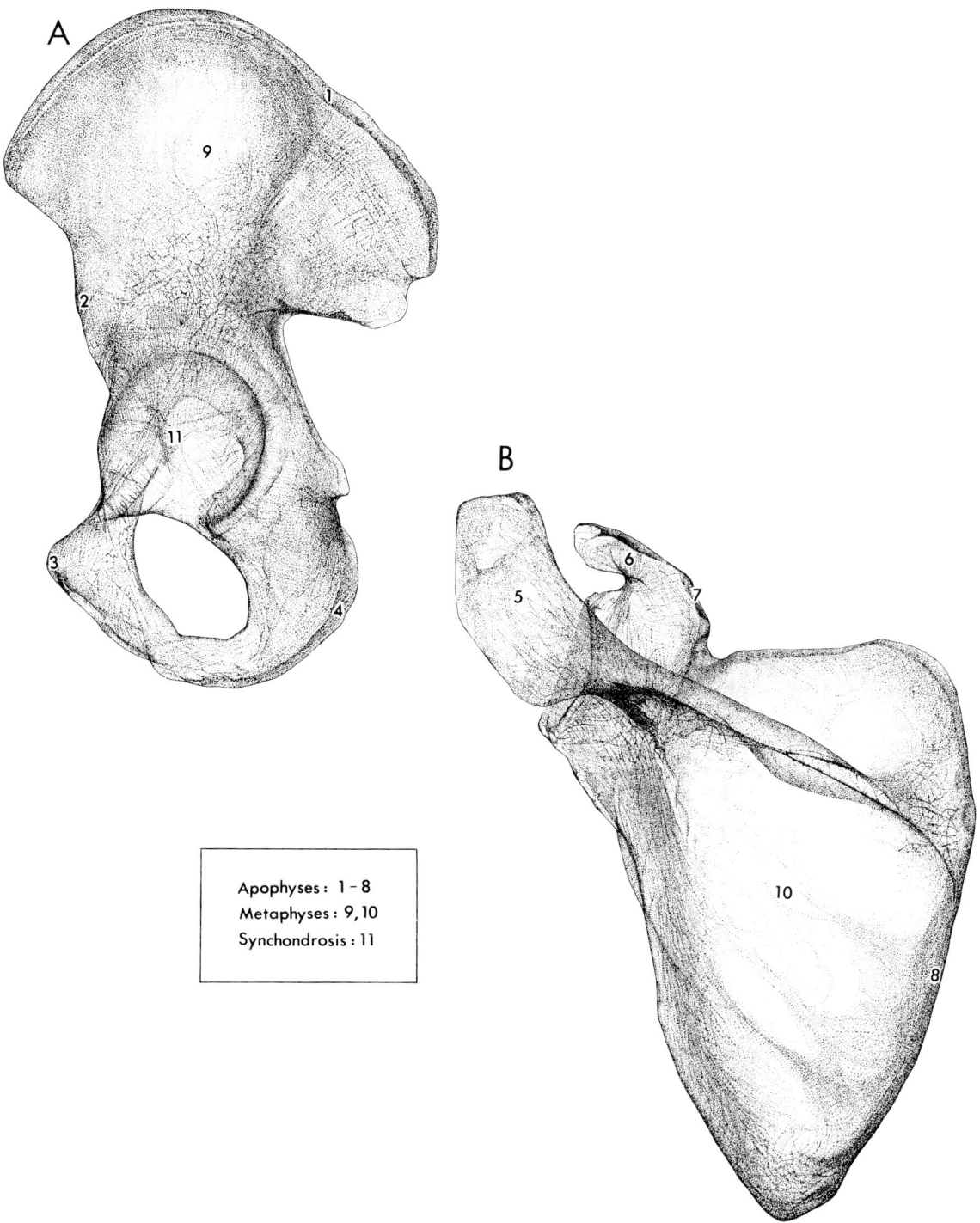

Figure 5.—Tumor locations in special bones. **A,** pelvis; **B,** scapula. Locations 9 and 10 are not true metaphyses but rather should be regarded as the analogue of the metaphysis of a long bone. (*Continued.*)

The Public Model / 19

B. Spine (51) 1.____Cervical
                2.____Dorsal
                3.____Lumbar
                4.____Sacrum
                5.____Coccyx

Lesion Centers on
Which Vertebral Body? (fill in one to twelve)_____(52–53)

	Center of Lesion— Check one (54–55)	Extends into— Check as Many as Applicable
Centrum	01____	(56) 1____
Pedicle	02____	(57) 1____
Neural Arch	03____	(58) 1____
Dorsal Process	04____	(59) 1____
Lateral Process	05____	(60) 1____
Soft Tissues		
Anterior	06____	(61) 1____
Lateral	07____	(62) 1____
Posterior	08____	(63) 1____
Disc Space	09____	(64) 1____

Disc Space(s) narrowed? (65) 1. Yes____
                                2. No ____

Identification of the specific elements of the *vertebral body* (Fig. **5, E** and **F**) is a recent addition to the radiographic protocol, so that little experience has been had with this parameter. The problem of including the elements of the spine and the paraspinous soft tissues was brought into focus in the diagnosis of chordoma.

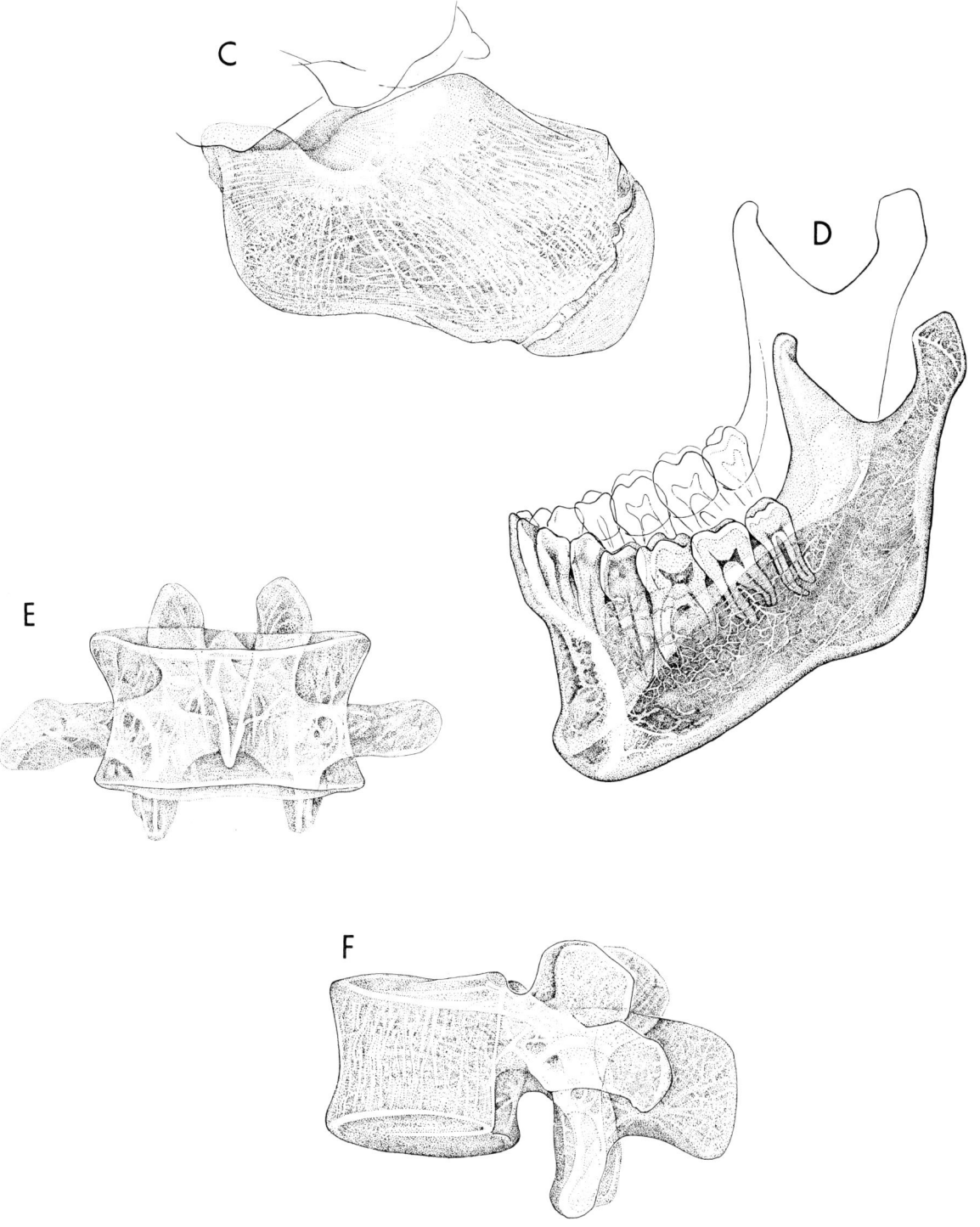

Figure 5 (cont.).—Tumor locations in special bones. **C,** os calcis; **D,** mandible; **E** and **F,** vertebral body. (*Continued.*)

C. Skull

	Center of Lesion- Check one (66-67)	Extends into- Check as Many as Applicable
Frontal	01 ___	(68) 1 ___
Parietal	02 ___	(69) 1 ___
Occipital	03 ___	(70) 1 ___
Vertex	04 ___	(71) 1 ___
Parasagittal	05 ___	(72) 1 ___
Ant. Basal	06 ___	(73) 1 ___
Mid. Basal*	07 ___	(74) 1 ___
Post Basal	08 ___	(75) 1 ___
Suture	09 ___	(76) 1 ___
Paranasal Sinus	10 ___	(77) 1 ___

Lesion Supplied by
Internal Circulation? (78)

1 ___ yes
2 ___ no
3 ___ unknown

Lesion Supplied by
External Circulation? (79)

1 ___ yes
2 ___ no
3 ___ unknown

* Includes sella and clivus

The geographic subdivisions of the *skull* have recently been listed in the radiographic protocol (Fig. **5, G** and **H**). This became necessary to improve identification of a number of tumors including osteoblastoma, cholesteatoma and chondroma, and tumors of the sinuses. The internal and external circulations are added to assist in distinguishing between meningiomas and primary tumors of the calvarium. Much more specific information is needed.

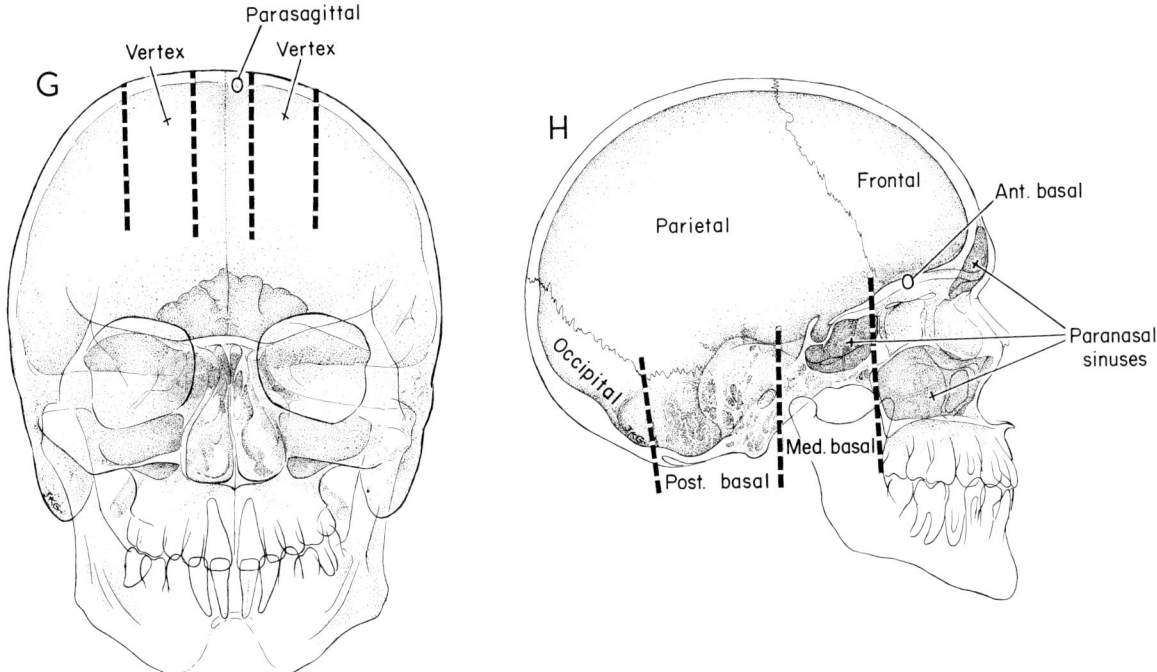

Figure 5 (cont.).—Tumor locations in special bones. **G** and **H,** the skull.

The relationship between histologic type and specific locations in these special bones is relatively unknown. With further detailed analysis of interrelationships, we hope to make the logic of radiologic decision-making more exact. Casual observation indicates that the natural laws which hold for giant cell tumor, chondroblastoma and location in long bones may hold also for apophyses, growth plates and synchondroses in other bones. The present form of the model makes it possible to relate center and extent of tumors to specific geographic areas in these special bones.

The boundaries and areas identified in **G** and **H** are being used for further study.

    V. SIZE OF LESION
        A. (11–13) Length_____mm
        B. (14–16) Width _____mm
        C. (17–19) Depth _____mm

SIGNIFICANCE OF SIZE IN PRIMARY BONE TUMORS.—The size of a primary tumor of bone is critical in predicting both behavior and histologic type (Fig. **6**).

First let us look at behavior. Two generalizations can be made. (1) Primary malignant tumors of bone usually are larger than 6 cm in greatest dimension at the time of discovery and often are larger than 9 cm. (2) Although many benign or slowly growing lesions may in time become

The Public Model / 23

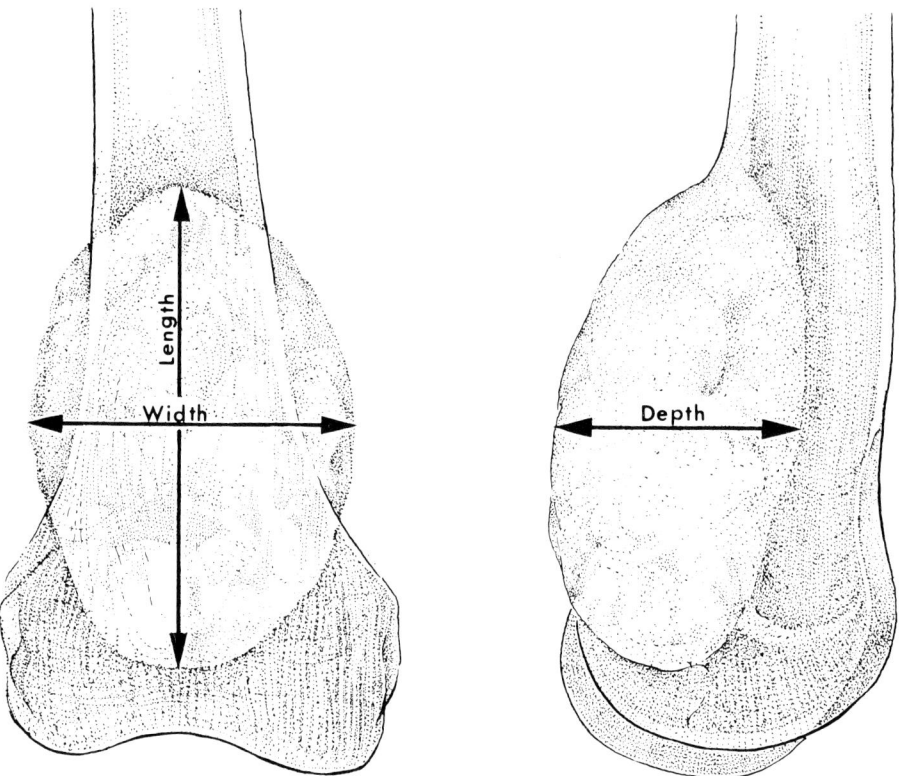

Figure 6.—Size and shape of the lesion. A matter of critical importance in estimating growth rate. There are upper limitations of size for certain histologic types such as osteoid osteoma.

very large, when first observed most are 6 cm or less in diameter and many are less than 3 cm. Consider such examples as the following benign lesions: a cortical defect is rarely larger than 2 or 3 cm; fibroxanthoma is usually 3 cm or less; nonossifying fibroma is a bit larger, but less than 6 cm; the nidus of osteoid osteoma is usually no larger than 1 cm, almost invariably smaller than 2 cm; chondroblastoma is usually 3 cm or less, rarely more than 6 cm; chondromyxoid fibroma is rarely more than 6 cm.

In connection with size, it is interesting to experiment with the computer. If we take a typical chondroblastoma of 3 cm diameter, which rates a probability of .99, and change the size to 6 cm, the probability drops to .85. Change the size to 9 cm, and the probability for chondroblastoma almost disappears, and giant cell tumor becomes the favorite choice.

On the other hand, some of the more slowly growing malignant lesions which metastasize late, such as chondrosarcoma, may continue to grow for years until they achieve an enormous size.

Even today, when early diagnosis is the rule, the usual highly malignant tumor of bone is 6–9 cm or larger when initially discovered. The principal exception is metastatic malignancy, which for some reason is often much smaller, perhaps because it is suspected earlier.

SHAPE AS A PREDICTOR VARIABLE.—Most tumors tend to grow in all directions at the same rate, and therefore are round or globular. This is not, however, invariably true, particularly in the long bones, where certain tumors tend to grow along the shaft to a greater degree. On the whole, shape of the tumor cannot be regarded as a powerful predictor variable, but is rather one to be used when clutching at straws.

The differentiation between a round and an elongated tumor is based on a simple measurement: where the greatest dimension is one and a half or more times the least, the tumor is regarded as elongated. All others are regarded as round. Tumors which commonly are elongated are Ewing's sarcoma, reticulum cell sarcoma, chondrosarcoma and angiosarcoma.

FACTORS RELATED TO INCREASED DENSITY

Three major processes lead to deposition of additional mineral in and around focal lesions of bone. These are: (1) dysplastic or neoplastic diseases with mineralization of tumor matrix; (2) proliferative or reparative response to injury, with the addition of normal new bone or callus, and (3) degeneration or death of tissues, with the addition of mineral. Mineralized tumor matrix is discussed here, the others (2 and 3) follow later in the chapter.

VI. TUMOR BONE (20) Tumor Bone
1_____Present
2_____Absent

If Absent, Skip to Section VII

A. Appearance of Bone

Appearance of Bone	Fraction of Tumor Inside Bone	Fraction of Tumor Outside Bone
Radiolucent	(21) /9	(22) /9
Ground Glass	(23) /9	(24) /9
Flocculent	(25) /9	(26) /9
Fleck	(27) /9	(28) /9
Solid	(29) /9	(30) /9
Lumpy	(31) /9	(32) /9
Cloudy	(33) /9	(34) /9
Veil-Like		(35) /9

B. Distribution of Tumor Bone (36) 1. Central
2. Peripheral
3. Uniform

TUMOR MATRIX MINERALIZATION.—Tumors which form bone and cartilage may be differentiated from other types of tumors by the radiographic evidence of their mineralized tumor matrix (Table 1). Mineralization within tumor substance is of special diagnostic value in identifying connective tissue tumors, since it is found so infrequently in others. The

TABLE 1.—MATRIX-FORMING LESIONS WHICH CALCIFY

BONE	CARTILAGE
Fibrosarcoma	Chondroblastoma
Fibrous osteoma	Chondroma (en-; periosteal)
Ossifying fibroma	Chondromyxoid fibroma
Ossifying hemangioma	Chondrosarcoma
Myositis ossificans	Chondrosarcoma, synovial
Osteoblastoma	
Osteochondroma	
Osteoid osteoma	
Osteosarcoma	
Parosteal sarcoma	

principal exceptions are hypernephroma of the kidney, where calcification may develop in hemorrhagic or necrotic tumor, and in carcinoma of the breast, and the ovary. As a rule, when calcification is of great volume and density, the likelihood is that the tumor is forming either cartilage or bone, or both.

In neoplastic cartilage, matrix mineralization is characterized by (1)

Figure 7.—Tumor matrix mineralization. **A** and **B,** calcific circles in a cartilaginous tumor. These circles are characteristic of endochondral bone formation in neoplastic cartilage. (**B** is AFIP Case No. 1044761; see Fig. 100.) (*Continued.*)

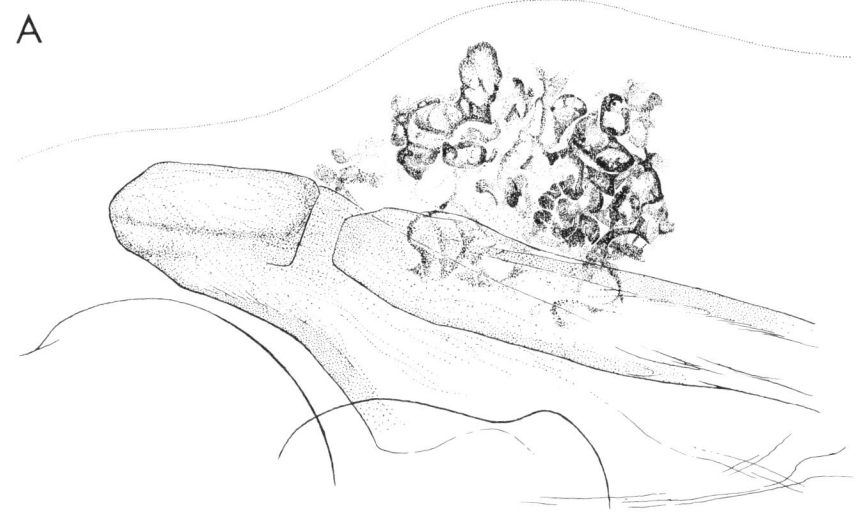

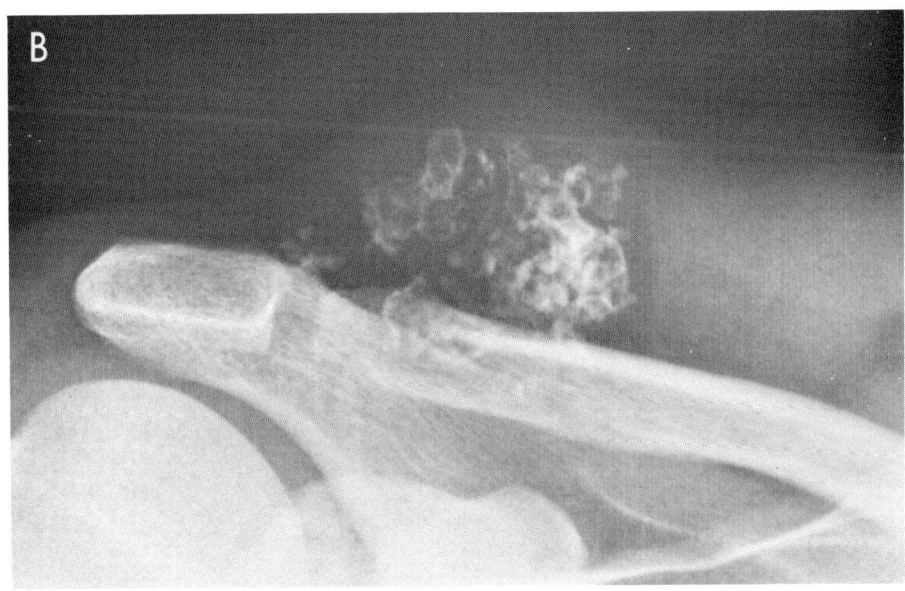

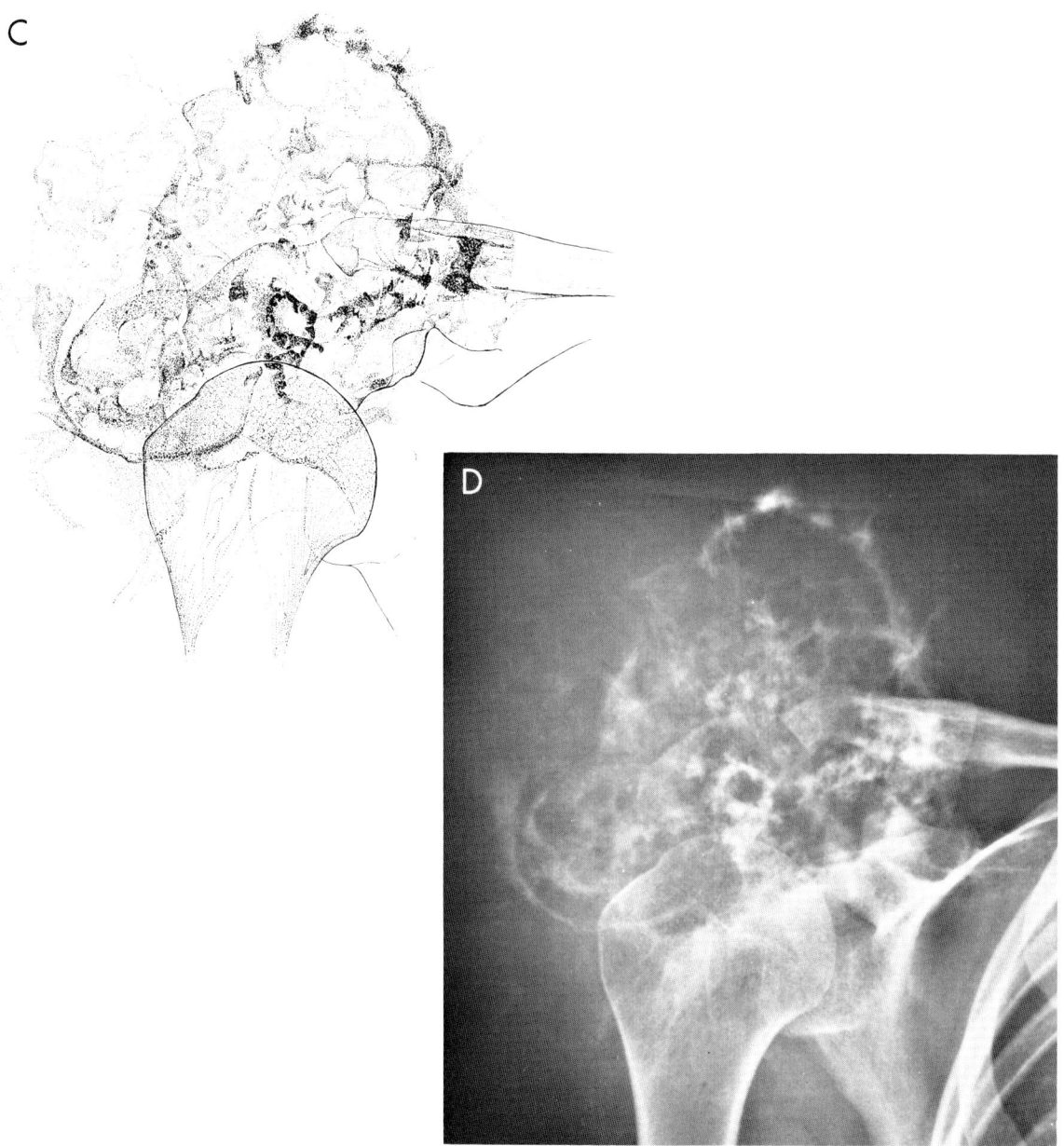

Figure 7 (cont.).—Tumor matrix mineralization. **C** and **D,** soft fluffy floccules in a large cartilaginous tumor. Note the prominent arcuate marginal calcifications. (*Continued.*)

rings of calcium (Fig. **7, A** and **B**); (2) floccules (**C** and **D**), any one or combination of which is called the *flocculent* pattern, or (3) multiple small, sharply defined, crystalline appearing collections (**E** and **F**). Since this calcification usually occurs in the most mature cartilage, it is found with greatest frequency in the center of a cartilaginous tumor. The central location of calcification in cartilage contrasts with that of bone infarct, where the calcium lies almost entirely in the perimeter of the lesion and is a reflection of the reparative reaction.

Matrix mineralization in neoplastic bone often takes a more organized appearance than it does in cartilage. In the highly mature tumor, such as parosteal sarcoma, the tumor bone will be heavily mineralized or *solid* to the very edge of the tumor (Fig. **7, H**), and often this mature neoplastic bone has a coarse trabeculated reticular pattern resembling spongy bone (Fig. 112, *A* and *B*). This spongy appearance and the sharp delineation of the edge of the tumor may be taken as evidence of mature differentiation.

Figure 7 (cont.).—Tumor matrix mineralization. **E** and **F**, tiny crystalline flecks of calcium in a benign lesion. (**F** is AFIP Case No. 1135669; see Fig. 99, *A*.) **G**, the fleck of osteoid osteoma, often unnoted unless carefully sought. (*Continued.*)

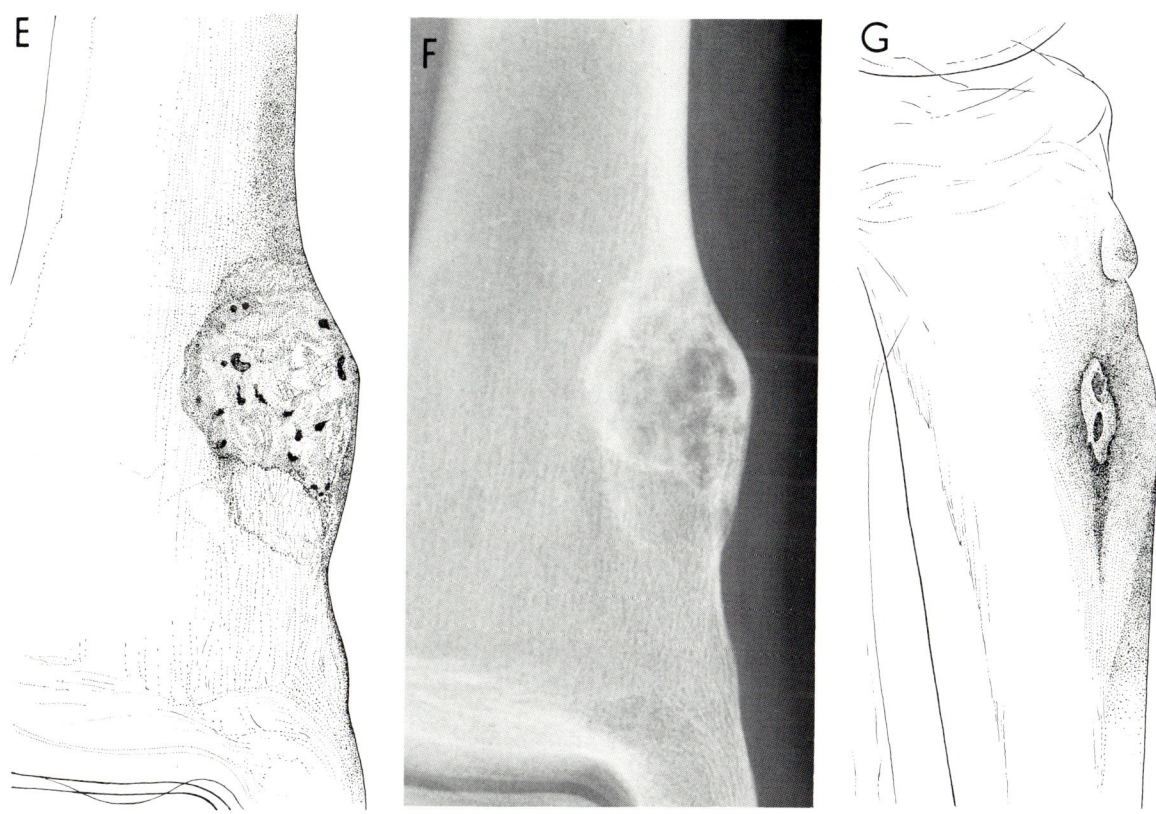

With the more rapidly growing tumors, the mineralization of the neoplastic bone is usually less well organized. *Lumps* (Fig. **7, I**) or *clouds* (**K** and **L**) of tumor bone with ill-defined edges and lack of structured appearance reflect poor differentiation. Occasionally in the extraosseous extension of a bone-forming tumor, neoplastic bone may form rays or spicules which are impossible to distinguish from the spicules formed from proliferative bone (Fig. 118). As with neoplastic cartilage, mineralization of neoplastic bone is usually observed first in the center of the tumor. Occasionally neoplastic bone is seen in the extraosseous part of an osteosarcoma and not in the intraosseous part, or vice versa. This may be attributed to the influence of skeletal metabolic fields.

Myositis ossificans, almost invariably centered parosteally, may be responsible for patterns of calcific density indistinguishable from the cloudy tumor bone seen in osteosarcoma. Alternatively, myositis, particularly in the smaller of the long bones, commonly produces ill-defined but regular spicular patterns (Fig. 123). However, myositis in time rapidly progresses either to a regular, dense hyperostosis attached to the cortex (Fig. 124) or to a *veillike* configuration (Fig. **7, J**) which is specific for this lesion.

Skeletal tumors may form both bone and cartilage and the radiograph will correspondingly reflect both patterns (Fig. 106). This combination is seen particularly in the rapidly growing osteosarcomas which contain both osteogenic and chondrogenic elements; also, the cartilage of a relatively mature chondrosarcoma may undergo typical endochondral type of conversion to bone. Certain osteoblastomas, particularly the massive lesions which lie on the surface of a flat bone, produce a kind of matrix which both calcifies and ossifies (Figs. 133 and 134). Oddly enough, our limited experiences with osteoblastomas arising *within* bone have shown them to be either completely radiolucent or to contain matrix which mineralizes very uniformly, a kind of *ground-glass* pattern (Figs. 135, *A*, and 136). Some of the ossifying fibromas around the mandible and maxilla produce a similar uniformly calcified ground-glass matrix (Fig. 72, *B*). The osteoid osteoma is characterized by one or more small distinct *flecks* of tumor matrix mineralization (Fig. **7, G**) in the center of the lesion, or the nidus.

Figure 7 (cont.).—Tumor matrix mineralization. **H,** solid tumor bone, often so well differentiated that both trabecular and cortical bone are present. **I,** lumps, often reflecting poor differentiation. **J,** veillike configuration, typical of myositis ossificans, reflecting a moderately advanced stage of organization of hematoma in soft tissues, finally consolidating into dense bone. **K** and **L,** clouds, in osteosarcoma, reflecting poor differentiation or relatively immature area of tumor.

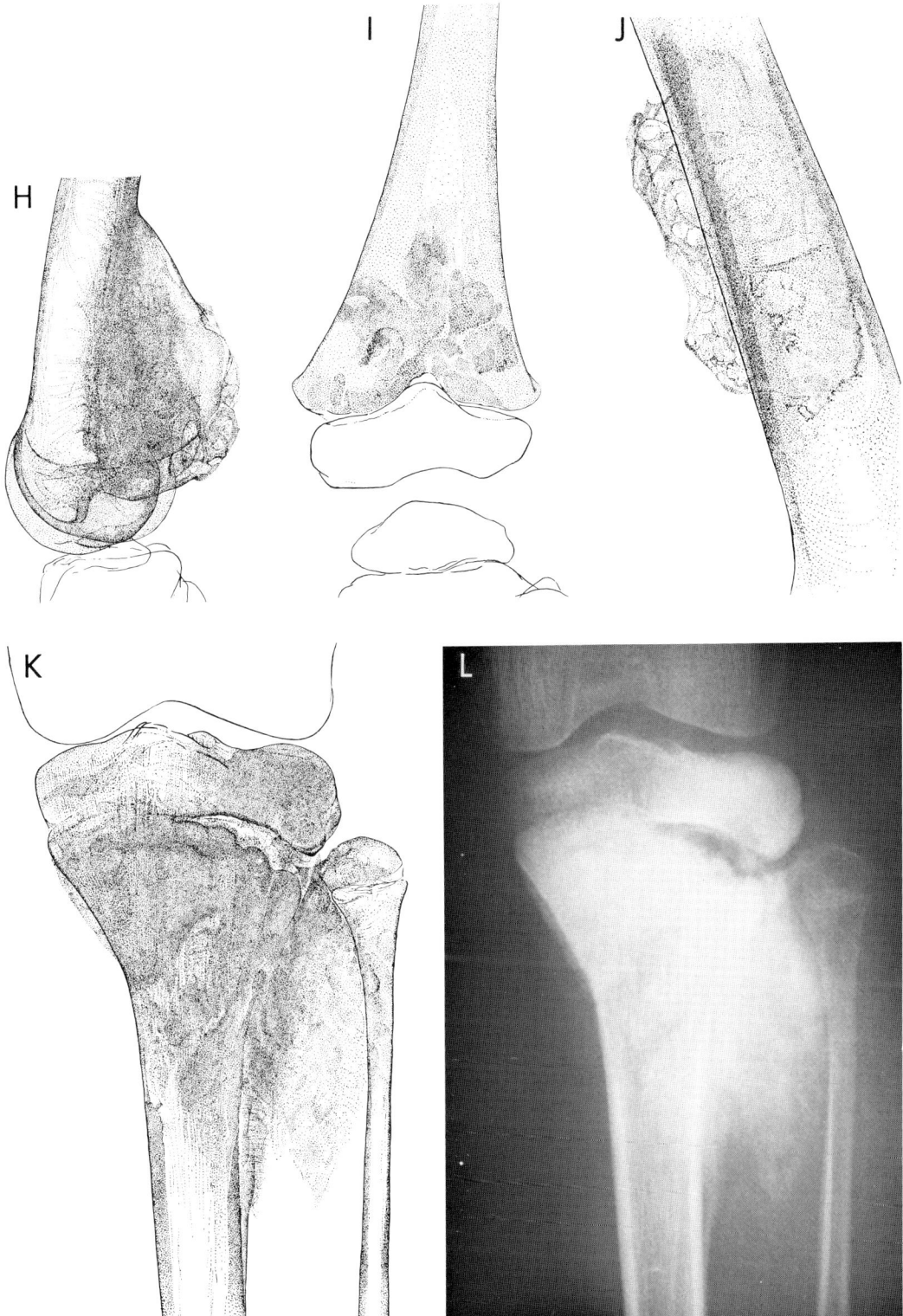

Figure 7 (cont.).—See legend on facing page.

These six patterns of tumor matrix mineralization (flocculent, fleck, solid, lumpy, cloudy, veillike) are powerful predictor variables. Flocculent calcification within a tumor strongly favors chondrosarcoma or chondroma. The only other tumor which contains flocculent calcification alone in significant amount is chondroblastoma, which can usually be identified conclusively on other grounds.

MINERALIZATION OF NECROTIC TISSUE.—Calcification in necrotic tumor, degenerative tissue or scar is a well-known phenomenon. Examples are the calcification in atheromatous intimal disease of the arteries, in chronic granulomatous disease in the lungs and in necrotic hypernephroma. Calcification in primary bone tumors is usually limited to lesions associated with the formation of a calcifiable matrix of cartilage or bone. Because of its consistency, such calcification is a highly dependable diagnostic sign.

Rarely, however, certain primary bone tumors that are not associated with matrix production will calcify. Myeloma is often associated with the local deposition of amyloid, which rarely may calcify heavily. Ewing's sarcoma and reticulum cell sarcoma, both highly cellular tumors without matrix production, may uncommonly contain finely scattered calcification throughout their soft tissue substance which is apparent on the radiograph (Figs. 146 and 159). Because it is so rare, this finding can be extremely misleading.

One other source of degenerative calcification is the lesion within bone which results in the necrosis of fat. In this situation, the liquefied fat at the edge of the lesion may saponify and calcify heavily.

C. (37) Fraction of Extraosseous
Mass with Ossified Edge
——/9

OSSIFIED EDGE.—Occasionally tissues at the margin of a slowly enlarging extraosseous mass ossify heavily enough to produce a crescentic or circumferential pattern of tumor bone at the edge of the lesion (Fig. **8, A;** see also Figs. 78, 82 and 131, *A* and *B*). This pattern may develop even when the center of the lesion is completely radiolucent. The crescentic pattern does not have the dense linear appearance of an expanded periosteal shell, but rather seems to have a structured appearance of mature tumor bone. This pattern is seen most often in chondrosarcoma, osteoblastoma and fibrosarcoma.

CLEAVAGE PLANE.—With parosteal sarcoma, the extraosseous mass of solid tumor bone often appears to lie rather loosely against the cortex and separated from cortex at the edges by a wedgelike zone of soft tissue

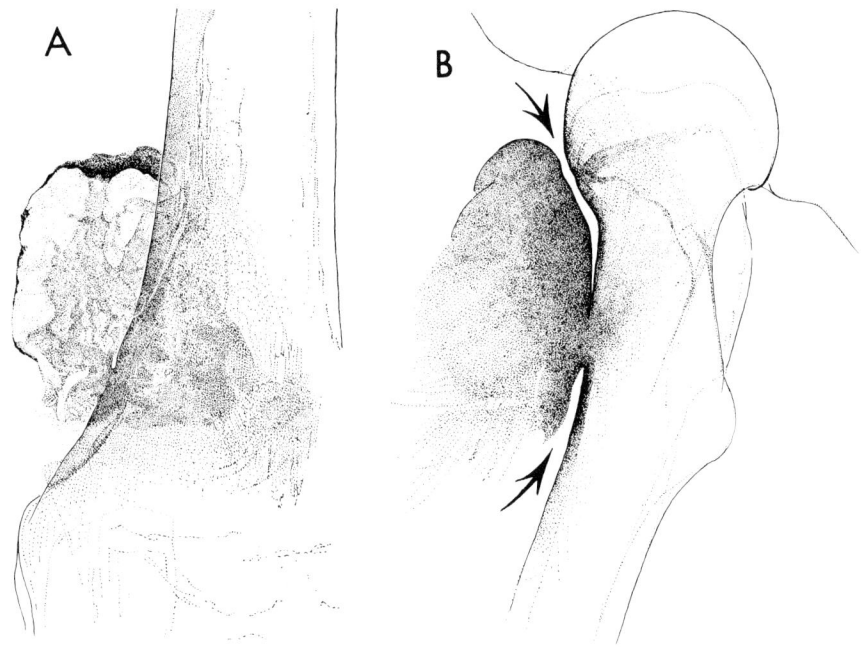

Figure 8.—**A,** ossified edge of extraosseous mass. **B,** cleavage plane.

density (Fig. **8, B**). This apparent cleavage plane between the tumor and the normal appearing cortex suggests that the tumor may be treated by wedging it loose from the cortex. This maneuver should not be attempted, however, since radiographically it is not always possible to distinguish between this tumor and normal bone. Also, this tumor often extends through the cortex into the medullary cavity. Despite its benign appearance, parosteal sarcoma is a malignant tumor.

BONE DESTRUCTION

VISIBILITY.—Destruction of bone is ordinarily the first response to local injury of bone. Occasionally it is the sole radiographic evidence of disease, although reactive proliferation often occurs with it. Destruction itself is a reactive phenomenon; it is not a direct effect of infection or neoplasm on the calcified osteoid matrix but rather is mediated through stimulation of osteoclasts which destroy bone. Although the details of osteoclastic resorption of bone are still debated, the evidence suggests that the mineral salts are first dissolved from the matrix by a chelating agent secreted by the osteoclast, followed closely by enzymatic reduction of the remaining osteoid.

Regardless of the cause, there is a delay between the initial stimulus to destroy bone and its actual roentgen appearance. The duration of this latent period is variable, being dependent to a considerable extent on the structural characteristics of the bone being destroyed. In spongy bone of the pelvis, ribs or ends of long bones, large amounts of cancellous bone may be removed with little or no reflection of change in the radiograph (Fig. **9, A–D**). Minor alterations of the structure of cortical bone are easily discernible, however, owing to the compactness of the cortex (**D**). The generalized loss of bone substance concurrent with aging makes the detection of destructive change in the elderly more difficult than in the young (**E–H**). The effect of these variations is such that the smallest destructive lesions of cortex are readily seen; but in spongy bone, when not accompanied by reactive proliferation in bone or periosteum, even advanced disease may go undetected.

In optimal circumstances for detection (alteration of dense cortical bone in a thin part) the minimal latent period between the stimulus and visualization of destruction is ten days, based on the observed delay in the appearance of bone destruction following the onset of symptoms of osteomyelitis. This period of latency must vary greatly in other diseases such as neoplasia in bone in which, in some circumstances, there is no apparent destruction of bone despite widespread presence of neoplasm (Fig. **9, I** and **J**). This is especially likely in metastatic lung cancer of the oat cell type.

Figure 9.—Visibility of bone destruction. **A,** bisected distal femur with trabecular bone and inner cortex removed. Edges of hole in trabecular bone are perpendicular, but those in area of cortical destruction are sloping. **B,** radiograph of **A** after halves were fitted together and submerged in water phantom. None of the edges of bone destruction are evident, in spongy bone because relative density is small and in cortex because of lack of sharp edges. The pattern of trabecular bone is gone. **C,** bisected proximal tibia with drill holes penetrating trabecular bone and partially penetrating the cortex. **D,** radiograph of **C,** showing that with sharp edges, even slight erosions of cortical bones are easily detected. (*Continued.*) ⟶

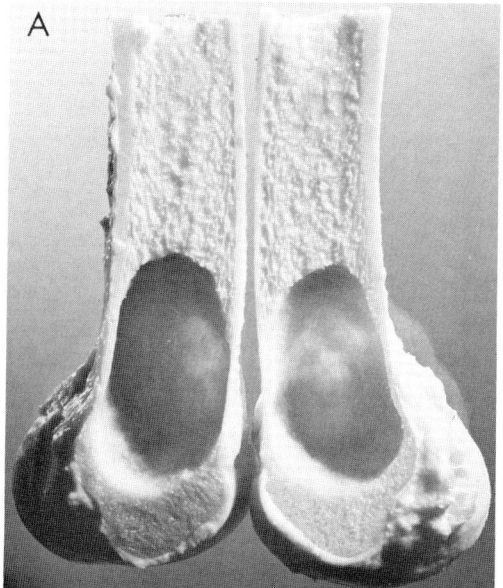
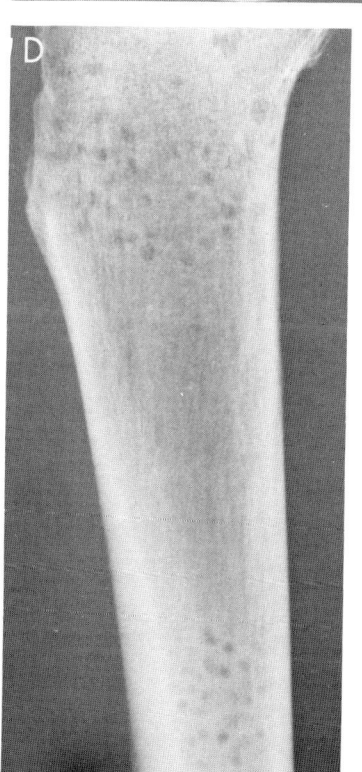

Figure 9.—See legend on facing page.

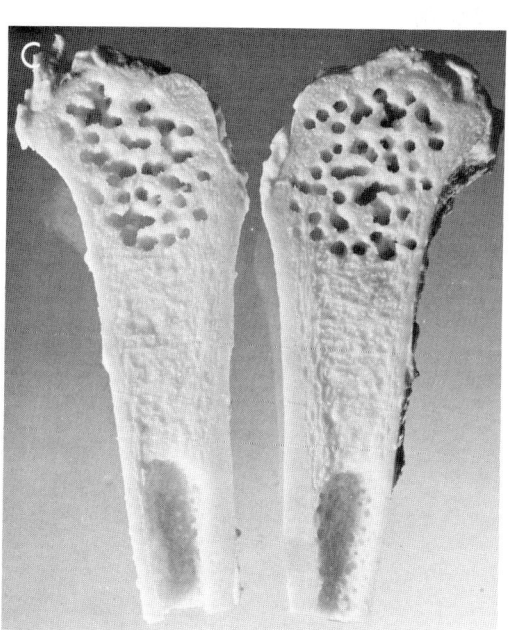

The Public Model / 35

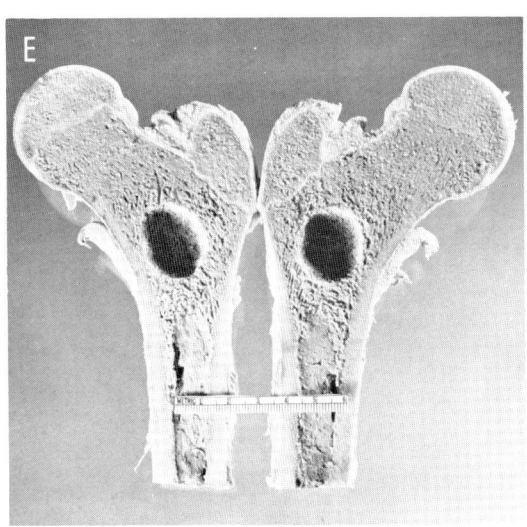
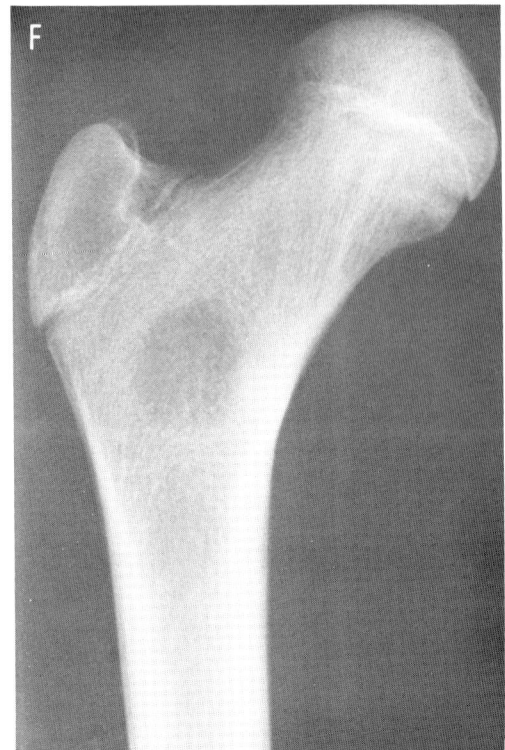

Figure 9 (cont.).—See legend on facing page.

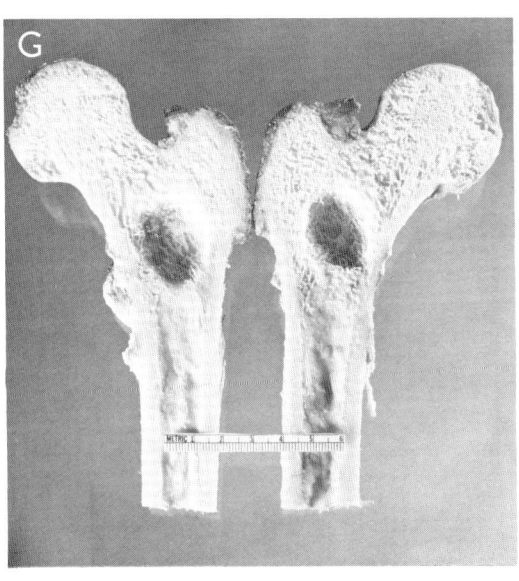
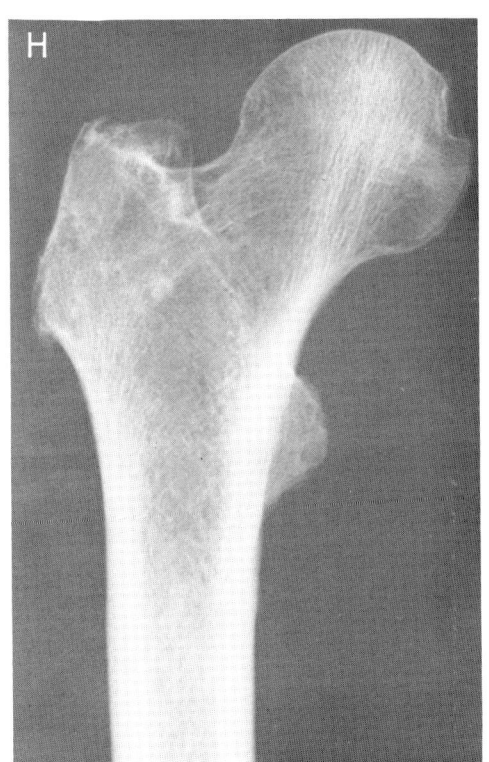

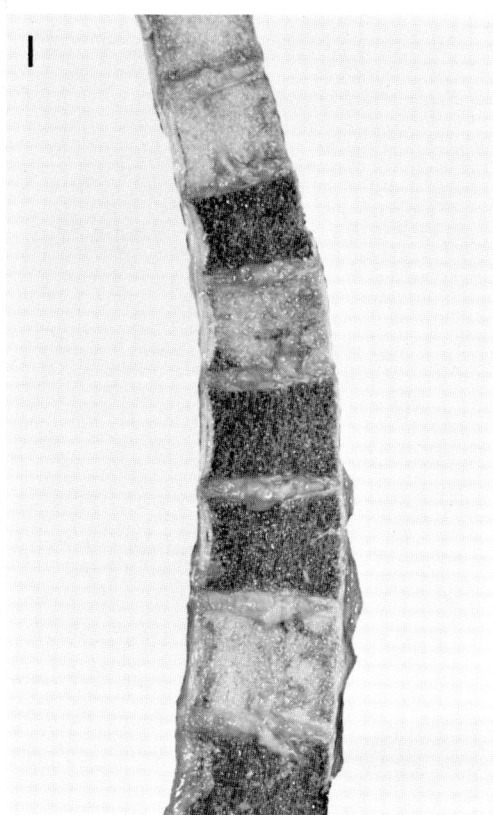 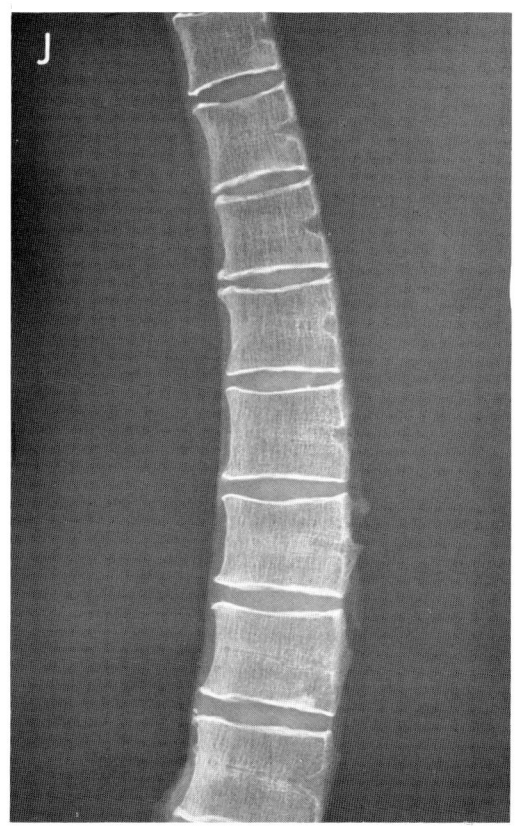

Figure 9 (cont.).—Visibility of bone destruction. **I,** section of spine involved in metastatic carcinoma. **J,** radiograph of **I.** (From Lodwick, in M. D. Anderson Hospital: *Tumors of Bone and Soft Tissue* [Chicago: Year Book Medical Publishers, 1965].)

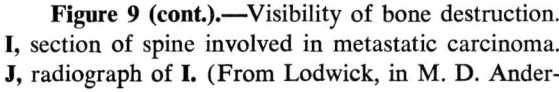

Figure 9 (cont.).—Visibility of bone destruction. **E,** bisected proximal femur of male, aged 14, with 2 cm defect in cancellous bone. **F,** radiograph of **E,** showing distinct density because of compactness of trabecular bone. **G,** bisected proximal femur of male, aged 72, with 2 cm defect in cancellous bone. **H,** radiograph of **G;** alteration of density is undetectable because contribution of atrophic cancellous bone to total radiographic density is slight. (**A–H** from Lodwick, Radiol. Clin. North America 2:209, 1964.) (*Continued.*)

VII. BONE DESTRUCTION (38) 1____Present
                             2____Absent

If Absent, go to Section VIII

A. Measurements of Destroyed Area

TYPE OF DESTRUCTION

	Geographic	Motheaten	Permeated
Diameter of Central Zone (or Entire Zone, if uniform)	(40-41) ____ ____ cm	(42-43) ____ ____ cm	(44-45) ____ ____ cm
Width of Marginal Zone, if present		(46-47) ____ ____ mm	(48-49) ____ ____ mm

KINDS AND SIGNIFICANCE OF BONE DESTRUCTION.—Holes in bone range from very large to very small. Large holes have many qualitative differences from small holes and signify something quite different in terms of rate of growth. Furthermore, large holes tend to be single, while small holes are multiple. Middle-sized holes are like neither the small nor the large.

We call the single large hole in bone *geographic* bone destruction. It is characterized in its pure form by a very sharp line of transition from no bone (completely destroyed bone) to intact bone. This line of distinction is often as sharp as if it were punched out or sheared by a sharp instrument (Fig. **10, A–E**). Although not always apparent radiographically, it is an integral feature of pure geographic bone destruction.

B. (50) For exclusively geographic destruction only—
Contour of Boundary between Intact Bone and Destroyed Area

1——Regular
2——Lobulated
3——ME
4——Not seen
5——Ragged
6——Reticulate

Another variable peculiar to geographic bone destruction is the contour of the edge. In some instances the edge is quite regular (Fig. **10, F**). In others the edge may be *lobulated* (**G**), others ragged and irregular (Figs. 10, C and D, and 12), and in still others there may be small *nibbled* (ME) irregularities (**H** and **I**). Occasionally the edge is *ill-defined* because it has a long sloping undercut (Fig. 18, upper margin).

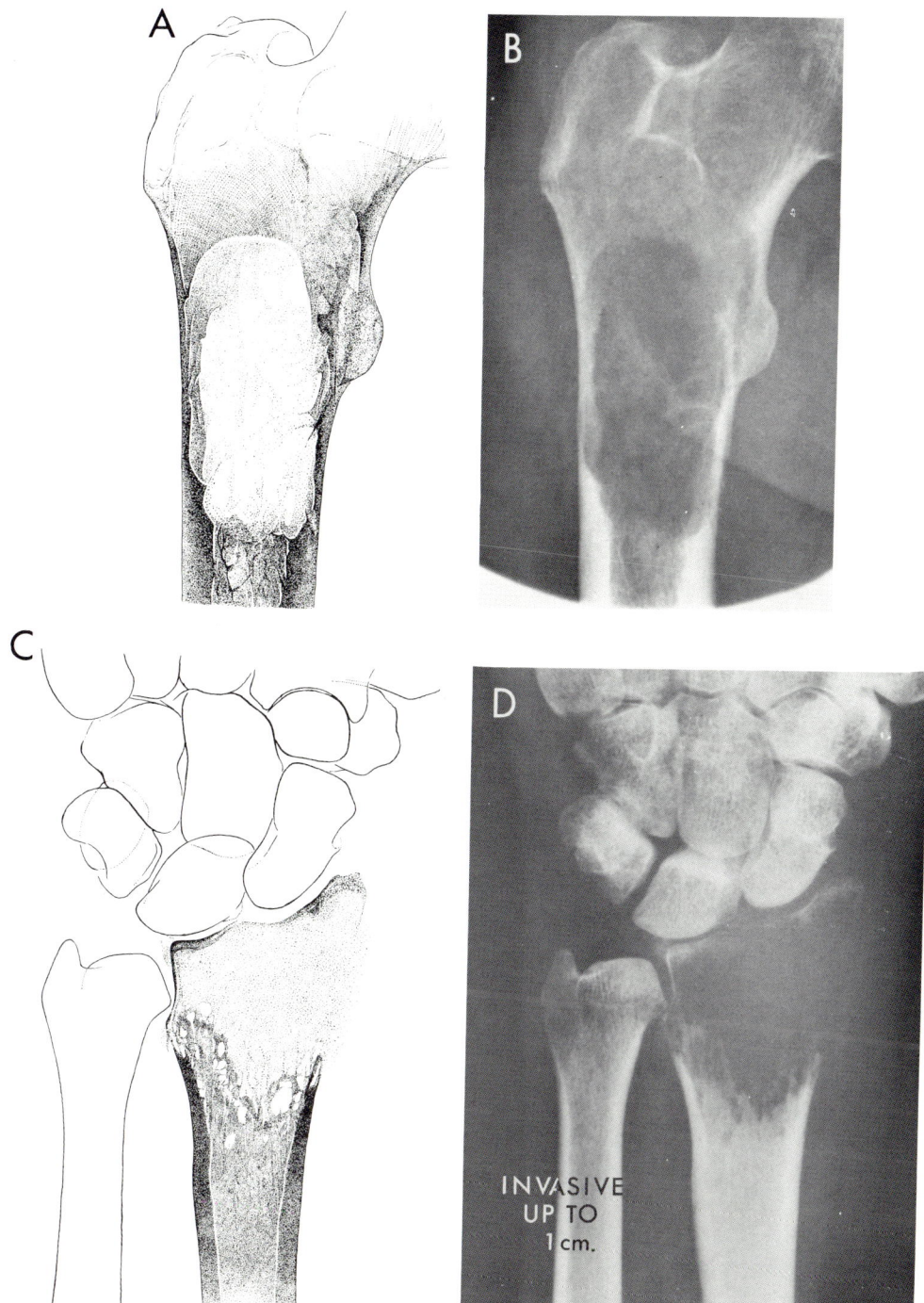

Figure 10.—Bone destruction. **A** and **B**, geographic destruction, where present, is complete, with sharp linear transition between destroyed area and intact bone. (**B** is AFIP Case No. 1067267; see Fig. 167.) **C** and **D**, combined geographic and moth-eaten, with the latter a transition zone (about 1 cm wide) between total geographic destruction and intact bone; giant cell tumor, growth rate IC. (*Continued.*)

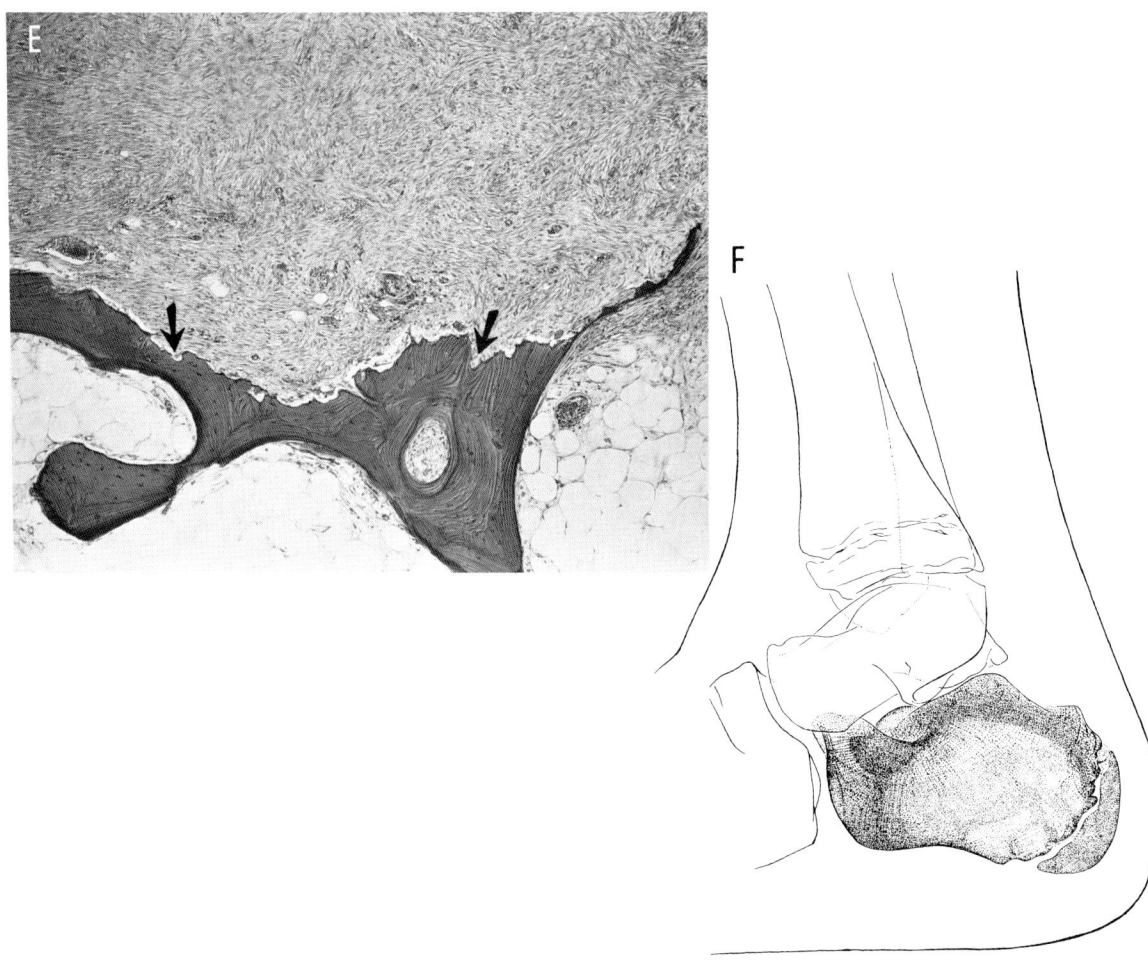

Figure 10 (cont.).—Bone destruction. **E**, geographic, with osteoclasts **(arrows)** destroying bone in an advancing front of fibrosarcoma. Linear conversion between tumor and intact bone is responsible for the edge typical of this pattern. (From Lodwick, Radiol. Clin. North America 2:209, 1964.) **F**, geographic, with regular contour of margin. (*Continued.*)

RELATION BETWEEN CONTOUR AND CONSISTENCY.—Some primary slowly growing tumors are extremely soft or semiliquid in consistency (giant cell and cystic tumors). Such tumors are usually globular and have a regular, a gently lobulated or a *reticulate* contour (Fig. **10, J**). This is usually seen in the expanded tumors of the rays of the hands and feet. Other slowly growing tumors (chondrosarcoma and chondromyxoid fibroma) are rubbery and may be elongated and irregularly lobulated to a degree that many areas of tumor seem to be growing independently of each other (Fig. **10, H** and **I**). These differences in contour may be due to variations in growth rate related to focal pressure differences in cystic and solid tumors, the pressure being more equally applied in the former.

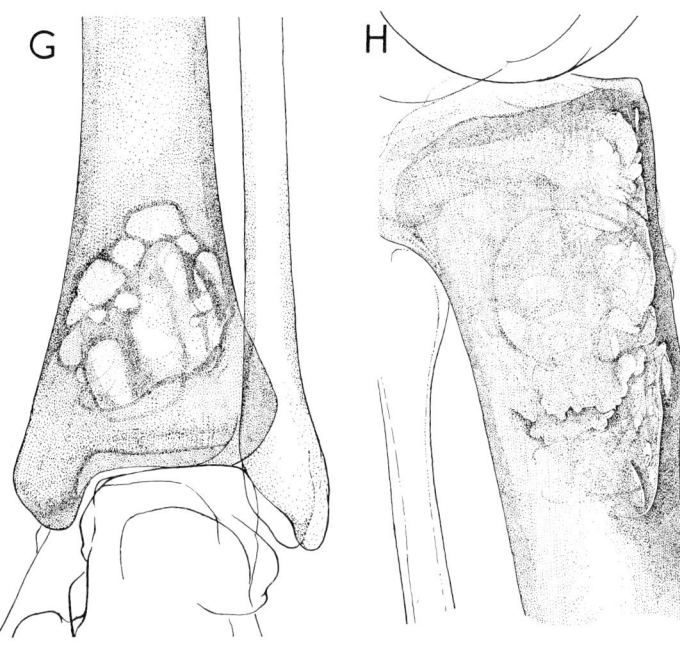
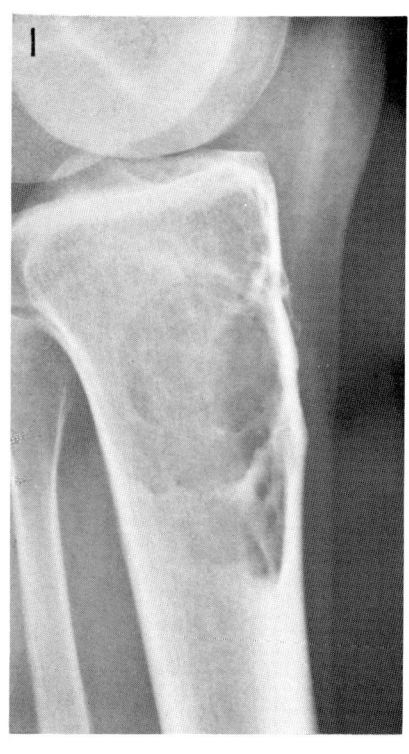
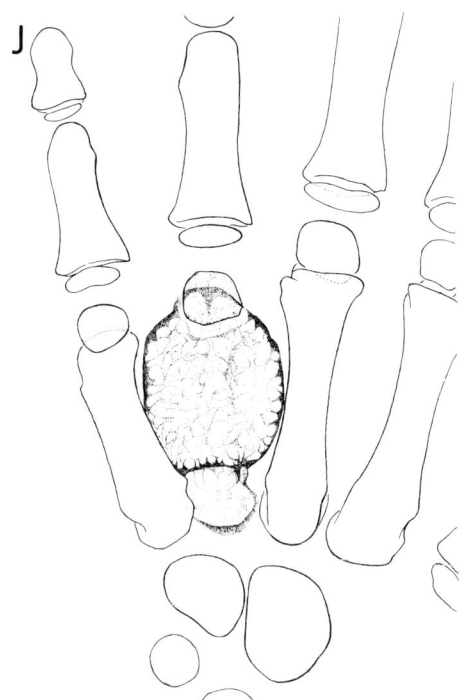

Figure 10 (cont.).—Bone destruction. **G,** geographic, with lobulated or scalloped contour plus a rim of reparative sclerosis. **H** and **I,** geographic, with ME contour; such scalloping is most common in tumors containing cartilage. (**I** is AFIP Case No. 1004844; see Fig. 63, *B* and *C*.) **J,** reticulate pattern, finely lobulated; seen usually in tumors of small bones, principally giant cell tumors and osteoblastomas.

The *permeated pattern* of bone destruction (small holes) is characterized by numerous elongated slotted holes which run parallel to the long axis of a bone (Fig. **11, A** and **B**). They are reasonably uniform in size but tend to become smaller and more scattered toward the periphery of the lesion to the point where they are no longer present. For this reason the margin of a zone of permeated bone destruction is *broad* and cannot be defined with accuracy. There is no sharp line of demarcation between intact bone and destroyed bone, in contrast to the geographic pattern. Permeated bone destruction may extensively involve the cortex yet leave it structurally almost intact but with greatly reduced density. In contrast, with geographic destruction, when it involves the cortex, the entire cortex often is cleanly removed.

The middle-sized holes, which comprise the *moth-eaten* pattern, are always multiple and, being large, often are confluent (**C** and **D**). The edges are rarely punched out, being irregular and not defined with the same degree of sharpness observed in geographic bone destruction. When the moth-eaten pattern is present, the cortex may be totally destroyed or may have multiple areas of discontinuity.

Both moth-eaten and permeated bone always entail total penetration of the cortex by the tumor. Although both patterns have their identifying characteristics, sharp distinction between them may be difficult if not impossible. This is not critical, as will be evident later when the decision tree and the logic of diagnosis are discussed. *What is very important* is that one distinguish the geographic pattern of destruction from the permeated and moth-eaten patterns, all of which have prime significance in diagnosis, prognosis and therapy.

There are yet other patterns of bone destruction which relate to scattered neoplastic disease, particularly the punched-out lesions of multiple myeloma. This kind of destruction is almost never seen in solitary lesions of bone and is mentioned only to exclude it. Additionally, the destructive process may be limited essentially to cancellous bone alone, in which case, if it is seen at all, there may be only a vague, ill-defined *reduction* of cancellous density which often cannot be further classified (see Fig. 41).

Thus there are three basic patterns of bone destruction, geographic, moth-eaten and permeated. Each may occur alone in pure form, or two or all three may be found together. Perhaps the most common combination is geographic and moth-eaten destruction (Fig. 10, *C* and *D*); here the geographic pattern is always the more central of the two, the moth-eaten portion usually forming a rim around the central geographic area. To define variations in growth rate we measure the width of the rim of moth-eaten bone destruction, the dividing line between narrow and wide zones of moth-eaten

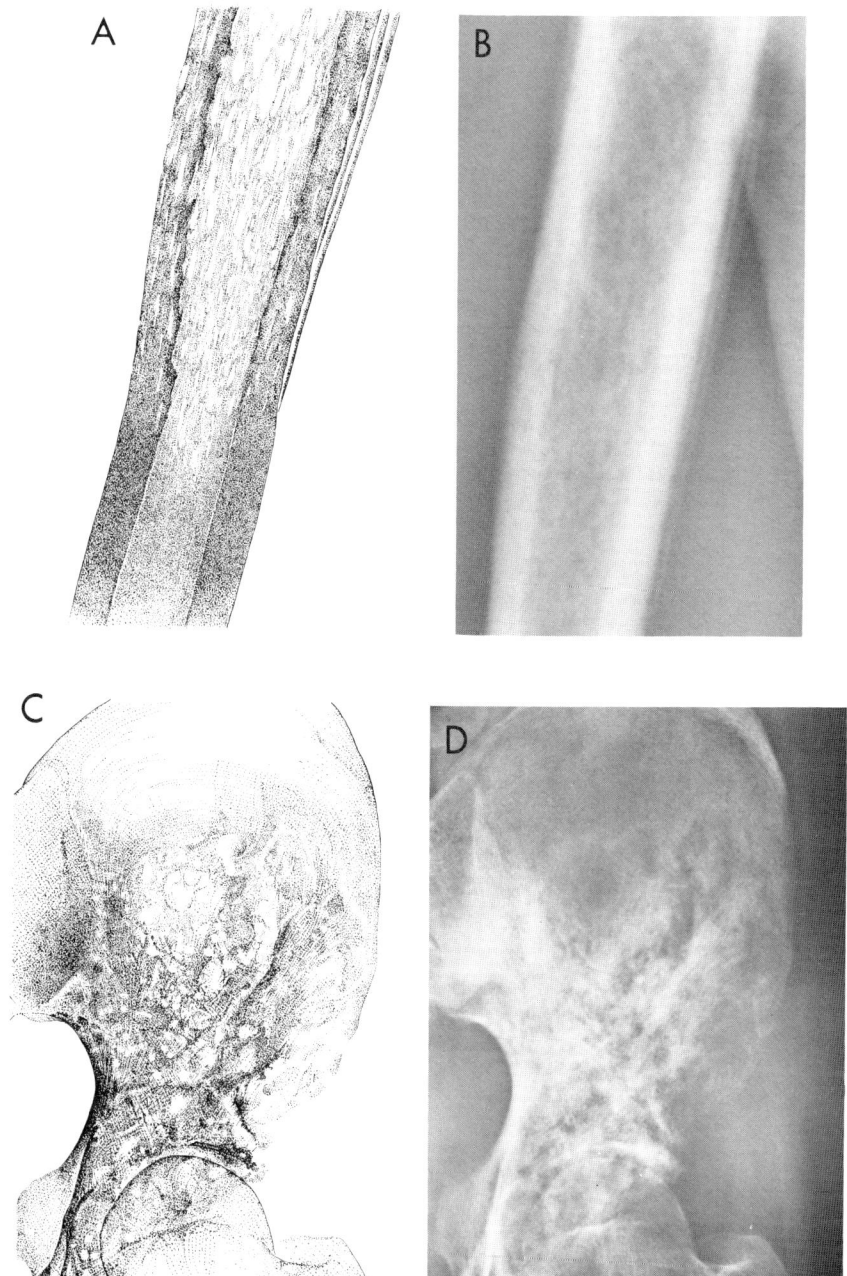

Figure 11.—Bone destruction. **A** and **B,** permeated pattern, with holes fading imperceptibly into intact bone without well-defined margin. Although greatly diminished in density in most involved areas, the cortex retains its structural dimensions. (**B** is AFIP Case No. 1062430; see Fig. 147.) **C** and **D,** moth-eaten pattern, with circular holes of varying size large enough to create substantial defects in the cortex. (**D** is AFIP Case No. 1178414; see Fig. 162.)

destruction being less than 1 cm for the narrow, and 1 cm or more for the wide. Permeated and geographic destruction are not measured.

The recognition of geographic, moth-eaten and permeated bone destruction and their permutations is exceedingly important in evaluating primary tumors because each is associated with a statistically significant different rate of growth. Geographic patterns suggest a slow rate of growth, permeated the most rapid, and moth-eaten an intermediate rate. Combinations of geographic and moth-eaten patterns tend to straddle the boundary between slow and intermediate growth rates. Apparently these three patterns of bone destruction comprise the most radiologically significant evidence that can be found to evaluate the rate of growth in a single roentgen examination of a bone lesion. Indeed when a lesion does not involve bone (therefore no bone destruction) the lack of this significant index of growth rate is sorely felt.

To summarize, the patterns of destruction of bone are (1) geographic, (2) moth-eaten, and (3) permeated. Margins in geographic destruction may be regular, lobulated, ME, ragged, ill-defined and reticulate. Margins of moth-eaten and permeated destruction are broad.

C. (51) Penetration of Cortex in Flat Bone
   1_____Partial
   2_____Total

D. Penetration of Cortex in Tubular Bone

Quadrant of Cortex	Partial	Total
(52) Anterior	1___	2___
(53) Medial	1___	2___
(54) Posterior	1___	2___
(55) Lateral	1___	2___

PENETRATION OF CORTEX.—When geographic bone destruction is present, the degree of cortical penetration by tumor arising within bone or even outside of the cortex may vary from no penetration to total penetration. The degree is usually assessed by looking at a lesion in at least two projections to see (1) whether there is a visible breach in the cortex as it is observed tangentially and (2) whether a part of the tumor protrudes through the cortex into the soft tissues. We have accepted the presence or absence of cortical penetration as an important point in the classification of growth rate in bone tumors, described later. For moth-eaten and permeated bone destruction, total penetration of the cortex is assumed, whether or not it is visible in the radiograph.

To summarize, the cortex may be intact, partially penetrated or totally penetrated.

> E. (56) Special Signs
> 1____Fracture
> 2____Displacement
> 3____Sequestrum

SPECIAL SIGNS.—*Fracture.*—Pathologic fracture is common in primary bone tumors. When present in benign lesions the fracture is of little prognostic significance because ultimately such fractures heal, often with healing of the underlying lesion. In malignant bone tumors pathologic fractures are serious events, since they commonly cause local hemorrhage with opening of vascular spaces and increased opportunity for seeding. Thus in the assessment of rate of growth the presence of a pathologic fracture automatically moves the radiologic grade one step in the direction of more rapid growth.

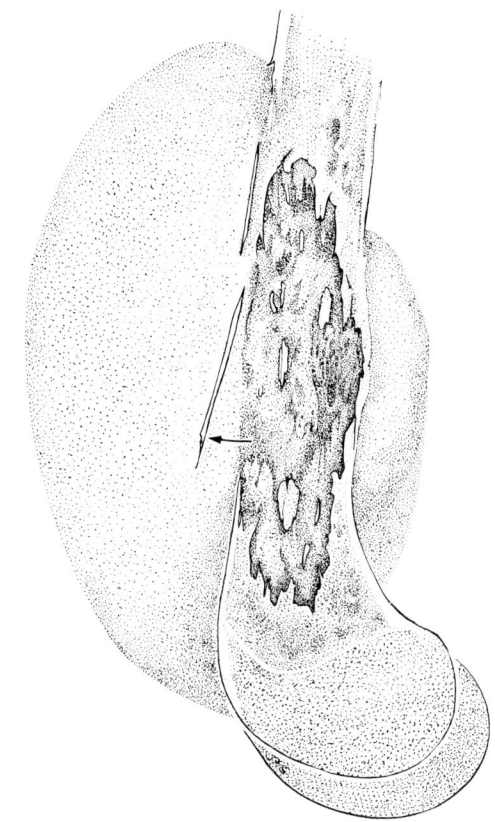

Figure 12.—Displacement phenomenon, in which pressures from a tumor expanding within the medullary cavity break loose and dislodge a fragment of bone into the soft tissues. Geographic bone destruction; ragged contour.

Displacement.—Rarely, in the presence of a destructive tumor of intramedullary origin, and particularly when no significant amount of tumor matrix mineralization is present, the growing tumor appears to burst out through the cortex carrying with it a separated fragment of bone (Fig. **12**). This phenomenon has been observed principally in primary fibrosarcoma. It must be distinguished from pathologic fractures with bone fragments displaced due to motion. Displacement is an interesting but uncommon finding.

Sequestrum.—This is rarely, if ever, observed in primary tumors of bone. Sequestrum is a provision in the model for subsequent differentiation of inflammatory lesions of bone.

PROLIFERATIVE RESPONSE

When bone is injured, ultimately some new bone may be added within either the endosteal or the periosteal envelope. In some instances the addition of new bone is clearly reparative: trabeculae are thickened, the cortex is shored up within and/or without, new bone may be added on the outer surface of the cortex to replace the bone removed from the inner surface, or a wall may be interposed between normal and abnormal structure. In other instances the deposition of new bone, although occurring in the same general locations, is of a more disorganized, random reactive distribution. In either instance the increased density is due to the deposition of normal new bone, by normal osteoblasts, in an apparently normal physiologic process. This process may be contrasted to the deposition of mineral in tumor bone or tumor cartilage and the deposition of calcium or new bone in necrotic tissue whether of normal or neoplastic origin.

Proliferative bone as seen by the radiologist is nearly always deposited at the interface between the endosteal or the periosteal envelope and normal structure. The kinds of proliferative response seem related to the rate of tumor growth and are identified here as *rate factors* (Fig. **13**). Another kind of proliferative response seems to be peculiar to particular types or groups of tumors, identified as *qualitative factors* (Fig. **14**). This separation cannot always be clearly made.

VIII. BONE PROLIFERATION   (11) 1_____Present
                                 2_____Absent

If Absent, go to Section IX

	Size, Thickness, or Height	Fraction of Total, or Tumor Area	Number of Units	Structure Coarse	Structure Delicate
A. RATE FACTORS:					
1. Codman's Triangle	(12-13) ___ ___ mm		(14) ___	(15) 1 2	
2. Buttress	(16-17) ___ ___ mm		(18) ___		
3. Expanded Shell	(19-20) ___ ___ mm				
4. Sclerotic Rim (Spongy Bone)	(21-22) ___ ___ mm	(23) ___ /9			
5. Mottling (Spongy Bone)		(24) ___ /9			
6. Septa	(25-26) ___ ___ mm			(27) 1 2	

PROLIFERATION IN THE ENDOSTEAL ENVELOPE.—Although proliferative responses are universal in all forms of bone disease, our particular reference is to neoplasms in bone.

The endosteal envelope (endosteum) is a thin continuous layer of connective tissue which covers the inner surface of the cortex and envelops each trabecula in the spongy bone. Structurally it is not nearly so apparent as the thick, tough periosteal envelope (periosteum) and functionally is not nearly so reactive.

As with bone destruction, 10–12 days are required after the inciting stimulus before sufficient bone has been laid down for it to be visible in the radiograph. As a result, proliferative response may be expected to lag about two weeks behind the stimulus in reflecting the actual status of a progressing or healing disease process.

The Public Model

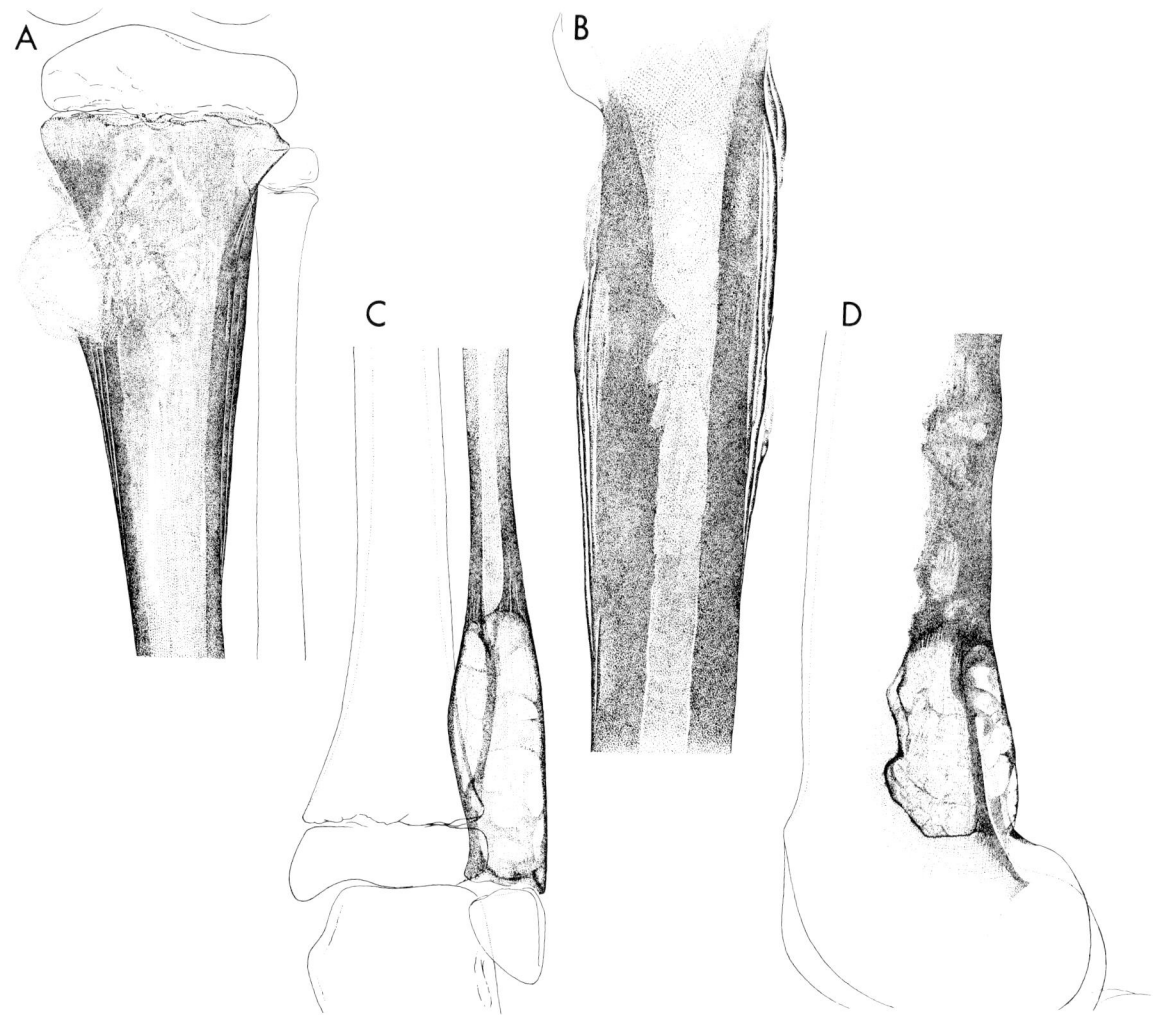

Figure 13.—Rate factors. **A,** coarse lamination and Codman's triangle; osteosarcoma. Periosteal response is coarse in that thickness of individual layers of bone is greater than that of the interleaved soft tissues. **B,** delicate periosteal lamination and Codman's triangle; Ewing's sarcoma. Periosteal response is characterized by layers of new bone, thinner than interleaved soft tissue layers. Tumor in the medullary canal has stimulated formation of endosteal new bone, thus narrowing the canal. **C,** buttress; chondromyxoid fibroma. Angle between cortex and expanded shell is filled with a triangle of solid new bone, the analogue of Codman's triangle. **D,** sclerotic rim; fibroxanthoma. The segment of tumor circumference in contact with spongy bone is sealed off by a thin layer of dense reparative bone that is continuous with the periosteal shell. (*Continued.*)

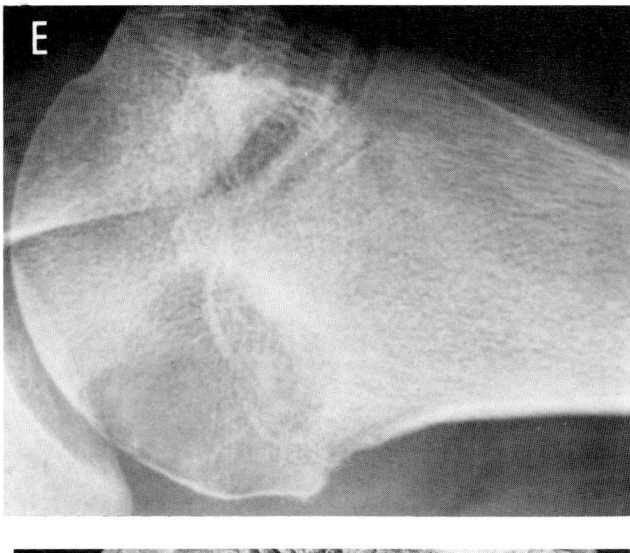

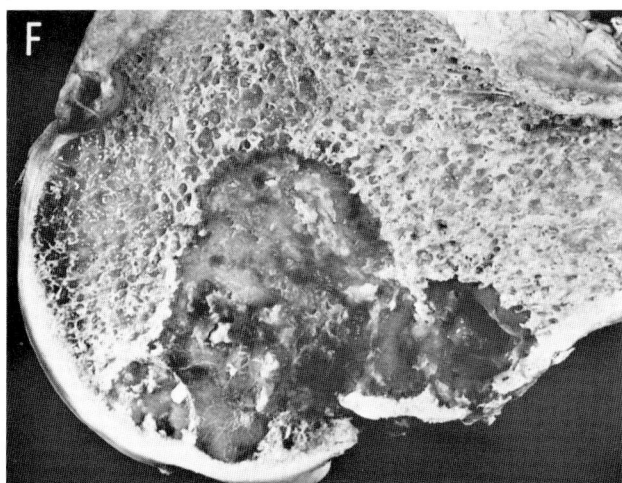

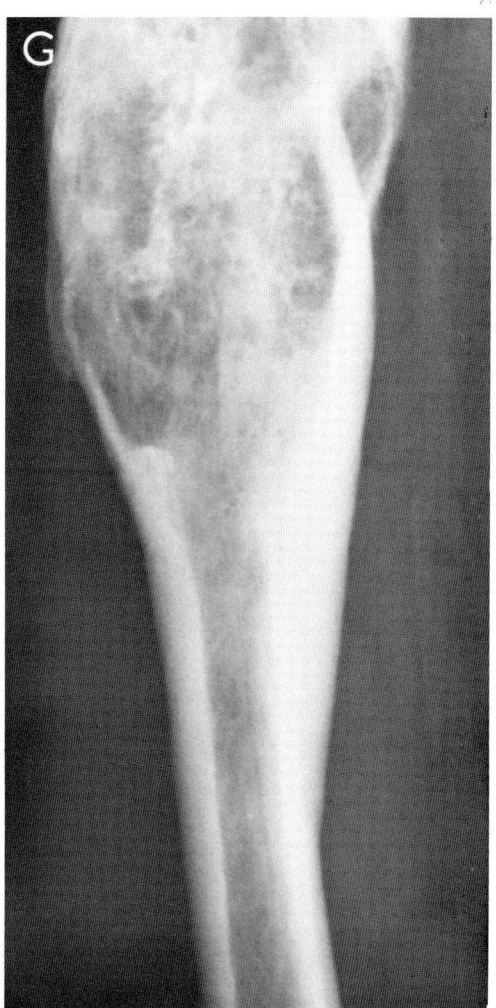

Figure 13 (cont.).—Rate factors. **E,** geographic destruction with marginal sclerosis; chondroblastoma of humeral head. Note layering of periosteal new bone remote from tumor site. **F,** hemisection of **E,** showing thickening of trabeculae at edge of hole produced by tumor. **G,** functional proliferation of bone in presence of slowly growing chondrosarcoma. The periosteal new bone serves to encapsulate the tumor and meet weight-bearing stress despite destruction of original cortex by tumor. (**E–G** from Lodwick, Radiol. Clin. North America 2:209, 1964.) (*Continued.*)

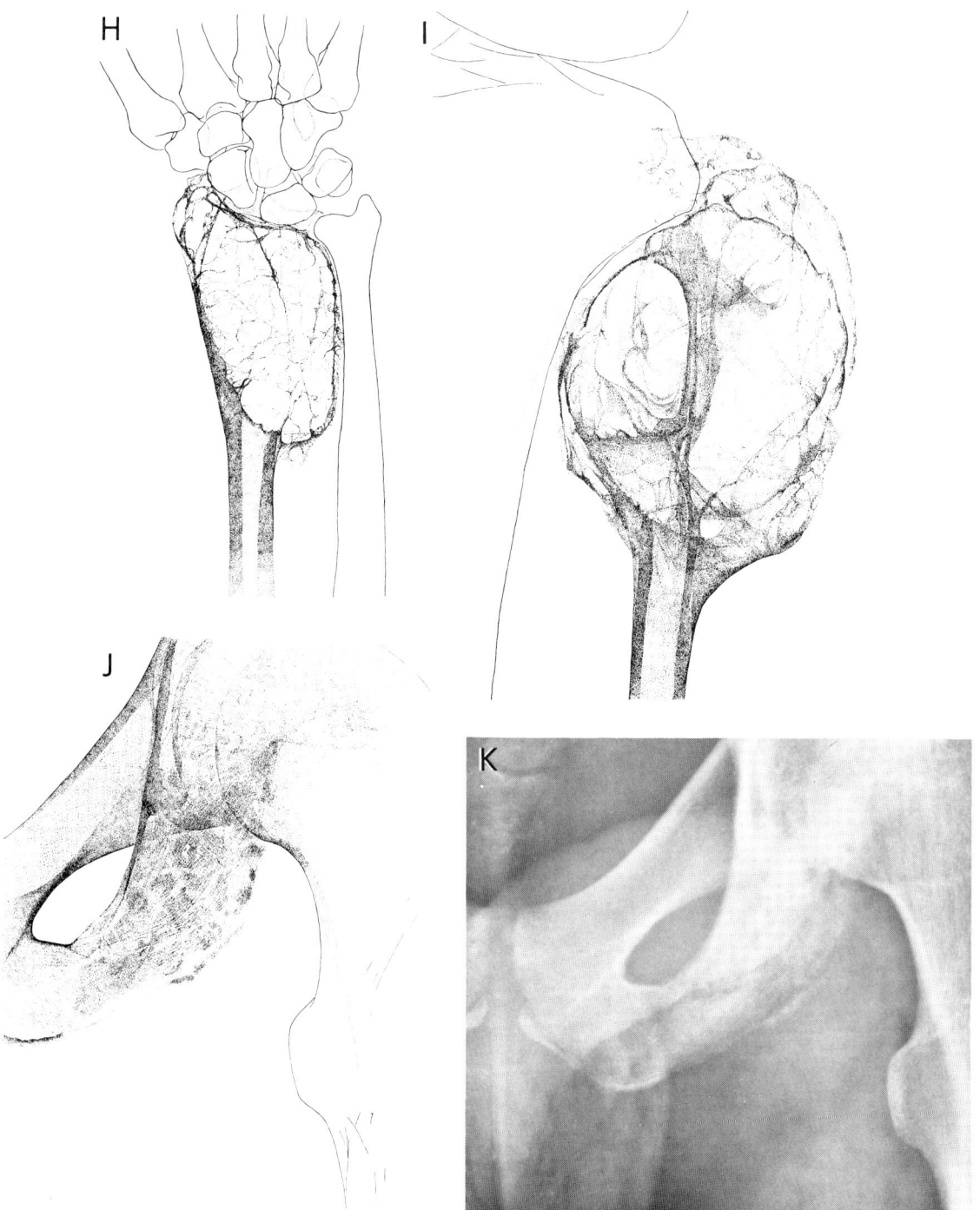

Figure 13 (cont.).—Rate factors. **H,** expanded shell, exceptionally delicate septa; giant cell tumor. Continuous with the sclerotic rim within, is the external shell of periosteal new bone which completes encapsulation. **I,** expanded shell, coarse septa; giant cell tumor. Because the fibula is so narrow, nearly all of the encapsulation is provided by the periosteal shell. **J** and **K,** mottled proliferation;

→

B. QUALITATIVE FACTORS:

1. Endosteal New Bone	(28-29) ___ mm				
2. Amorphous Periostosis	(30-31) ___ mm				
3. Laminated Periostosis	(32-33) ___ mm		(34) ___	(35) 1 2	
4. Spiculation	(36-37) ___ mm			(38) 1 2	
5. Honeycombed		(39) /9			
6. Hyperostosis	(40-41) ___ mm				
7. Diffuse Sclerosis (Spongy Bone)	(42-43) (44-45) ___ X ___ cm	(46) /9			

Time appears to play another important role in the development of endosteal proliferative response. We have already seen that a neoplasm growing slowly within bone may be expected to have a sharply delineated line of conversion between destroyed bone and intact bone. As the tumor slowly enlarges, the edge of the zone of bone destruction moves slowly as a front (see Fig. 10, *E*). Tumors which stimulate proliferative response will do so largely in the zone of contact with normal bone. As a result, in the presence of slow growth, new bone is deposited along the edge of the destroyed area on the surfaces of the preexisting normal trabeculae, thickening their structure and narrowing the intertrabecular spaces (Fig. **13, F**) to the point where ultimately a solid wall may be formed. This wall is reflected radiographically as a sclerotic rim (Fig. **13, E–G**). Usually this reactive rim is narrow. However, certain tumors, such as osteoid osteoma stimulate a vigorous reactive response in a broad zone around the central destroyed area which may be far more prominent in terms of its density and total area of involvement than the active tumor itself (see Fig. 14, *F*). In some instances the only clue to the presence of a tumor may be a large zone of *diffuse sclerosis* of cancellous bone.

The rapidly advancing tumor does not allow sufficient time for structuring of an organized front of reactive sclerosis; radiographically it appears to have no linear front at all. Rather, the tumor grows in depth through the intertrabecular spaces of the spongy bone (Fig. **13, L**) and through multiple tunnels and slots in the cortex, providing a broad zone of contact between

---

Ewing's sarcoma. Reparative new bone is present, but instead of being concentrated at the tumor edge, as in sclerotic rim, it is scattered randomly throughout the tumor. This pattern depends on presence of spongy bone, which provides the structural framework on which most such new bone is deposited. Close observation reveals the increased density to be due to thickening of trabeculae. (*Continued.*)

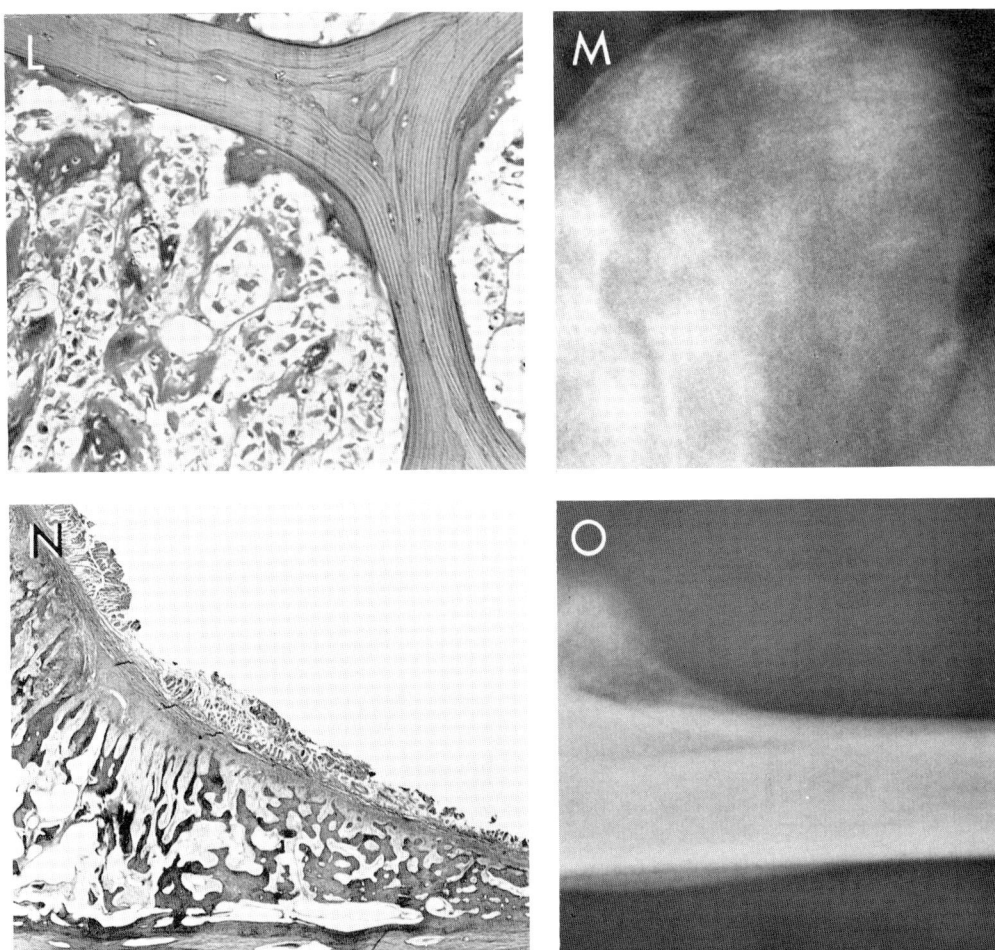

Figure 13 (cont.).—Rate factors. **L**, new bone being formed on surface of trabeculae and in space formerly occupied by marrow; lung carcinoma metastatic to trabecular bone. **M**, increased density due to thickening of trabeculae without alteration of trabecular pattern; prostate carcinoma metastatic to ilium. **N** and **O**, periosteal proliferation; osteosarcoma. Both vertical and horizontal layering of bone is apparent histologically, but only horizontal layering radiographically. (**L–O** from Lodwick, Radiol. Clin. North America 2:209, 1964.)

the tumor and the normal bone. In this circumstance newly formed bone is scattered throughout the broad zone of contact in many discrete or confluent foci. These are deposited on residual spongy bone and on the endosteal surface of the cortex which has been bypassed by the tumor. Through this mechanism reparative response in a rapidly spreading lesion is reflected as a broad zone of *mottled* increased density usually intermixed with a permeative or moth-eaten pattern of destruction (Fig. **13, J, K** and **M**).

With certain tumors, especially Ewing's sarcoma, proliferative new bone may be formed more or less uniformly on the inner surface of the cortex.

This localized thickening of the inner surface is reflected radiographically as an *endostosis* (see Fig. 14, *A*) and seems to be the result of bone proliferation exceeding bone destruction.

To summarize, the patterns of endosteal proliferation of new bone are: sclerotic rim, mottled, diffuse sclerosis, and endostosis.

PROLIFERATION IN THE PERIOSTEAL ENVELOPE.—As with endosteum, the principal radiographic evidence of periosteal envelope activity is the formation of new bone. Periosteal new bone may form as a result of neoplasm growing through the cortex from within bone or of neoplasm arising in the soft tissues and invading the periosteum from without. The former mechanism is much the commoner. As with the endosteum, the radiographic evidence of periosteal new bone formation lags some two weeks behind the stimulus.

When tumor grows through the cortex it elevates the periosteum and stimulates periosteal response. If the tumor is growing slowly, the periosteum has time to consolidate a thick layer of new bone on the surface of the cortex over the tumor. Typically the tumor attacks and destroys the inner surface of the cortex, while additional layers are being formed on the outer surface, with the effect of shifting the cortex outward to form an *expanded cortex* or shell (Fig. **13, I**). Expanded cortex ultimately may become strong enough to assume the supportive function of bone destroyed by tumor (Fig. **13, G**). Where the growth of tumor is uneven, the cortical shell is thin over nodules of relatively rapidly growing tumor and thick in the intervening areas, forming a *septate* radiographic pattern (Fig. **13, H** and **I**). Rarely, with certain tumors, especially hemangiomas, the cortex is penetrated by relatively large holes framed by a coarse reticulate pattern of periosteal new bone, the *honeycomb* appearance (Fig. 56, *A* and *B*). More rarely, the honeycomb pattern may be combined with low uniform spicules of new bone which arise and extend outward from the septal network (Fig. **14, E**).

With slow growth the obtuse angle between normal cortex and the expanded portion tends to fill in with dense new bone to produce a thick wedge that acts as a *buttress* to the margin of the expanded portion (Fig. **13, C** and **G**). Occasionally, and especially with chondroblastoma, multiple layers of periosteal new bone simply consolidate to form a smooth thickness of bone or *hyperostosis* on the outer surface of the cortex (Fig. **14, B**).

With rapid growth the process of periosteal new bone formation is the same. The end product is different, however, because there is insufficient time for the periosteum to produce the organized response characteristic of slow growth. In rapidly growing aggressive tumors the periosteum is elevated to produce a thin layer of *laminated* new bone. Certain tumors, principally

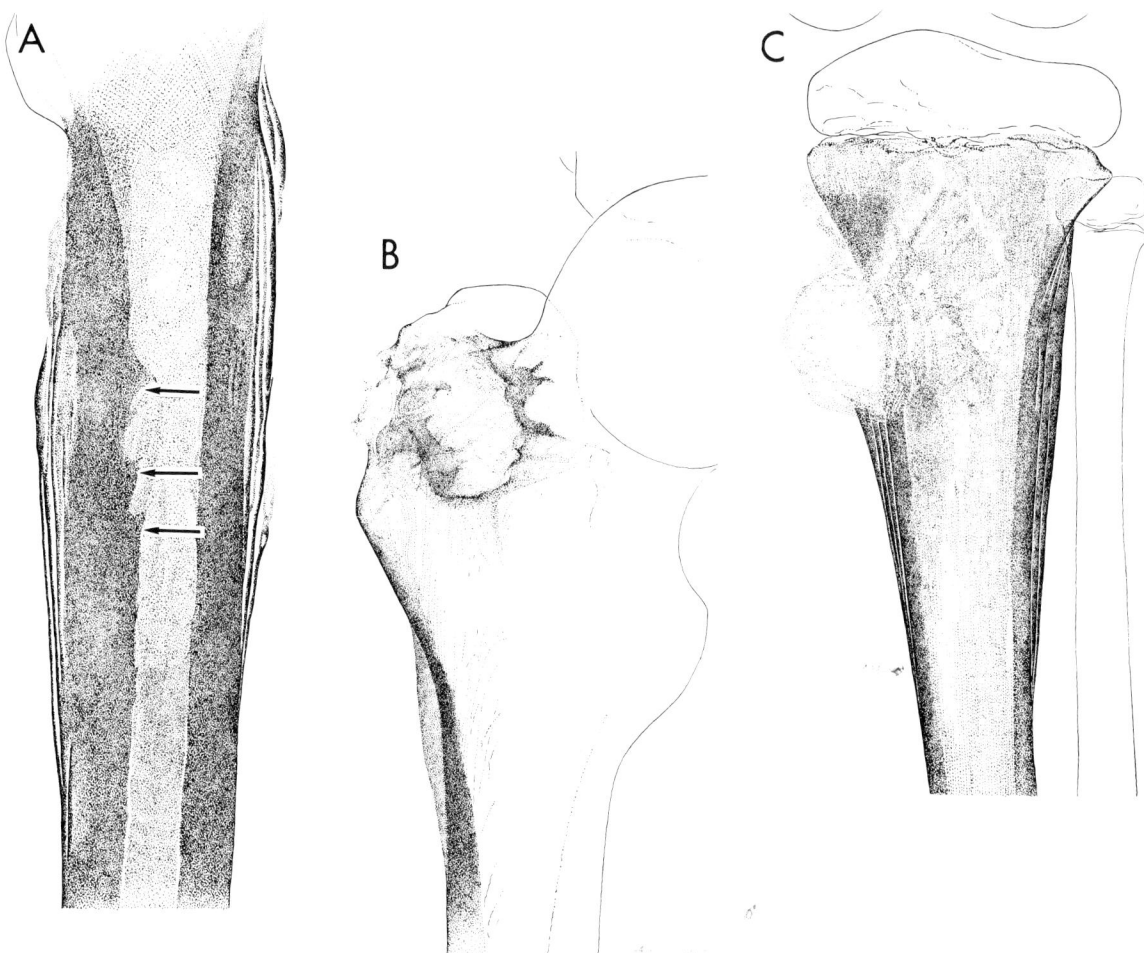

Figure 14.—Qualitative factors. **A,** endostosis and delicate lamination; Ewing's sarcoma. Reparative bone has been deposited on inner surface of cortex, increasing its total thickness and narrowing its medullary canal, while multiple thin layers of new bone have been deposited on the external surface by the periosteum. **B,** hyperostosis; chondroblastoma. A thick wedge of hyperostotic new bone has been deposited on the lateral surface of the femoral cortex, remote from primary site. **C,** coarse periosteal lamination; osteosarcoma. Multiple coarse layers of new bone have been deposited on the outer surface of the cortex. (*Continued.*)

Ewing's and osteosarcoma, may grow in spurts, in which case the periosteum may respond by producing multiple concentric layers of periosteal new bone in a laminated *onion-peel* pattern (Fig. **14, A** and **C**). But inevitably, however, the central thrust of the rapidly growing tumor overcomes the capacity of the periosteum to form bone and penetrates it to grow directly into the soft tissues surrounding the bone. In this situation the periosteal response nearest the center of the tumor is completely disorganized or destroyed, leaving only cuffs of periosteal new bone at the margin of the tumor where it is just penetrating the cortex. These cuffs or *Codman's triangles* are well-known evidence of aggressive tumor behavior (Fig. **13, A** and **B**). They represent the analogue of the buttress in the slowly growing tumor.

Instead of producing smooth laminations of uniform density some tumors produce a single nonuniform layer of new bone, irregular and undulating in contour and *amorphous* in appearance (Fig. **14, D**). This is seen most often in reticulum cell sarcoma and fibrosarcoma. Parenthetically, it can be said

Figure 14 (cont.).—Qualitative factors. **D,** amorphous periostosis. New bone is irregular in thickness and outer contour, presenting a lumpy, rough appearance in profile. Codman's triangles are uncommon with this type of periosteal response. **E,** honeycomb pattern, with highly structured combination of holes in bone, marginal sclerosis and spicular periosteal response. Usually, honeycomb refers to a pattern of holes of uniform size and relationship. **F,** diffuse sclerosis. In contrast to marginal sclerosis, a broad (more than 5 mm) zone of increased density is seen around a focal lesion, usually in spongy bone. It may have no visible central nidus of disease and may be the only evidence of osteoid osteoma; infection is also a common cause. It may result from broad areas of endosteal or periosteal deposition of dense new bone.

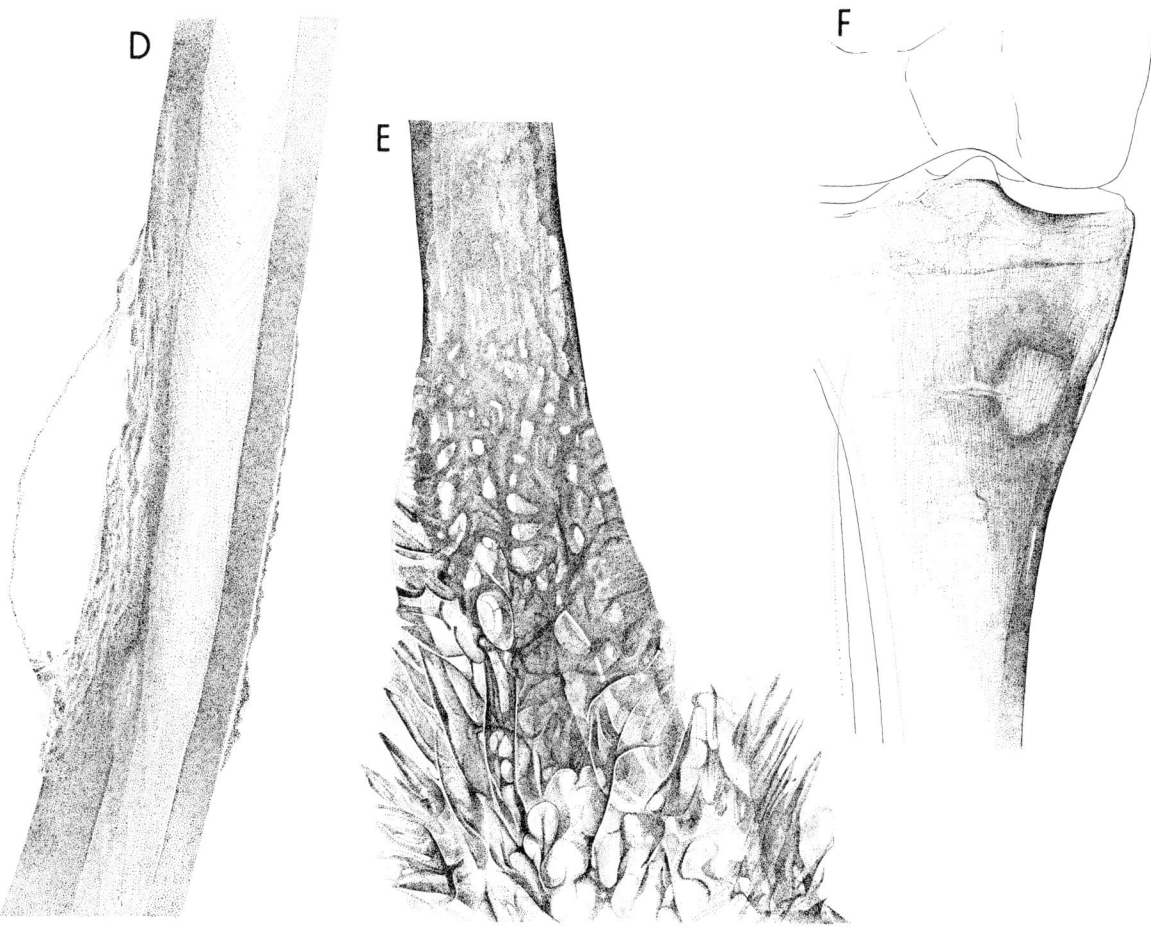

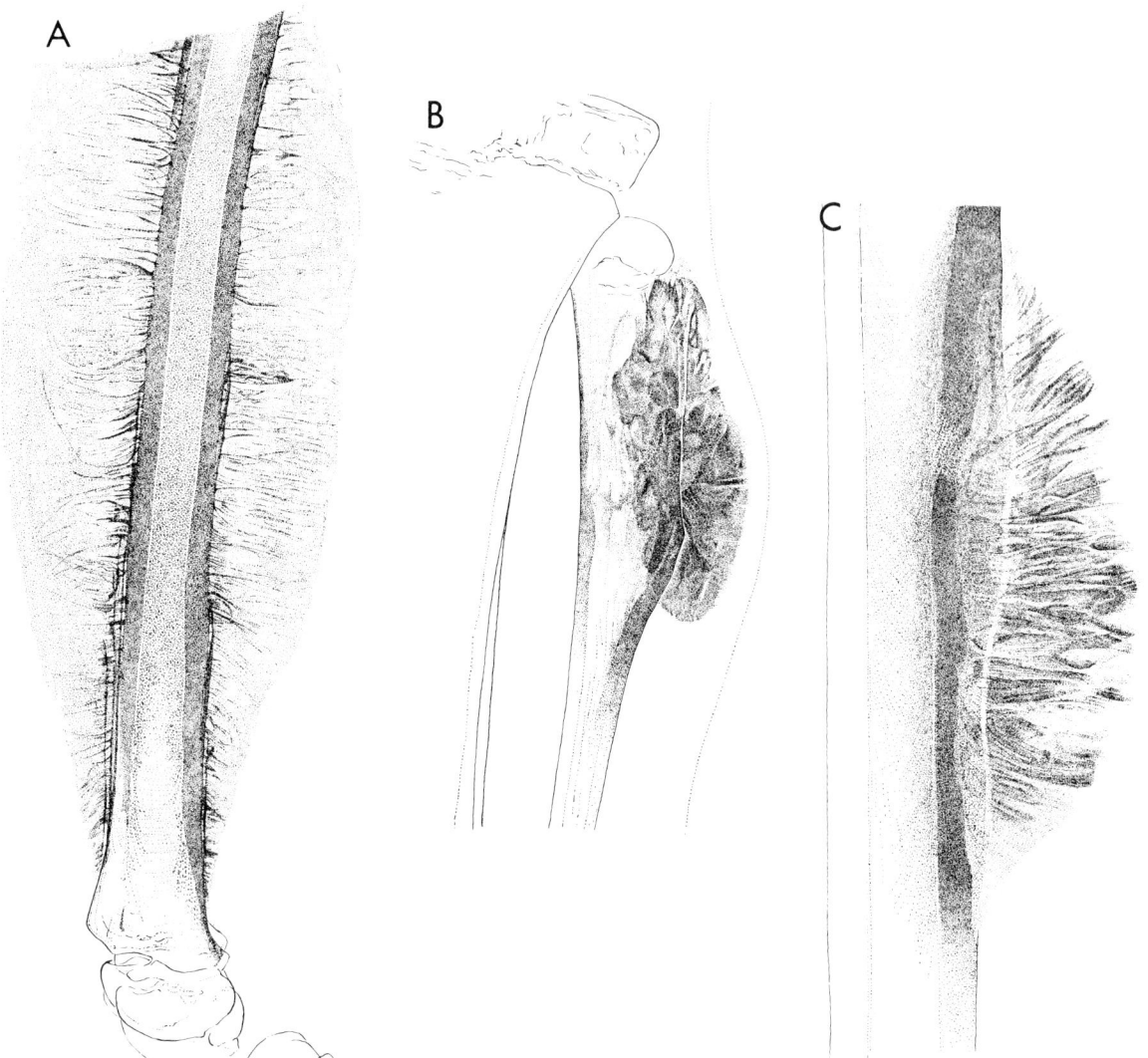

Figure 15.—Spiculation. **A,** hair-on-end. Spicules of new bone are delicate, more widely spaced than other spiculations and mostly perpendicular to the cortical surface; common in Ewing's sarcoma. **B,** regular. Spicules are coarse, closely packed, usually radiate from a point source and are almost uniform in length, providing a regular contour to their outer surface; usual in parosteal sarcoma. **C,** sunburst. Spicules are coarse, radiate from a point source and are essentially nonuniform in length. They reflect a less well differentiated tumor than the regular spicular pattern, usually an osteosarcoma. This and nondescript (see Fig. 15, *E*) are the patterns most often seen in metastatic and nonneoplastic diseases. (*Continued.*)

that in the presence of infection the periosteum usually responds by producing a single solid lamina of new bone, quite different from the patterns observed when neoplasms are the inciting cause.

> C. (47) Kind of Spiculation
> 1_____Regular
> 2_____Sunburst
> 3_____Nondescript
> 4_____Hair on End
> 5_____Velvet

When periosteum is elevated by tumor, multiple vertical *rays* of new bone commonly form between the cortex and the active surface of the periosteum. The spaces between these delicate rays contain blood vessels. Usually the rays are so delicate that they cannot be demonstrated radiographically. Sometimes, for unknown reasons, the striations become thick and long enough to be seen in the radiograph. In tumors that tend to spread along the long axis of a bone, especially Ewing's sarcoma, the spiculations are perpendicular to the cortex, as *hair-on-end* (Fig. 15, **A**). In tumors with a globular pattern of growth, such as osteosarcoma, the calcified spicules often radiate along lines emanating from a point source at the center of the tumor, giving a *sunburst* effect (**C**). *Velvety* spiculation is a low, slanting pattern of spicules, unequal in length and fuzzy in outline; it is particularly likely to be seen in chondrosarcoma (**D**). A few very slowly growing lesions incite a spicular response which is quite uniform and *regular* (**B**). The rest are so *nondescript* as to defy classification (**E**).

> D. (48) Does Expanded Shell of Bone
> Completely Encapsulate the
> Tumor
> 1_____Yes
> 2_____No

Does periosteal new bone form an intact shell around the tumor, or are there areas where the tumor and the periosteal soft tissues lie in direct contact? The diagnostic and prognostic significance of this finding has never been evaluated.

Coarse and delicate periosteal response and spiculation.—Some tumors, principally Ewing's sarcoma, produce a very delicate septation, lamination and spicules, whereas others, such as osteosarcoma, parosteal sarcoma and metastatic cancer, excite a much coarser response. The qualifications of coarse and delicate are difficult to define. Generally speaking, in a delicate periosteal response the thickness of the layer of periosteal new bone is less

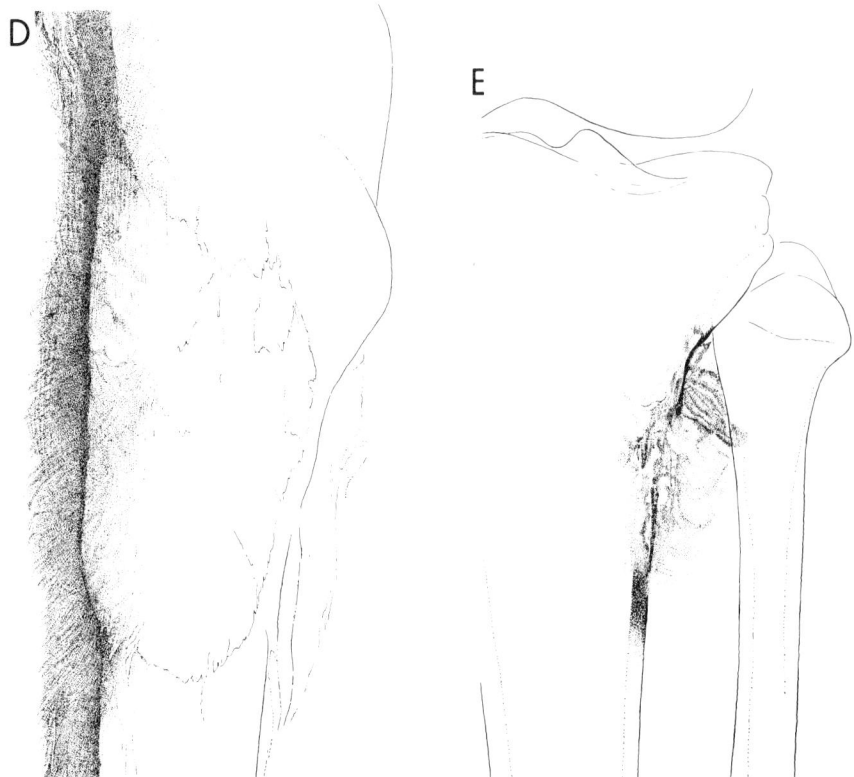

Figure 15 (cont.).—Spiculation. **D,** velvet. A low slanting pattern, fuzzy in outline, most often seen in slowly growing chondrosarcoma. **E,** nondescript. This irregular pattern cannot be classified in any of the other spicular patterns.

than the thickness of the soft tissue layer between it and the cortex. In contrast, in coarse periosteal response the thickness of the soft tissue layer is equal to or less than that of the laminae of new bone.

The qualities of coarse and delicate relative to spiculation are even more difficult to define. In delicate spiculation the individual spicules are quite straight and narrow to the point of being linear, like hair standing on end. Coarse spicules appear to be heavy, have width, often are tapered from the base and are more likely to radiate.

To summarize, periosteal proliferation of new bone leads to expanded cortex, septation, buttress formation, hyperostosis, laminated response, amorphous response and spiculation (regular, sunburst, nondescript, hair-on-end, velvety) which may be delicate or coarse.

C. Assessment of Growth Rate

MOST EXPERIENCED RADIOLOGISTS develop an intuitive feeling as to whether the radiographic image is of a benign or a malignant bone tumor. Based on the criteria already described under tumor size, bone destruction, reparative response and tumor matrix mineralization, it is clear that most components of the radiographic image are related more to the aggressiveness or slowness of tumor growth than to histologic type. Indeed, one reason why identification of histologic type from the radiograph is so difficult is that it is a diagnosis made by inference. That is, Ewing's sarcoma is Ewing's sarcoma because of its typical location and size, its scattered permeated pattern of bone destruction, its nonencapsulative periosteal response, the absence of any evidence of tumor matrix mineralization and, last, the age of the patient. There is nothing which permits a radiologist to evaluate the particular kinds of cells which identify a tumor as being Ewing's sarcoma. The pathologist, on the other hand, in looking at biopsy material, sees only an abnormal, highly cellular structure characteristic of Ewing's sarcoma and little or none of the characteristics of growth rate which substantially form the radiographic image. The two kinds of evidence, radiographic and histologic, complement each other extraordinarily well, yet neither may be regarded as a total substitute for the other.

In short, the radiograph reflects growth rate, whereas histologic sections reflect cellular structure. This the radiologist must constantly appreciate, for if he focuses entirely on trying to identify the cell type of a tumor, he may well deprive the patient and the referring physician of the kind of evidence (growth rate) which he is most competent to offer.

In recognition of this direct relationship between the radiographic image and the growth rate of a tumor, we grade *rate of growth* into three major divisions: I, *slow*; II, *moderate*; and III, *rapid*. Since slow growth rate (I) comprises a rather major segment of the total spectrum of growth rate, it has been further subdivided into IA, IB, and IC, based on variations in the radiographic pattern.

  C. (74) Growth Rate (Circle One)
      IA IB IC II III
      (1) (2) (3) 4 5

The criteria used in radiographic estimation of growth rate are: (1) destruction of bone; (2) proliferation of bone; (3) tumor matrix mineraliza-

TABLE 2.—TRUTH TABLE FOR GRADING OF PRIMARY BONE TUMORS

	IA	IB	IC	II	III
Bone destruction pattern					
Absent	1000	1000	1000	1000	1000
Geographic w/reg. margin	1000	1000	1000	0	0
Geographic w/lob. margin	1000	1000	1000	0	0
Geographic w/me margin	1000	1000	1000	0	0
Geog. w/rag. or unseen marg.	0	0	1000	0	0
Geog. and moth-eaten $>$ 1 cm	0	0	0	1000	0
Geog. and moth-eaten $<$ 1 cm	0	0	1000	0	0
Moth-eaten	0	0	0	1000	0
Permeated included	0	0	0	0	1000
Penetration of cortex					
Absent	1000	1000	0	0	0
Partial	1000	1000	0	0	0
Total	0	0	1000	1000	1000
Sclerotic rim					
Present	1000	1000	1000	1000	1000
Absent	0	1000	1000	1000	1000
Expanded shell					
Absent	1000	0	1000	1000	1000
$<$ 1 cm	1000	0	1000	1000	1000
$>$ 1 cm	0	1000	1000	1000	1000
Buttress					
Present	1000	1000	1000	0	0
Absent	1000	1000	1000	1000	1000
Mottling					
Present	0	0	0	1000	1000
Absent	1000	1000	1000	1000	1000
Codman's triangle					
None	1000	1000	1000	1000	1000
One	0	0	1000	1000	1000
Two	0	0	0	1000	1000
Three or more	0	0	0	0	1000
Tumor bone pattern					
Absent	1000	1000	1000	1000	1000
Cloudy	0	0	0	0	1000
Cloudy and lumpy	0	0	0	1000	0
Lumpy	0	0	0	1000	0
Lumpy and solid	0	0	1000	1000	0
Cloudy, lumpy, solid	0	0	0	1000	0
Solid	1000	1000	1000	0	0
Cloudy and solid	0	0	0	1000	0
Flocculent					
Present	1000	1000	1000	1000	0
Absent	1000	1000	1000	1000	1000
Flecks					
Present	1000	0	0	0	0
Absent	1000	1000	1000	1000	1000
Ground-glass					
Present	1000	1000	1000	0	0
Absent	1000	1000	1000	1000	1000
Size					
$<$ 6 cm	1000	1000	1000	0	0
$>$ 6 cm	1000	1000	1000	1000	1000

tion, and (4) size, and in that order. This is not to say that in every instance the pattern of bone destruction is more significant as to rate of growth than the pattern of proliferative response. To develop a decision scheme which consistently arrives at the same decision, given a certain set of information about a tumor, there must be a rank order of priority for each particular kind of information. In other words, to arrive at a consistent decision, one must always follow the same logic. The logic which we employ is shown in Table 2.

In the Truth Table (Table 2) the factors used for estimating rate of growth are listed in the order of their importance. The process of decision begins at the top of the table and proceeds downward until only one possibility of grade remains. The number 1000 means that a particular grade is still in the running for that particular finding unless it has been eliminated above; zero means that the grade has been eliminated from further consideration. In this scheme, destruction of bone is obviously the most powerful grading tool. Reactive new bone is of next greatest importance. When neither destruction nor proliferation of bone is present, the decision ultimately hinges on the extent of tumor matrix mineralization and its combinations, plus the size of the tumor. In this situation, more than one grade are commonly reported.

In essence, this decision scheme recognizes the following possibilities for intraosseous tumors. *Growth rate IA*, slowest growth (Fig. **16, A**): geographic bone destruction with incomplete penetration of the cortex, a sclerotic rim and, at most, expansion of the cortex 1 cm or less beyond the projected surface of the original cortex. *Growth rate IB*, a bit more aggressive (**B**): geographic pattern, incomplete penetration of the cortex, but with expansion of the cortex greater than 1 cm beyond the projected surface of the original cortex, and permissible sclerotic rim. *Growth rate IC*, even more aggressive (**C** and **D**): still geographic pattern; there may be a marginal zone of moth-eaten bone destruction, but if so, the transition of the moth-eaten zone from complete destruction to none must be 1 cm or less in width as viewed en face. There is complete penetration of the cortex with extension of tumor into the soft tissues beyond the projected surface of the cortex. A buttress or one Codman triangle is permissible. *Growth rate II*, moderate growth (**E**): moth-eaten destruction, or geographic pattern with a marginal rim of moth-eaten bone destruction, the transition from complete destruction to intact bone being more than 1 cm wide as viewed en face; in either situation, total penetration of the cortex is inferred. There may be one or more Codman triangles. *Growth rate III*, the most aggressive (**F**): permeated destruction, alone or in combination with moth-eaten or geographic pattern,

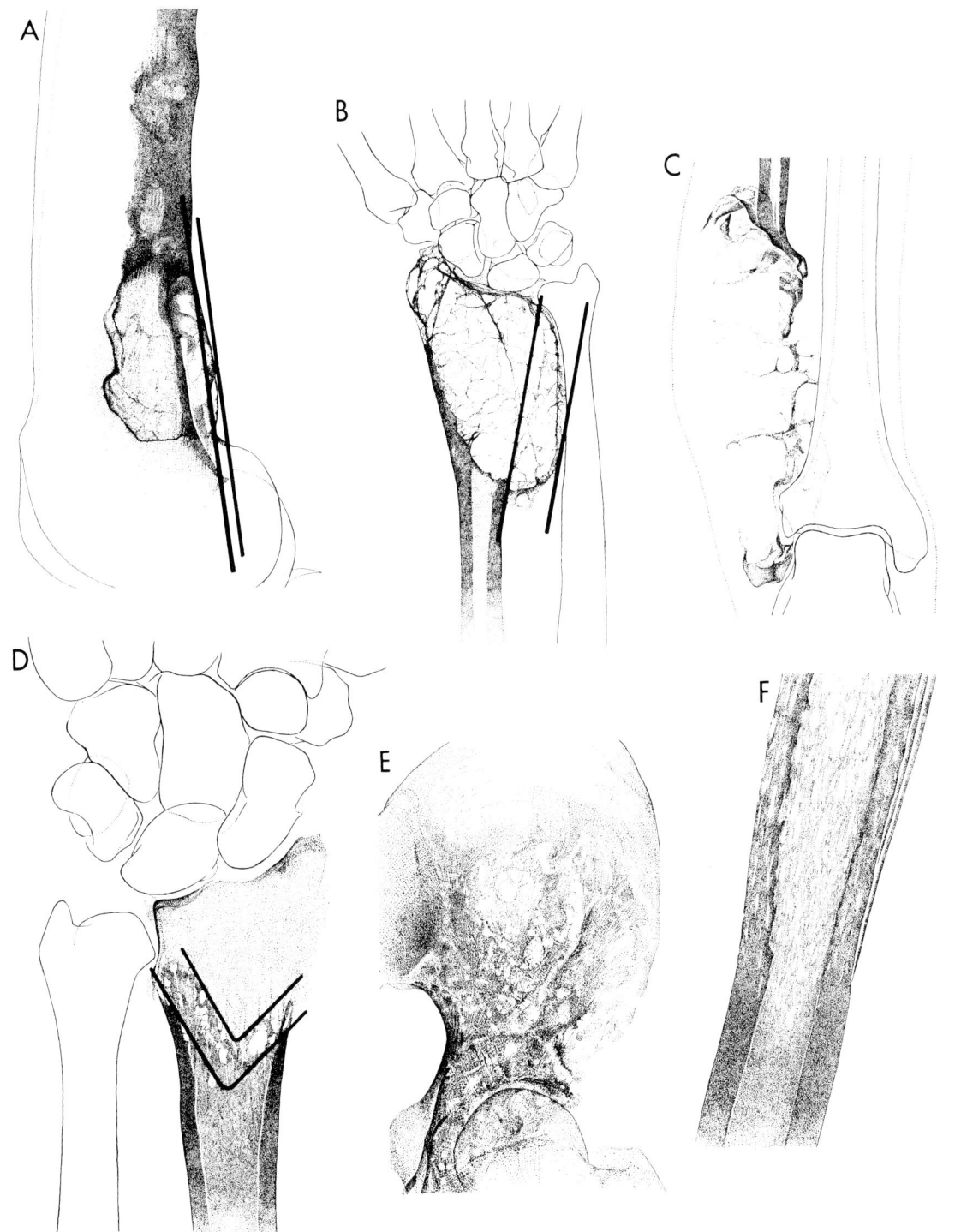

Figure 16.—Rates of growth. **A,** grade IA. **B,** grade IB. **C** and **D,** grade IC. In **C,** an adamantinoma, no marginal zone of moth-eaten bone destruction is present; **D** represents a giant cell tumor. **E,** grade II. **F,** grade III.

or both; complete penetration of the cortex is inferred. There may be two or more Codman triangles.

One occasionally encounters a tumor with geographic destruction, incomplete penetration of the cortex, no significant degree of expansion and absence of sclerotic rim. This peculiar combination most resembles the pattern for IA but, lacking the sclerotic rim, is classified in the next step upward as IB.

If there is a fracture, for prognostic purposes the classification is moved one step toward the more rapidly growing end of the spectrum in recognition of the unfavorable influence of fractures on malignant and potentially malignant tumors.

Nearly all tumors which arise inside of bone are characterized by some pattern of destruction of bone. If destruction of bone is not visible, evidence for determining growth rate rests first on additional reactive phenomena, then on the patterns of tumor matrix mineralization, and then on size. In the computer-mediated mechanism for this evaluation the evidence is examined and grades are eliminated until only one remains. In a few cases a final decision will not be reached because of inadequate information. In such instances the computer reports that the growth rate may be two or more of five possible choices. In no instance has the computer reported two or more possible choices which did not occupy immediately adjacent portions of the spectrum of growth rate. This fact speaks for the strength of the internal logic of the system. As a measure of overall performance, the computer has successfully graded between 90 and 95% of most series submitted for examination.

When finding growth rate is based on reparative phenomena, generally the lower grades are characterized by the components of reparative new bone formation which reflect slow growth, such as buttress formation, expanded cortex and septation, while the more aggressive grades are characterized by components which reflect lack of encapsulation, such as Codman's triangles and mottling of spongy bone.

In tumors which arise in a parosteal location, neither destruction nor repair of bone may be present, thus depriving the evaluative mechanism of two of the most useful tools for estimation of growth rate. Here one must rely on the less satisfactory pattern of tumor matrix mineralization for grading. When large solid masses of tumor bone are present, the assumption is that there is a good deal of differentiation. When clouds of tumor bone are visualized, poor differentiation is assumed. When the soft tissue tumor is completely radiolucent without evidence of tumor matrix mineralization and there is neither bone destruction nor proliferation, the situation for grading from a radiograph is hopeless.

	IA	IB	IC	II	III	% Graded
TABLE 3.—Results of Grading of Growth Rate of 143 Fibrosarcomas						
Distribution of tumor graded	19	15	50	32	27	94.1
Average delay in diagnosis (months)	50.0	15.3	15.2	14.3	6.6	
Absolute 5 yr. survival (%)	52.6	46.7	36.0	15.6	7.4	

Table 3 shows an application of the technique for grading of growth rate to 143 fibrosarcomas from the Codman Registry. Note that the distribution of cases is normal with a slight skewing toward the right—the more aggressive growth rates. The duration of symptoms before diagnosis falls off evenly as the more aggressive growth rates are examined, and the absolute five year survival follows the same trend. Examination of this evidence gives a rather complete picture of the character of fibrosarcoma, and one quite different from osteosarcoma, where the peak incidence is in the most rapidly growing end of the spectrum. Fibrosarcoma, however, is an ideal tumor for grading rate of growth because it is distributed throughout the full spectrum of malignancy and because in fibrosarcoma it is less likely that the radiographic image of destruction and repair will be obscured by tumor bone or massive proliferative response.

D. Prediction of Histologic Diagnosis

THUS FAR we have looked at the decision-making process in relation to the kinds of tools we use in the diagnosis of bone disease. In particular we have examined a model of bone disease which includes the parameters of age, size, shape, location, bone destruction, reparative response and tumor matrix mineralization. These tools are most useful for estimating the growth rate of neoplasms, for the image of bone disease is dynamic in that it is possible to evaluate rate of growth from a single film rather than requiring several examinations on different dates. We have also examined a system for placing a tumor in one of five different growth rates for purposes of identification, treatment and prognosis. We now come to the most difficult problem—that of predicting histologic type from radiographic patterns of disease. Prediction of histologic type is of greatest usefulness (1) when such a prediction is of a high enough order of statistical accuracy that it matches that of the pathologist, or (2) when, if there is an error in prediction, the kind of error is such that it probably will not affect future management. An example of the first situation is fibroxanthoma, where the probability of diagnostic error should be less than 5%. Fibroxanthoma is a good example for the second situation as well; an error in diagnosis would not be likely to affect management since, whatever you called the lesion, its rate of growth would be so slow, probably IA, that aggressive management would not be called for. Another example is the rapidly growing osteosarcoma (growth rate III) because, even if called something else, such an error should not affect the speed with which a biopsy is obtained and management decided upon.

Our present model and earlier editions of it have been used to analyze the radiographs of more than 1,400 tumors. The considerable volume of data thus collected reflects the frequency of each of the elements of the model, in each type of tumor. Such data may be conveniently presented in the form of a prior probability matrix, the X axis representing symptoms and signs, and the Y axis tumors. Each of the interstices contains the raw probability that a certain sign will be found in a certain kind of tumor. From the statistical point of view, the best probability matrix is one based on an infinite number of examples, but since an infinite number of examples is impossible to collect, our experience has been far from theoretically ideal.

There is another type of probability matrix, the *personal* one. In this, each of the interstices contains a probability figure supplied from the memory of the investigator; if the investigator has had broad experience, his personal

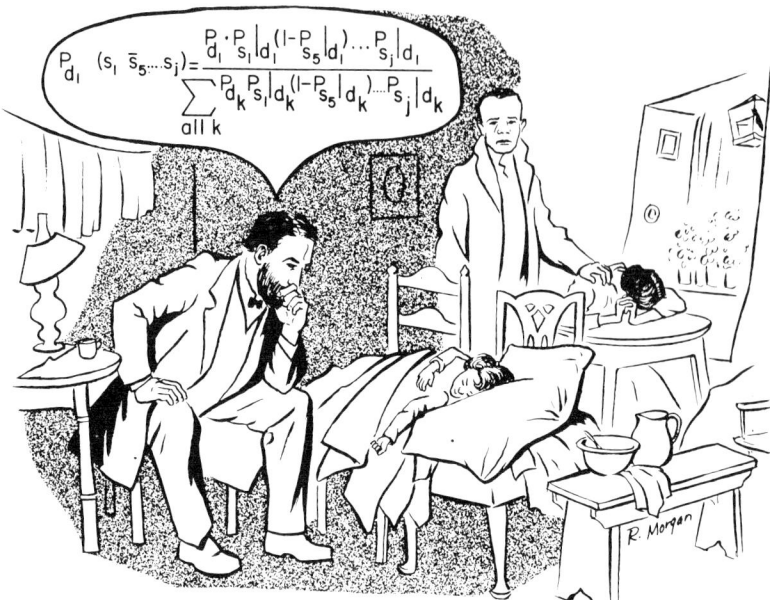

Figure 17.—Bayes's rule of inverse probability.

probability matrix should be excellent. In my experience, the personal probability matrix has provided for a more accurate program of computer diagnosis than one based on raw data. Considerable judgment is involved in building a personal probability matrix, principally regarding the natural incidence of specific findings in a particular disease as compared with all other pertinent diseases. In a probability matrix of the complexity required with this diagnostic situation, the personal probability matrix is grafted on one based on raw probabilities and represents a modification of the real world by personal experience. The most current matrix may be obtained by request from the author.

The mathematical model which we have used in the computer diagnostic decision scheme is Bayes's rule of inverse probability (Fig. 17). This rule has been highly controversial, particularly among statisticians who correctly argue that most symptoms are not independent of each other and that when large numbers of kinds of data are involved, the numbers of cases needed to provide a statistically valid probability matrix are astronomical. Despite these irrefutable criticisms of the Bayesian approach, it has a major virtue— it works.

Diagnostic principles have been discussed largely in the context of computer-assisted diagnosis. I believe that this is appropriate, since the entire decision scheme, including the public model, the probability matrix, the mathematical model and the final array of probabilities may be regarded as a model of the decision scheme which operates in one's own human built-in computer. Our experience has been that in modeling difficult problems, we arrive at solutions which are equally applicable to human-mediated decision schemes and to computer-mediated decision schemes. However, the goal of this text is not to teach computer-assisted diagnosis, although most of the tools for such are presented in detail. The goal is to demonstrate techniques for improving human-mediated diagnosis.

THE DECISION TREE

One of the most difficult problems in the differential diagnosis of a large array of lesions is knowing where to begin. With bone tumors, certain basic tools are available, including matrix mineralization, radiologic growth rate and location, size and shape of the lesion. One must begin with a criterion

TABLE 4.—DECISION TREE: TUMORS TO BE CONSIDERED IN DIFFERENTIAL DIAGNOSIS*

01	Adamantinoma	31	Lipoma, myxolipoma
02	Benign cartilaginous tumor (chondroma, enchondroma, periosteal chondroma)	32	Liposarcoma
		33	Meningioma
03	Chondroblastoma	34	Metastatic tumor
04	Chondromyxoid fibroma	35	Mucocoele
05	Chondrosarcoma, myxosarcoma	36	Myeloma
06	Chondrosarcoma of mesenchymal or synovial origin	37	Myositis ossificans
		38	Neurofibroma, neurolemmoma
07	Chordoma	39	Osteoblastoma
08	Cortical defect, benign	40	Osteochondroma, exostosis
09	Cortical desmoid	41	Osteoid osteoma
10	Cyst, unicameral and simple	42	Osteosarcoma
11	Cyst, dentigerous	43	Parosteal sarcoma
12	Cyst, periodontal	44	Pleomorphic sarcoma
13	Cyst, subchondral	45	Reticulum cell sarcoma
14	Epidermoid of skull	46	Sarcoma, postirradiation
15	Ewing's sarcoma	47	Sarcoma, soft tissue
16	Fibroma	48	Synovial sarcoma
17	Fibroma, desmoplastic	49	Villonodular synovitis
18	Fibroma, nonossifying; fibroxanthoma	50	Xanthoma of bone
19	Fibroma, ossifying	51	Aneurysm
20	Fibrosarcoma, including neural origin	52	'B' Tumor
21	Fibrous dysplasia	53	Carcinoma (including in sinus)
22	Fibrous osteoma	54	Hematoma
23	Giant cell tumor, benign or malignant	55	Hydatid disease
24	Glomus tumor	56	Pseudolipoma
25	Hemangioma	57	Pseudomalignant osseous tumor of soft tissue
26	Hemangioma, ossifying		
27	Hemangioendothelioma	58	Unclassified malignant cellular tumor
28	Hemangio-, angiosarcoma	59	Uncommitted metaphysial lesion
29	Histiocytosis X	60	Ameloblastoma
30	Infection (osteomyelitis, TBC, Brodie's abscess, chronic osteitis)		

* The numbers relate to computer entries and to the notations in the diagrams of decision trees which follow.

which applies to all lesions, and in bone disease the only such criterion is location. Every tumor has its location. As the result of this observation, the decision tree illustrated in Table 4 begins with location relative to the axis of bone.

The decision tree contains the basic rules for differential diagnosis. In a way, the immediate goal of this decision tree is data reduction, that is, the elimination of as many diagnoses as possible. In this context application of radiologic growth rate has provided an excellent data reduction technique, since there is a large group of lesions which are found only in grades IA, IB and IC (Table 5). Although some lesions have peak frequencies in grade III, such as osteosarcoma and Ewing's sarcoma, rare examples of these lesions fall in grade I. About the only lesion which seems consistently to fall in grade III alone is pleomorphic sarcoma, and our experience with this tumor is so limited that no probability values are known.

Grading of growth rate is not used for parosteal lesions because of lack

TABLE 5.—USUAL GROWTH RATES OF BONE TUMORS

LESIONS WHICH ARE GRADE I	LESIONS WHICH MAY BE ANY GRADE
Adamantinoma	Chondrosarcoma
Benign cartilaginous tumor (chondroma, enchondroma, periosteal chondroma)	Ewing's sarcoma
	Fibrosarcoma
Chondroblastoma	Hemangioendothelioma
Chondromyxoid fibroma	Hemangiosarcoma
Chordoma	Liposarcoma
Cortical defect, benign	Metastatic tumor
Cortical desmoid	Osteosarcoma
Cyst, unicameral and simple	Reticulum cell sarcoma
Cyst, dentigerous	
Cyst, periodontal	LESIONS DIFFICULT TO GRADE
Cyst, subchondral	Myositis ossificans
Epidermoid of skull	Parosteal sarcoma
Fibroma	Soft tissue sarcomas
Fibroma, desmoplastic	Synovial sarcoma
Fibroma, nonossifying; fibroxanthoma	
Fibroma, ossifying	
Fibrous dysplasia	
Fibrous osteoma	
Giant cell tumor, benign or malignant	
Glomus tumor	
Hemangioma	
Hemangioma, ossifying	
Lipoma, myxolipoma	
Mucocoele	
Myeloma	
Neurofibroma, neurolemmoma	
Osteoblastoma	
Osteochondroma, exostosis	
Osteoid osteoma	
Villonodular synovitis	
Xanthoma of bone	

of adequate evidence of growth rate in this location. Instead, matrix mineralization is used for data reduction since, when it is present, a number of diagnoses may be eliminated.

Circumstances can arise in which information not already present in the public model is needed to differentiate further between diagnoses. For example, with a giant cell tumor, blood calcium and phosphorus levels might point to an underlying hyperparathyroidism and the key question, appropriately asked, would provide the correct answer. Key questions have not yet been built into this decision tree, but are being developed in the on-line computer version.

The decision tree and its associated logic are most powerful in distinguishing between lesions in the long bones. Many of the subsections of the decision tree for other than long bones are introduced simply because the logic of diagnosis for long bones does not yet apply to these other areas. The exact relationship between location and tumor type needs additional work in several areas, particularly the pelvis, spine and skull. The model described in this Atlas has only recently been modified to accommodate description of such relationships, and further detailed application is required.

In the following diagrams, note that each branch of the decision tree terminates in two or more tumor choices. The lesions in circles are regarded as rare, and are *not* considered for further analysis except to be listed as possible differential, mainly because probability tables are not yet available for them. At this point, the user can examine the probability matrix (obtainable from the author) for incidence in specific bones and eliminate many other possibilities. With the computer, the tumor types which are survivors of this procedure are then subjected to Bayesian analysis; human beings at this point may use their built-in computer.

The selection of the kinds of disease at the end of each branch of the decision tree needs further testing by application of this decision scheme to other large groups of tumors, particularly comprehensive collections such as those of the Orthopedic and Radiologic Registries of the Armed Forces Institute of Pathology and the collection at the Royal National Orthopedic Hospital in London. It is frustrating to present this incomplete analysis, knowing that so much additional work must be done. It is hoped that others with access to these and other major collections will undertake to correct and implement further the decision tree and add to the probability matrix.

1. Is the lesion centered parosteally ?

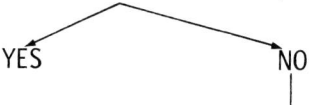

2. Is the lesion centered in the cortex ?

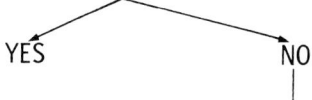

3. Is the lesion centered in medullary bone ?

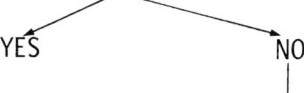

4. Is the lesion centered in a joint ?

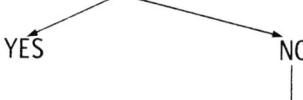

5. ERROR IN LOGIC

Decision Tree for axial location of tumor. 1. Axial location appears to be the best beginning point for analysis of bone tumors because each tumor inevitably can be classified according to this logic, and because, once classified, the number of diagnostic possibilities is narrowed sharply. In other words, identification of the location of a tumor according to the long axis of a bone is an excellent data reduction technique.

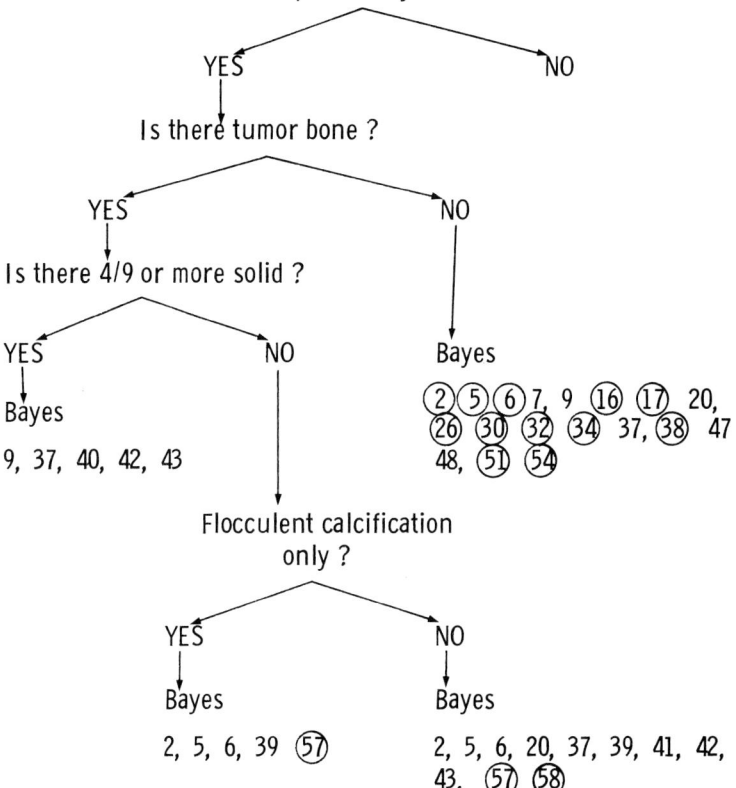

Decision Tree for lesions centered parosteally. Here the grading step is omitted because parosteal lesions often do not affect bone or periosteum, so that the information essential to proper grading is not available.

1. Is there 4/9 or more solid? A positive answer sharply limits the spectrum of parosteal lesions to cortical desmoid, myositis ossificans, osteochondroma and parosteal sarcoma (rarely osteosarcoma). Ordinarily, the parosteal portion of a cortical desmoid may be radiolucent, but an occasional lesion seems to contain a large dense segment of bone.

2. Flocculent calcification only? A positive answer sharply limits consideration to tumors of cartilaginous origin and osteoblastoma. With a negative response, a tumor may or may not contain flocculent calcification, and also any other possible combination of tumor bone.

Prediction of Histologic Diagnosis / 71

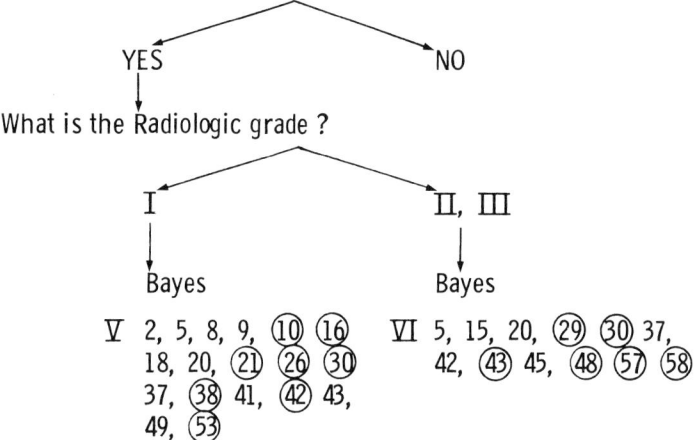

Decision Tree for tumors centered in the cortex. What is the radiological grade? In this location, sufficient information is usually present to accomplish significant data reduction. For cortical lesions the exact geographic location (epiphysis, metaphysis, etc.) does not seem to be of critical importance.

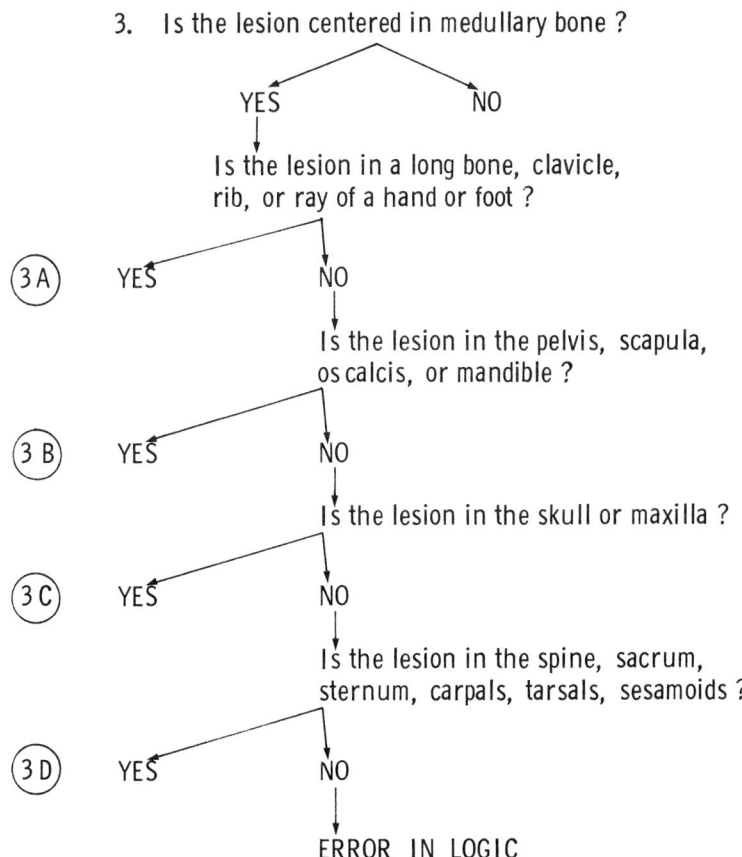

Decision Tree for lesions centered in medullary bone. This includes the majority of skeletal lesions. Since the organization to the approach to diagnosis is different for long bones, flat bones, skull, spine and small bones, four different decision trees are involved (3A, B, C and D).

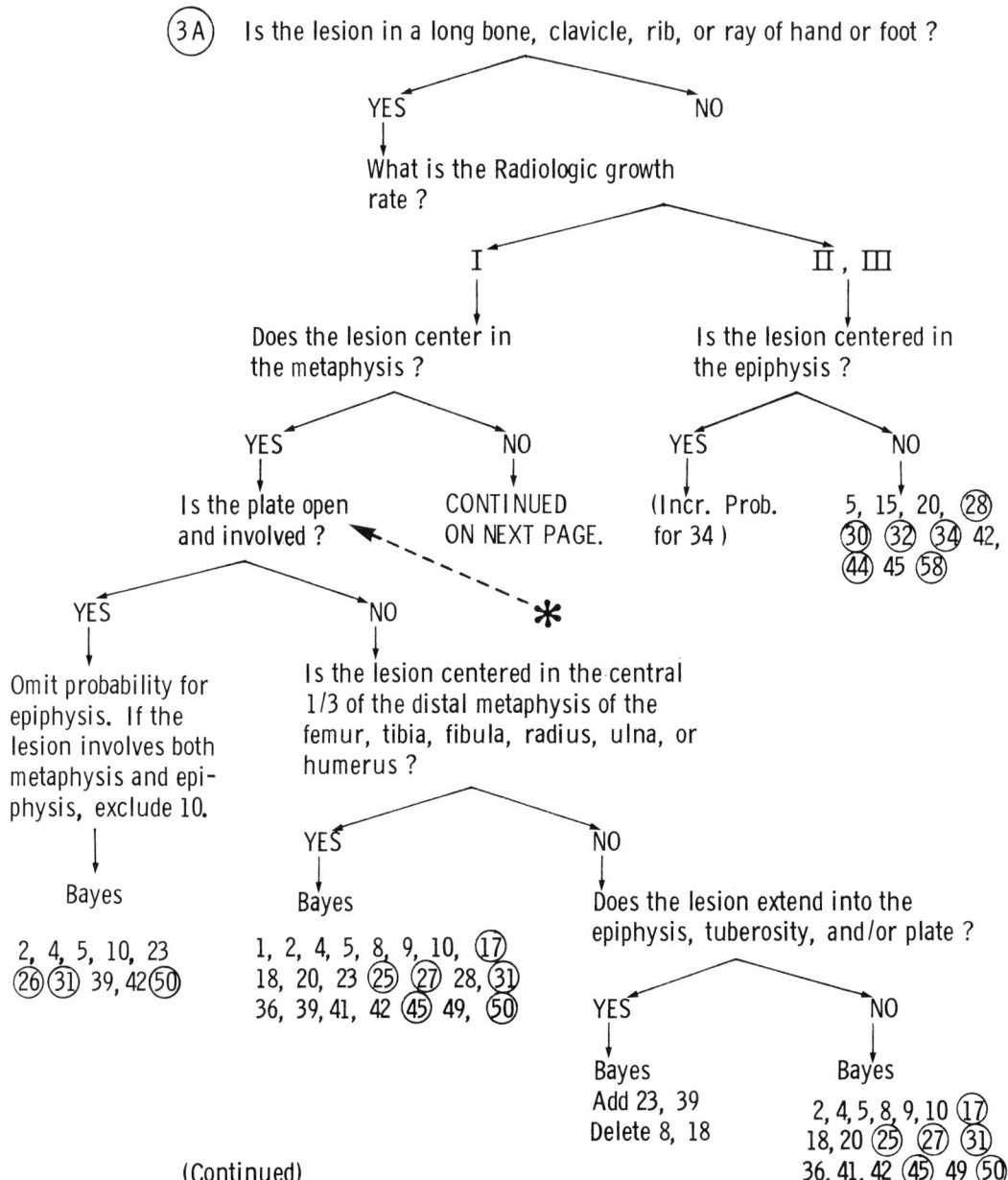

74 / Radiologic Concepts

Decision Tree 3A.

1. With lesions centered in medullary bone, use of the radiologic growth rate effectively reduces the number of diagnostic possibilities.

2. Does the lesion center in the metaphysis? The positive answer identifies lesions presumed to arise on the metaphysial side of the plate.

3. Is the plate open and involved? This is a double question. Involved in this instance means that the tumor and/or its immediate reactive change appear to lie in contact with the unfused plate. The giant cell tumor in this age group usually fulfills this criterion; fibroxanthoma almost never does. Thus a positive answer eliminates fibroxanthoma, but a negative answer does not eliminate giant cell tumor because it may imply that the plate is closed rather than not involved.

4. (*a*) Omit probability for epiphysis and articular cortex. If a lesion is centered in the metaphysis, and the plate is open and involved, the possibility that a growth rate I tumor will penetrate the plate to involve the epiphysis and articular cortex is remote. The probabilities for epiphysis and articular cortex should be omitted in calculating the diagnostic probabilities in this instance. These probabilities are used when a tumor, such as a giant cell tumor, *does* ordinarily involve these areas after the plate becomes fused.

(*b*) If the lesion involves both metaphysis and epiphysis, exclude 10. A number of lesions may penetrate the open plate, including giant cell tumor. We have never seen 10 (a cyst) which penetrated the plate, thus the special rule.

5. Is the lesion centered in the central third of the distal metaphysis of certain bones? The positive answer introduces the possibility of adamantinoma. The negative answer (for lesions centered in the metaphysis) excludes it.

6. Does the lesion extend into the epiphysis, tuberosity or plate? A positive answer adds giant cell tumor and osteoblastoma to the range of possibilities but excludes cortical desmoid and fibroxanthoma.

7. Does the lesion center in the epiphysis, tuberosity, trochanter or plate? The positive answer narrows the range of possibilities considerably. If the plate is open, cyst is excluded.

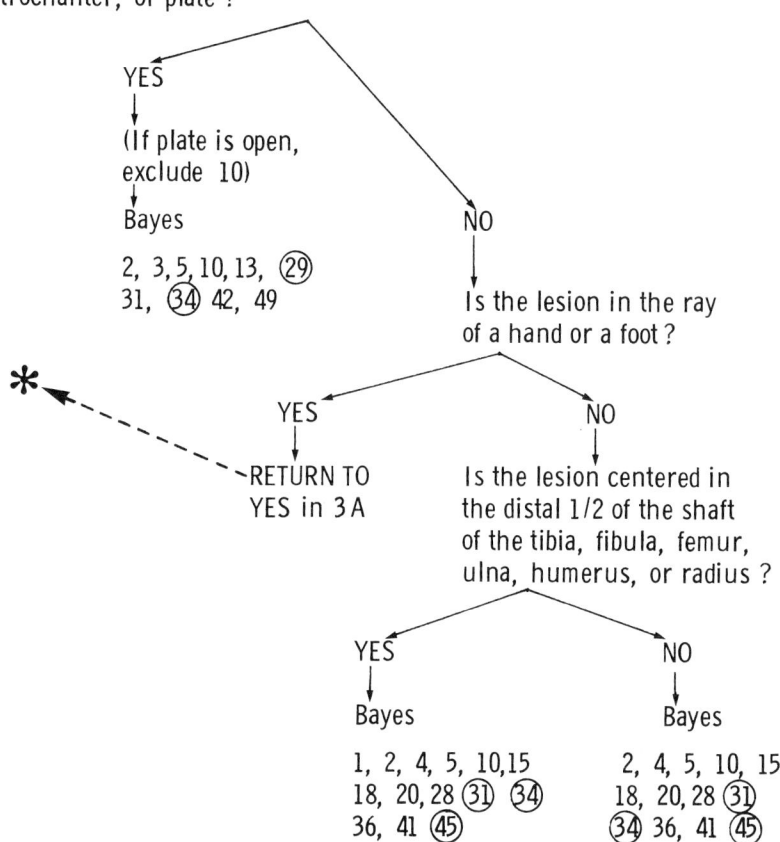

Decision Tree 3A (cont.).

8. Is the lesion in the ray of a hand or a foot? At this point we know that the lesion does not center in the metaphysis or epiphysis and must therefore center in the shaft. In a small bone, special rules for shaft are meaningless and the lesion is treated as if centered in the metaphysis.

9. Is the lesion centered in the distal half of the shaft of certain bones? The positive answer introduces the possibility of adamantinoma. I have seen an adamantinoma that appeared to center in the proximal shaft, but this must be a rare exception.

10. Is the lesion centered in the epiphysis under radiologic growth rates II and III? The positive choice increases the probability for metastatic tumor. The negative choice includes all other diagnostic possibilities that are listed. Note that the conventional rules relating to location largely are not applied to the rapidly growing malignant lesions.

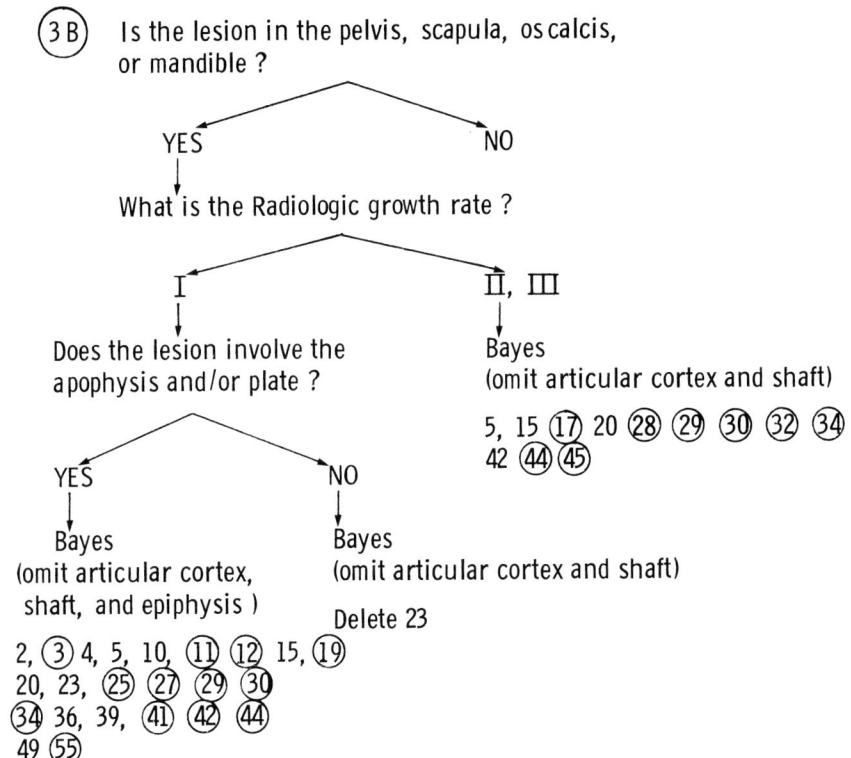

Decision Tree 3B.

1. Again, radiologic growth rate may be used as an effective data reduction technique.

2. Does the lesion involve the apophysis and/or plate? In these bones, the epiphysial and apophysial centers are so narrow that all lesions are assumed to arise on the side of the metaphysis analogue. The negative answer eliminates giant cell tumor from the range of possibilities. The probabilities for articular cortex epiphysis and shaft do not apply in this location and, if used, introduce diagnostic error.

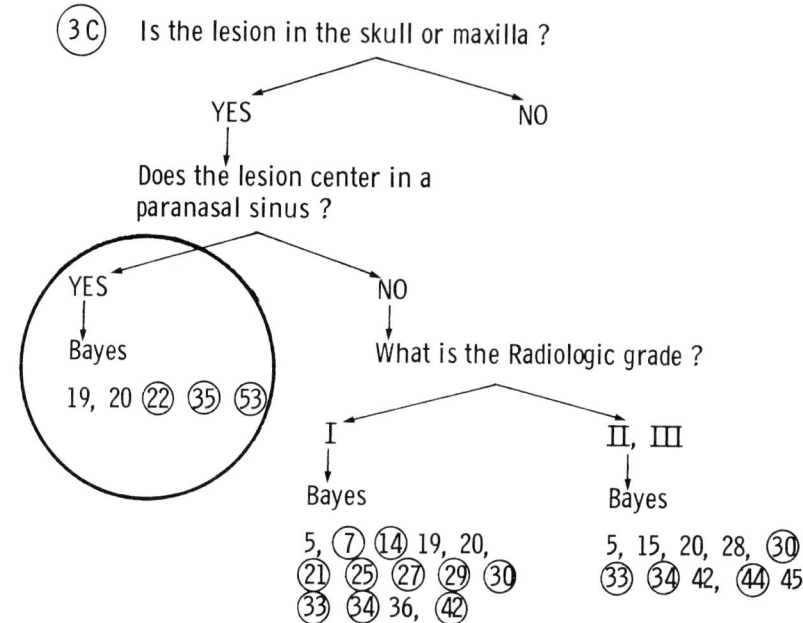

Decision Tree 3C.

1. Does the lesion center in a paranasal sinus? The positive answer introduces a special probability table which includes the lesions most likely to arise in a sinus.

2. Rate of growth is used to narrow the range of possibilities further.

3. This decision tree is incomplete because in the skull, other data reduction techniques are available. For example, if a slower growing, cystic appearing lesion crosses a suture, the possibility of epidermoid of the calvarium is greatly increased. This tree needs expert augmentation.

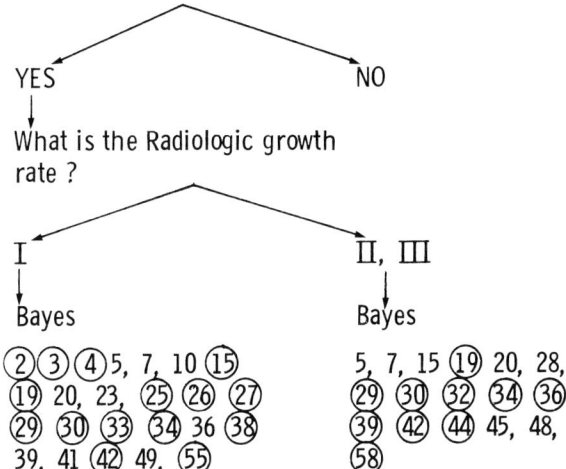

③D Is the lesion centered in the spine, sternum, sacrum, carpals, tarsals, or sesamoids?

YES → What is the Radiologic growth rate?

I → Bayes
②③④ 5, 7, 10 ⑮ ⑲ 20, 23, ㉕ ㉖ ㉗ ㉙ ㉚ ㉝ ㉞ 36 ㊳ 39, 41 ㊷ 49, ㊴

II, III → Bayes
5, 7, 15 ⑲ 20, 28, ㉙ ㉚ ㉜ ㉞ ㊱ ㊴ ㊷ ㊹ 45, 48, ㊽

NO

Decision Tree 3D. Radiologic growth rate is the best data reduction technique now available. The present model includes a modification which permits more detailed analysis of the relationship between location and histologic type. Such detailed information is not available; only with future application will we know the extent to which the location of a lesion in the spine affects diagnosis.

Decision Tree for joint. Is the lesion centered in a joint? A joint in this context means articulations through which a broad range of motion occurs, such as the knee, ankle and shoulder. Sutures in the skull and the intervertebral discs are not included.

Here again, further detailed analysis is needed, particularly of the relationship between exact location and diagnosis and also of the kinds of change observed when tumors arise within joints.

4. Is the lesion centered in a joint?

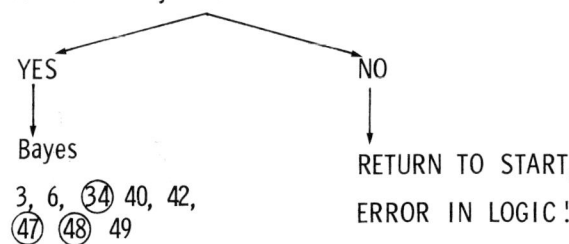

YES → Bayes
3, 6, ㉞ 40, 42, ㊼ ㊽ 49

NO → RETURN TO START, ERROR IN LOGIC!

Prediction of Histologic Diagnosis / 79

E. Classification System

THE TUMORS AND CYSTS illustrated in the following pages are presented in the following categories:

    Giant cell and cystic tumors
    Fibrous tumors
    Cartilaginous tumors
    Osseous tumors
    Round cell tumors
    Tumors of joints and soft tissues
    Miscellaneous tumors

With few exceptions, the histologic classifications of the tumors in this volume are straightforward. The principal exception is cystic tumors and lesions other than those arising in the mandible and maxilla.

1. *Cystic lesions.*—Experience has led Dr. Lent Johnson to regard many cysts as being cystic tumors or "cystomas." This classification generally includes the lesions commonly described as unicameral cyst of bone, aneurysmal cyst and simple cyst. A new concept has been postulated, based on his finding that while the lining of a cyst may be entirely fibrous with a thin lining membrane of mesenchyme cells, in the soft tissues and bone beneath this lining are frequently found nests of cells which appear to be of vascular, fibrous, cartilaginous or adipose origin. Simple curettage or stripping of the wall of the cyst does not eliminate these deeper nests of cells, which are responsible for the recurrence of the original cystic lesions. An example of the marked capability of a cyst to recur may be seen in the case shown in Figures 39 and 40, in which the cystic lesion was ultimately eliminated only by resection of the segment of bone which contained it.

To most radiologists, the idea of a cystic lesion having locally aggressive potential is foreign. I found the concept of aneurysmal bone cyst difficult to discard until I was shown that in many aggressive lesions with radiologic characteristics of aneurysmal bone cyst, none of the cellular characteristics ascribed to aneurysmal bone cyst were present. Dr. Johnson's scheme for classifying the cystic lesions of bone is one which works in practice, adequately explaining the curious ability of these lesions to recur and implying an appropriate method of treatment. I still believe that the "aneurysmal bone cyst" needs further consideration. There is growing evidence that this tumor, in a large number of instances, is a secondary reactive tumor of bone in the presence of a primary which initiates an osseous arteriovenous fistula. The primary may be nonossifying fibroma, chondroblastoma, giant cell tumor of bone, osteoblastoma, giant cell reparative granuloma, fibrous dysplasia, fibromyxoma, unicameral bone cyst and probably in some cases malignant primary and secondary tumors as well.[1] This conclusion is not inconsistent with Dr. Johnson's opinion.

2. *Fibrosarcoma.*—Although most pathologists agree on the histologic characteristics of fibrosarcoma, differences in interpretation are apt to arise when neoplastic tissues other than fibrosarcoma are present. For example, some pathologists are inclined to change a diagnosis from fibrosarcoma to osteosarcoma if neoplastic cells in the tumor are forming osteoid. Others may depend more on the radiographic image, in which case, if any neoplastic bone is apparent, the diagnosis becomes osteosarcoma. From the nonpartisan point of view of the radiologist, a change from one classification to another based on histologic findings should be meaningful in terms of treatment and survival. Generally speaking, the five year survival and even the method of treatment for osteosarcoma and for fibrosarcoma may be quite different. In my experience with material from the Codman Bone Sarcoma Registry, the five year survival for primary bone tumors having a predominantly fibrosarcomatous cell type but which may be interpreted from the radiographic image as containing large amounts of bone is not materially different from that for fibrosarcomas which contain no visible bone, and is much better than for the typical osteosarcoma. For this reason I am inclined to regard the tumor which radiographically resembles fibrosarcoma, and which histologically contains neoplastic bone, as fibrosarcoma rather than osteosarcoma, because its behavior is usually that of fibrosarcoma. In this volume, however, Dr. Johnson's classification of fibrosarcoma has been followed.

3. *Giant cell tumor.*—The radiologist may be thoroughly confused by the grossly divergent opinions of competent pathologists on giant cell tumor, one of whom even questions the very existence of this tumor.[2] When one talks about giant cell tumor, inevitably aneurysmal bone cyst and often villonodular synovitis are included in the differential diagnosis. Not only do the radiographs of these lesions tend to look alike, but apparently there must be very real histologic resemblances among these three lesions on some occasions. There is little likelihood for either pathologist or radiologist to become confused by a typical case. The atypical ones are the trying cases. Generally speaking, the decision rules for location, age and kind of proliferative response may be definite in differentiating these three lesions in the

---

[1] Biesecker, J. L., *et al.*: Aneurysmal bone cysts: A clinicopathologic study of 66 cases, Cancer 26:615, 1970.

[2] Aegerter, E. E.: *Orthopedic Diseases* (2nd ed.; Philadelphia: W. B. Saunders Company, 1963), p. 487.

typical case, but in some situations the radiologist is unable to distinguish between giant cell tumor, a cyst and villonodular synovitis.

4. *Myositis ossificans.*—Not ordinarily a problem, in some cases both pathologist and radiologist may have difficulty in distinguishing between myositis ossificans and parosteal sarcoma. Ordinarily the natural history is quite different, the myositis progressing rapidly to a definitive status within a month or six weeks and parosteal sarcoma growing slowly for years. However, if the lesion is first seen in an advanced stage, histologic distinction between the two may be very difficult. The radiologist can dependably but not invariably make this distinction based on the radiographic morphology of the lesion.

This volume contains an unusual collection of myositis ossificans of the fingers. The lesions appear to follow a rapid course which leads to complete healing even though in the active phase the radiologic patterns appear ominous. On occasion it is impossible to distinguish radiologically between myositis ossificans and ossifying hemangioma of the finger. The rapid sequence of fulmination and healing provides an early clue to myositis.

5. *Pleomorphic sarcoma.*—In the experience of any pathologist, this lesion is rare. It is apparently a highly malignant variant or mixture of fibrosarcoma, giant cell tumor and osteosarcoma. The radiologist finds it impossible to distinguish between pleomorphic sarcoma and a highly malignant fibrosarcoma or an osteosarcoma which is not producing a calcified matrix.

6. *Reticulum cell sarcoma.*—There is some confusion between primary reticulum cell sarcoma of bone and primary reticulum cell sarcoma of soft tissues. The histologic criteria of Parker and Jackson[3] are apparently not invariably followed. In this situation the radiologist has little to offer to resolve this distinction, since the gross radiographic morphology of reticulum cell sarcoma and lymphoma generally are quite similar if not identical.

---

[3] Parker, F., Jr., and Jackson, H., Jr.: Primary reticulum cell sarcoma of bone, Surg., Gynec. & Obst. 68:45, 1939.

PART 2

Giant Cell and Cystic Tumors

Figure 18.—Giant cell tumor of the femur.

AFIP Case No. 1190412: **A,** anteroposterior, and **B,** lateral views.

DIAGNOSIS AND GRADE.—Giant cell tumor, femur; growth rate IA.

LIFE INFORMATION.—Female, 15 years; last known to be well.

LOCATION.—A lesion centered in the midmetaphysis of the distal femur, extending down to the subarticular cortex of lateral condyle (**A, arrow**) and reaching the shaft above; no evidence of soft tissue extension.

SIZE.—9 × 6 × 5 cm.

MINERALIZATION OF TUMOR.—None.

DESTRUCTION.—Geographic; regular contour; thinning of cortex.

PROLIFERATION.—Several areas show sclerosis of the margin (**A, a**) and moderate septation (**b**). There is a single lamina of periosteal new bone.

DIFFERENTIAL DIAGNOSIS	PROBABILITY
Giant cell tumor	.64
Fibrosarcoma	.27
Cyst	.04
Chondrosarcoma	.04
Chondromyxoid fibroma	< .01

COMMENT: A rather passive appearing giant cell tumor which, as most do, reaches the subarticular cortex.

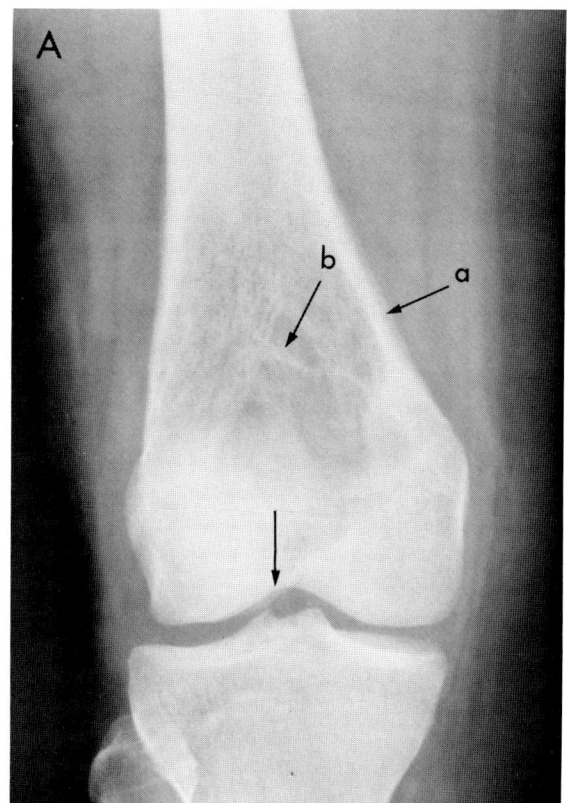
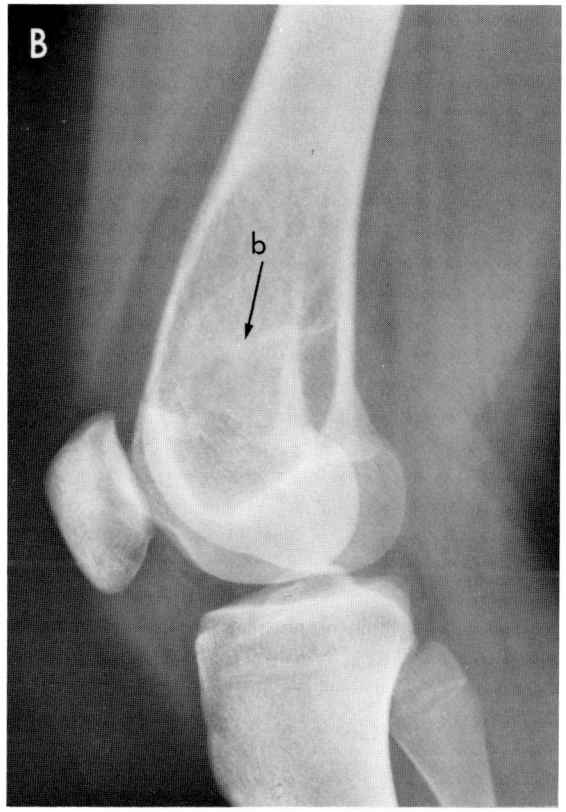

Figure 18 · Giant Cell Tumor of Femur / 85

Figure 19.—Giant cell tumor of the femur.

AFIP Case No. 1080027: **A,** anteroposterior, and **B,** lateral views.

DIAGNOSIS AND GRADE.—Giant cell tumor, distal femur; growth rate IB.
LIFE INFORMATION.—Female, 22 years; well three years after onset.
LOCATION.—A lesion centered eccentrically in the peripheral third of the distal femoral metaphysis, extending distally into the epiphysis and to the subarticular cortex, proximally into the middle and proximal thirds of metaphysis; no evidence of soft tissue extension.
SIZE.—8 × 5 × 5 cm.
MINERALIZATION OF TUMOR.—None.
DESTRUCTION.—Geographic; lobulated contour; pathologic fracture (**arrows**).
PROLIFERATION.—Entire margin slightly sclerotic (**b**); cortex expanded laterally for 1 cm; moderate septation (**a**); small buttress (**c**).

DIFFERENTIAL DIAGNOSIS	PROBABILITY
Giant cell tumor	.78
Villonodular synovitis	.19
Chondromyxoid fibroma	.01
Fibrosarcoma	< .01

COMMENT: The computer feels more strongly about villonodular synovitis than I do.

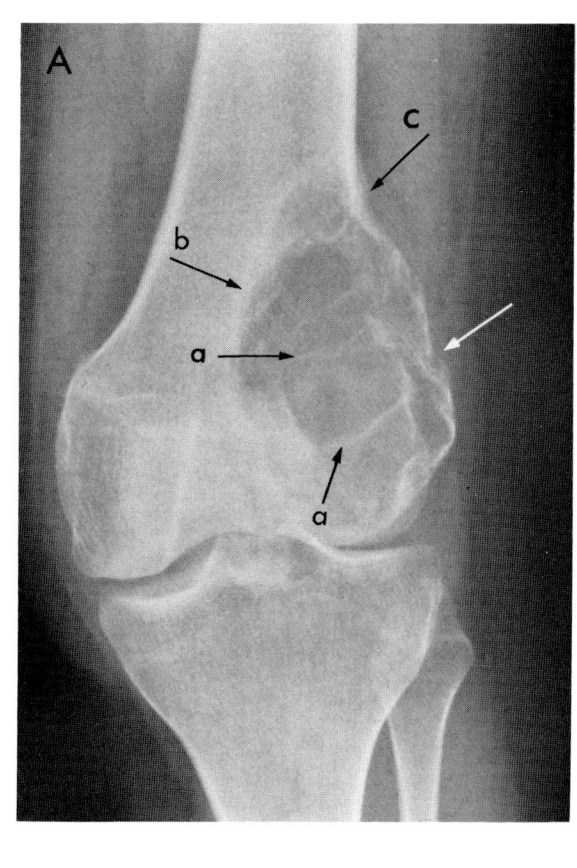
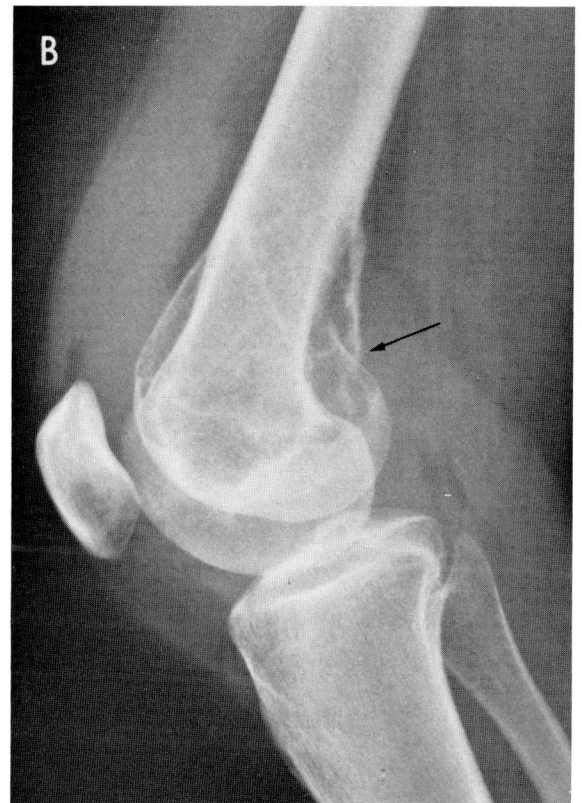

Figure 19 · Giant Cell Tumor of Femur / 87

Figure 20.—Giant cell tumor of the femur.

AFIP Case No. 1135211: **A,** anteroposterior, and **B,** lateral views.

DIAGNOSIS AND GRADE.—Giant cell tumor, femur; growth rate IC.
LIFE INFORMATION.—Male, 20 years; well three years after onset.
LOCATION.—An eccentric lesion in the peripheral third of the distal femoral metaphysis, penetrating the epiphysis to the subarticular cortex and extending up into the midmetaphysis; a small extraosseous extension.

SIZE.—8 × 5 × 6 cm.
MINERALIZATION OF TUMOR.—None.
DESTRUCTION.—Geographic; lobulated contour; cortex penetrated laterally and anteriorly (**b**).
PROLIFERATION.—Faint zone of marginal sclerosis (**A, a**); cortex expanded slightly anteriorly and laterally (**b**), but expanded portion does not completely encapsulate the tumor, which extends into the soft tissues laterally (**A, c**).

DIFFERENTIAL DIAGNOSIS	PROBABILITY
Giant cell tumor	.93
Villonodular synovitis	.05
Chondromyxoid fibroma	< .01
Fibrosarcoma	< .01
Cyst	< .01
Osteoblastoma	< .01

COMMENT: This degree of aggressiveness is characteristic of giant cell tumor. A large percentage of the malignant giant cell tumors are in growth rate IC. The computer agrees that this case is typical.

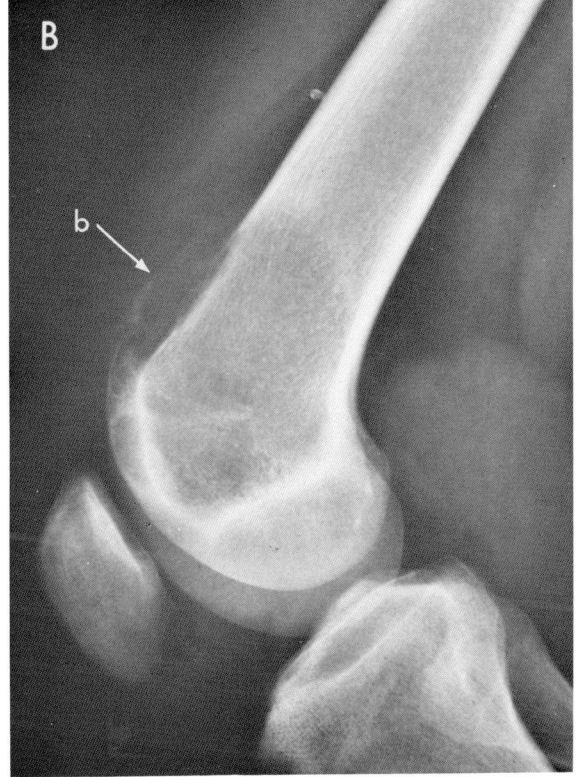
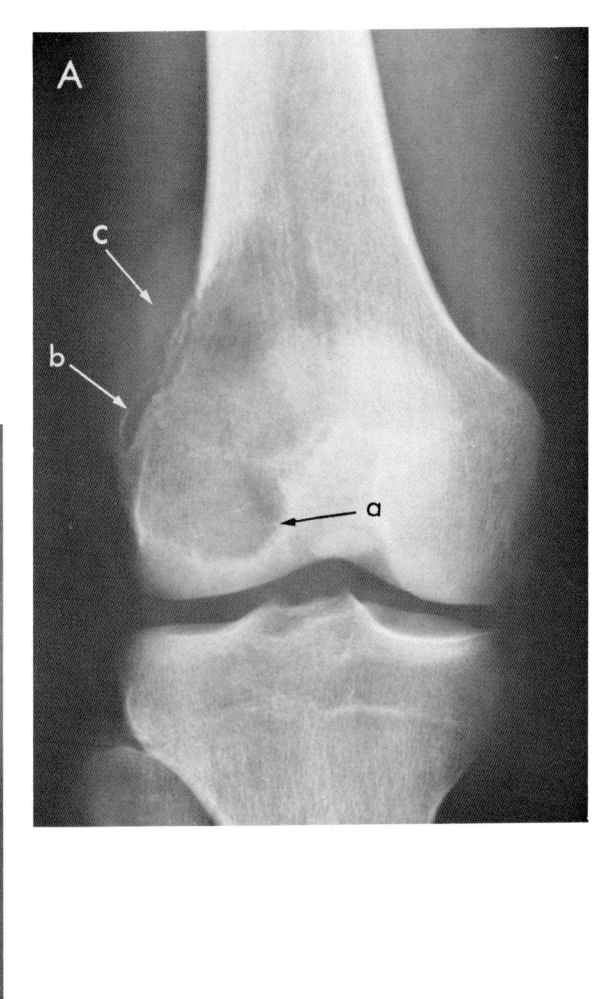

Figure 20 · Giant Cell Tumor of Femur / 89

Figure 21.—Giant cell tumor of the femur.

AFIP Case No. 1147238: **A,** anteroposterior, and **B,** lateral projections.

DIAGNOSIS AND GRADE.—Giant cell tumor, femur; growth rate II.

LIFE INFORMATION.—Male, 12 years; died of metastatic disease seven months after onset.

LOCATION.—An eccentric lesion in the mid-distal metaphysis, extending distally to the unfused epiphysial plate, proximally into the central third of the metaphysis and laterally into the soft tissues.

SIZE.—6 × 5 × 5 cm.

MINERALIZATION OF TUMOR.—None.

DESTRUCTION.—Centrally geographic with a 1 cm peripheral zone of moth-eaten bone destruction (**A, a**), ragged contour (**B, b**) and total penetration of cortex laterally (**c**).

PROLIFERATION.—Faint but broad zone of marginal sclerosis (**A, f**); two Codman triangles (**d**).

DIFFERENTIAL DIAGNOSIS	PROBABILITY
Osteosarcoma	.90
Ewing's sarcoma	.04
Fibrosarcoma	.03
Chondrosarcoma	.01

COMMENT: Few giant cell tumors fall in growth rate II. The differential diagnosis best begins at the more malignant end of the spectrum, such as osteosarcoma. Identification of the mineralized fragment (**A, e**) is difficult in this instance; a fragment of residual bone is the first choice because of its organized trabecular structure. Because this lesion falls in growth rate II, giant cell tumor is not even considered in the differential diagnosis.

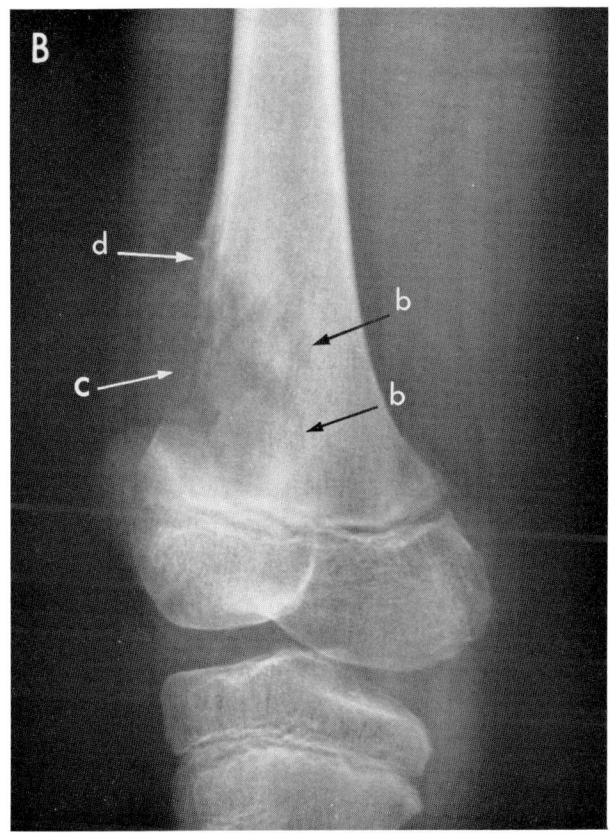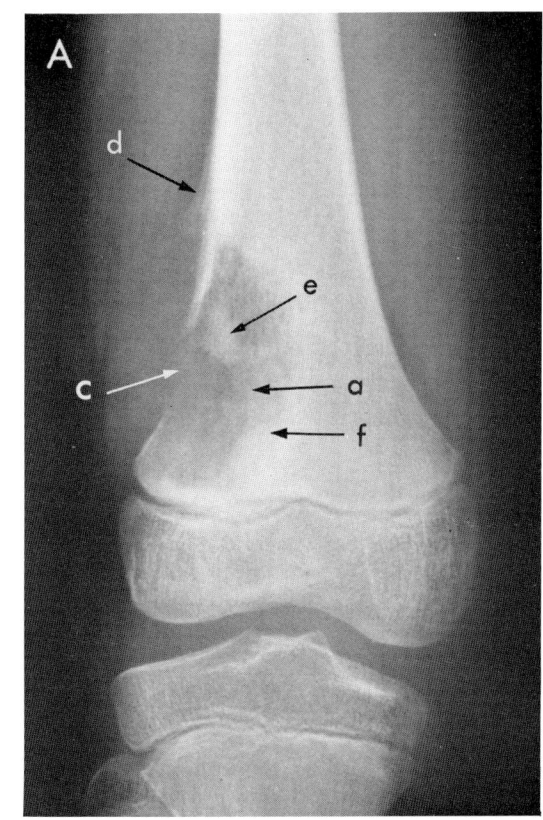

Figure 21 · Giant Cell Tumor of Femur / 91

Figure 22.—Giant cell tumor of the femur.

AFIP Case No. 1016356: Lateral views—**A,** initial study, **B,** seven months later.

Diagnosis and Grade.—Giant cell tumor, distal femur; growth rate IA.
Life Information.—Male, 34 years; last known to be well.
Location.—An eccentric lesion in the peripheral third of the distal femoral metaphysis, near the plate. On first examination (**A**), the tumor extends symmetrically into the epiphysis and metaphysis.

Size.—3 × 2 cm on initial examination.
Mineralization of Tumor.—None.
Destruction.—Geographic; regular contour; cortex penetrated anteriorly (**A, a**).
Proliferation.—In even the early stage of growth, there is a faint zone of marginal sclerosis (**A, b**), which qualifies the tumor for growth rate IA. In the more advanced stage, marginal sclerosis remains, yet the cortex is totally penetrated anteriorly.

Seven months later (**B**), the tumor has enlarged to 7 × 4 cm. The proportionate distribution of tumor is the same, but it now involves the subarticular cortex (**c**) and there is a small anterior soft tissue extension through an anterior penetration of the cortex (**x**). Note the secondary vascular changes in the patella. The tumor now has the characteristics of growth rate IC.

Differential Diagnosis	Probability
Giant cell tumor	.99
Fibrosarcoma	< .01

COMMENT: It is unusual to observe giant cell tumor this early. The site of origin appears to be very near the fused plate. The subarticular cortex becomes involved as growth extends. The differential diagnosis is based on the second examination.

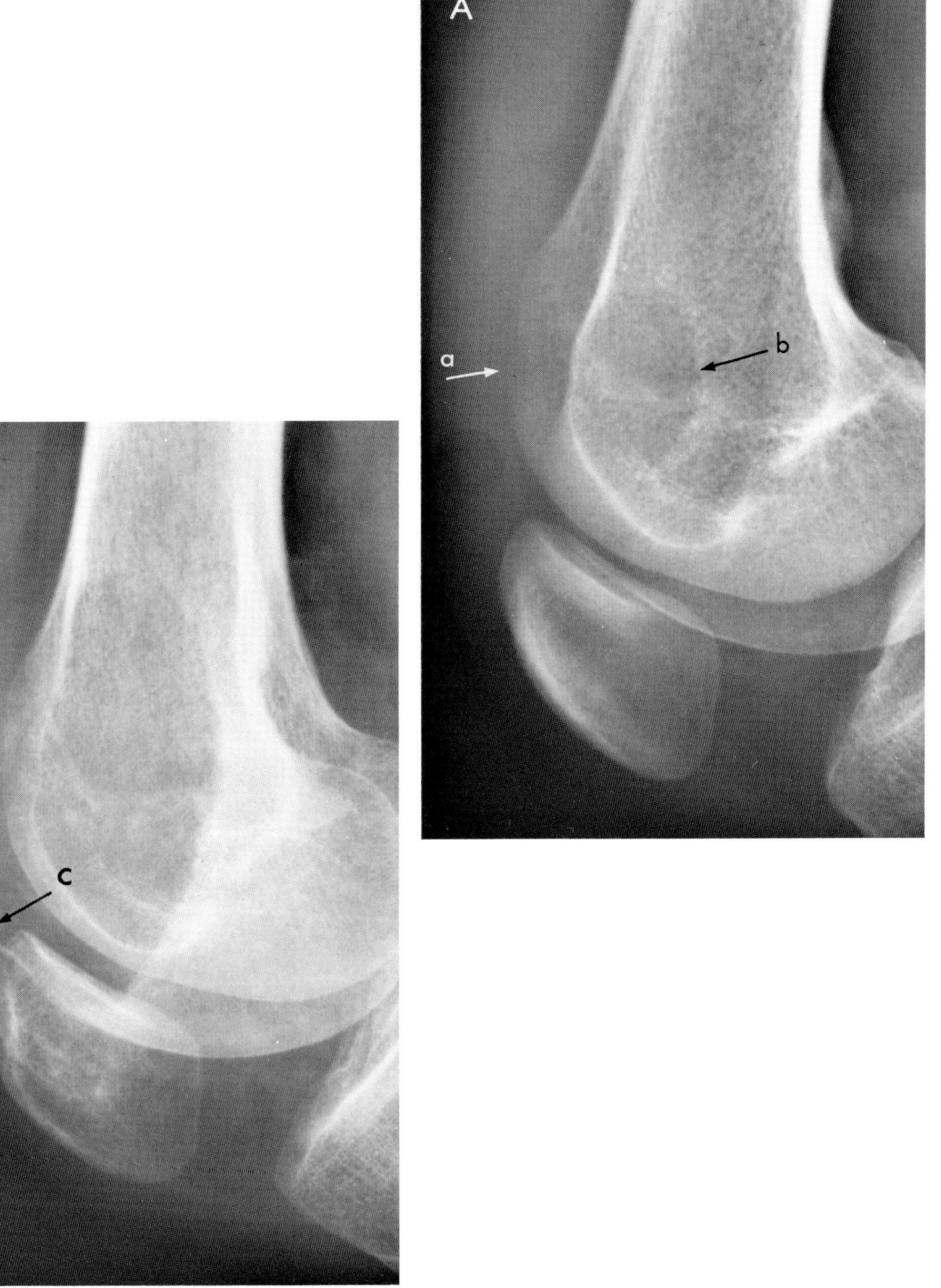

Figure 22 · Giant Cell Tumor of Femur / 93

Figure 23.—Giant cell tumors of the astragalus and metatarsal.

AFIP Case No. 996237: **A,** lateral projection.

DIAGNOSIS AND GRADE.—Giant cell tumor, astragalus; growth rate IA.
LIFE INFORMATION.—Male, 17 years; well six years after onset.
LOCATION.—The tumor is centered in the body of the astragalus and extends into subarticular cortex of the ankle and subtalar joint.
SIZE.—3 × 3 cm.
MINERALIZATION OF TUMOR.—None.
DESTRUCTION.—Geographic; regular contour; partial penetration of cortex.
PROLIFERATION.—Dense marginal sclerosis; faint septation.

DIFFERENTIAL DIAGNOSIS	PROBABILITY
Giant cell tumor	.99
Chondrosarcoma	< .01

COMMENT: A typical giant cell tumor in the astragalus.

AFIP Case No. 1163342: **B,** anteroposterior projection.

DIAGNOSIS AND GRADE.—Giant cell tumor, metatarsal; growth rate IB.
LIFE INFORMATION.—Male, 22 years; last known to be well.
LOCATION.—The tumor, centered in the distal shaft of the second metatarsal, extends distally to involve the metaphysis, epiphysis and subchondral cortex and proximally to involve the middle third of the shaft.
SIZE.—4 × 3 × 3 cm.
MINERALIZATION OF TUMOR.—None.
DESTRUCTION.—Geographic; reticulated contour; incomplete penetration of cortex.
PROLIFERATION.—More than 1 cm expansion of the cortex, with delicate septate pattern; small buttresses (**arrow**); tumor apparently completely encapsulated by expanded shell.

DIFFERENTIAL DIAGNOSIS	PROBABILITY
Giant cell tumor	.99
Osteoblastoma	< .01
Fibrosarcoma	< .01

COMMENT: A typical giant cell tumor in a small bone.

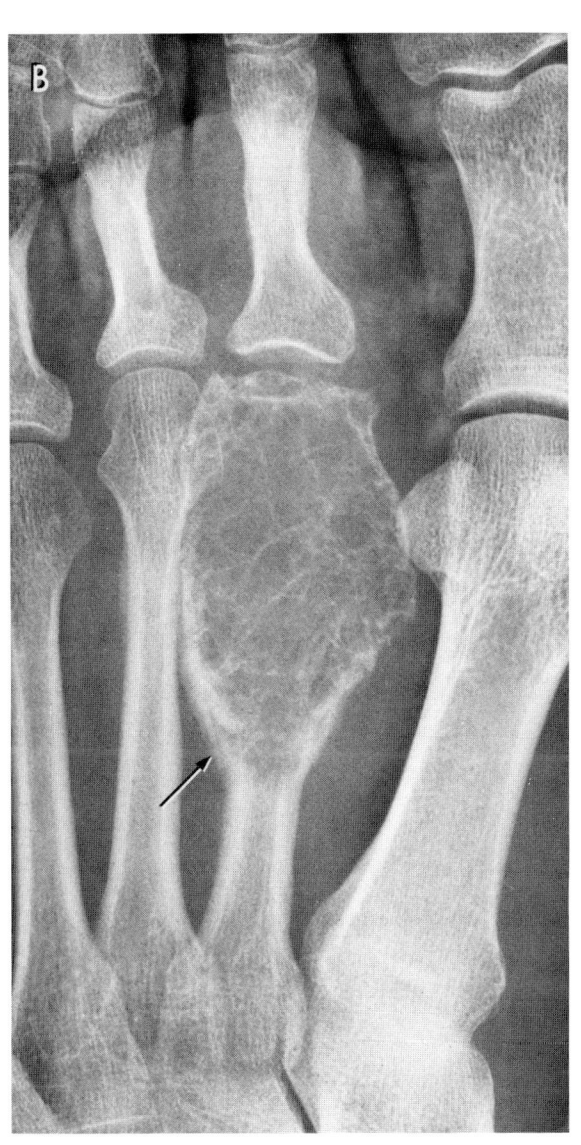
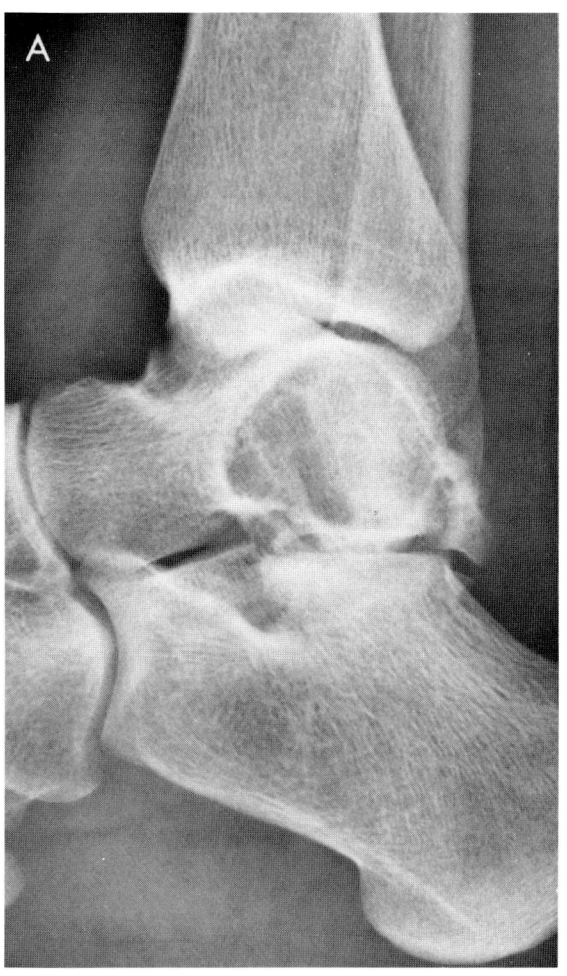

Figure 23 · Giant Cell Tumors of Small Bones / 95

Figure 24.—Giant cell tumor of the clavicle.

AFIP Case No. 1171403: Anteroposterior projection.

DIAGNOSIS AND GRADE.—Giant cell tumor, clavicle; growth rate IC.
LIFE INFORMATION.—Female, 11 years; survival unknown.
LOCATION.—If one regards the clavicle as a tubular bone, the tumor is centered in the distal metaphysis and extends distally to the end of the bone, proximally into the shaft and laterally into the soft tissues.
SIZE.—5 × 3 × 3 cm.
MINERALIZATION OF TUMOR.—None.
DESTRUCTION.—Centrally geographic; narrow moth-eaten marginal zone and ragged contour; total penetration of cortex superiorly.
PROLIFERATION.—Expansion of cortex greater than 1 cm inferiorly (**arrows**); faint septation; small Codman triangles (**a**).

DIFFERENTIAL DIAGNOSIS	PROBABILITY
Giant cell tumor	.98
Cyst	< .01
Fibrosarcoma	< .01

COMMENT: A tumor of moderate aggressiveness. When there is no growth plate, other diagnoses, such as hyperparathyroidism, should be strongly considered.

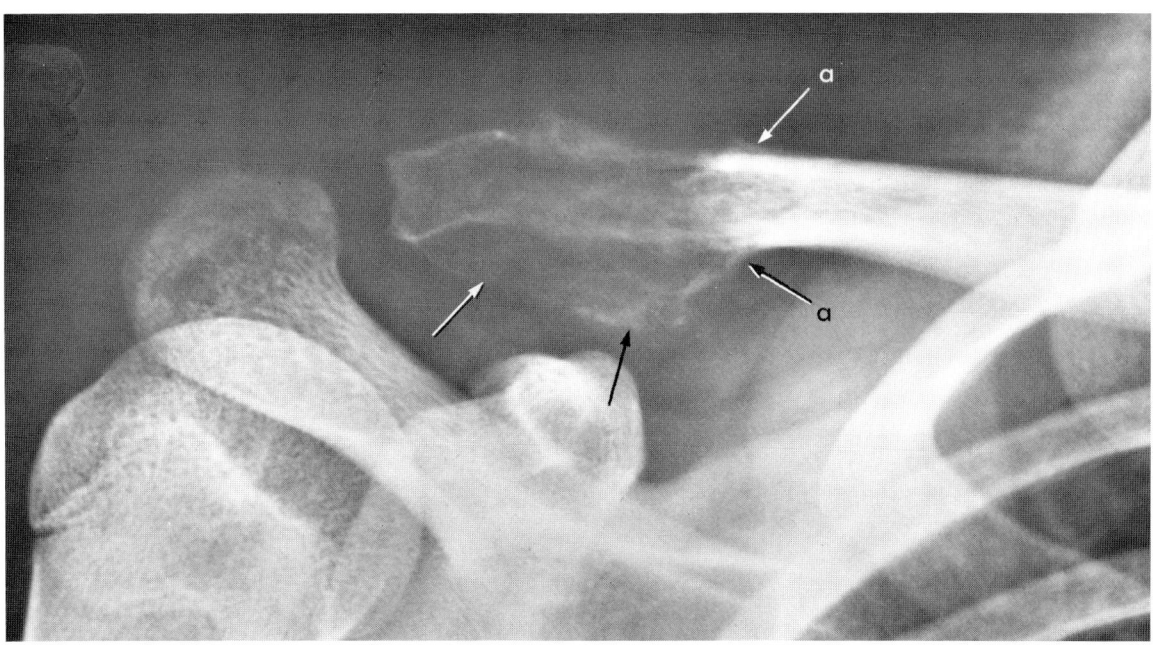

Figure 24 · Giant Cell Tumor of Clavicle / 97

Figure 25.—Giant cell tumor of the rib.

AFIP Case No. 1160108: Anteroposterior projection.

DIAGNOSIS AND GRADE.—Giant cell tumor, rib; growth rate IC.
LIFE INFORMATION.—Female, 27 years; last known to be well.
LOCATION.—A lesion centered in the proximal end of the left sixth rib, presenting sharply against the pulmonary background as a globular mass.
SIZE.—9 × 9 × 9 cm.
MINERALIZATION OF TUMOR.—None.
DESTRUCTION.—Geographic; contour of boundary not seen.
PROLIFERATION.—An expanded shell near the edge of the destroyed area (**arrows**); tumor not encapsulated by bone.

DIFFERENTIAL DIAGNOSIS	PROBABILITY
Giant cell tumor	.95
Chondrosarcoma	.02
Fibrosarcoma	.01
Myeloma	< .01
Osteosarcoma	< .01

COMMENT: Typical picture of a large tumor arising in a bone of narrow caliber in that the bone is completely overgrown with little or no structure remaining (see the adamantinoma of the fibula in Figure 179).

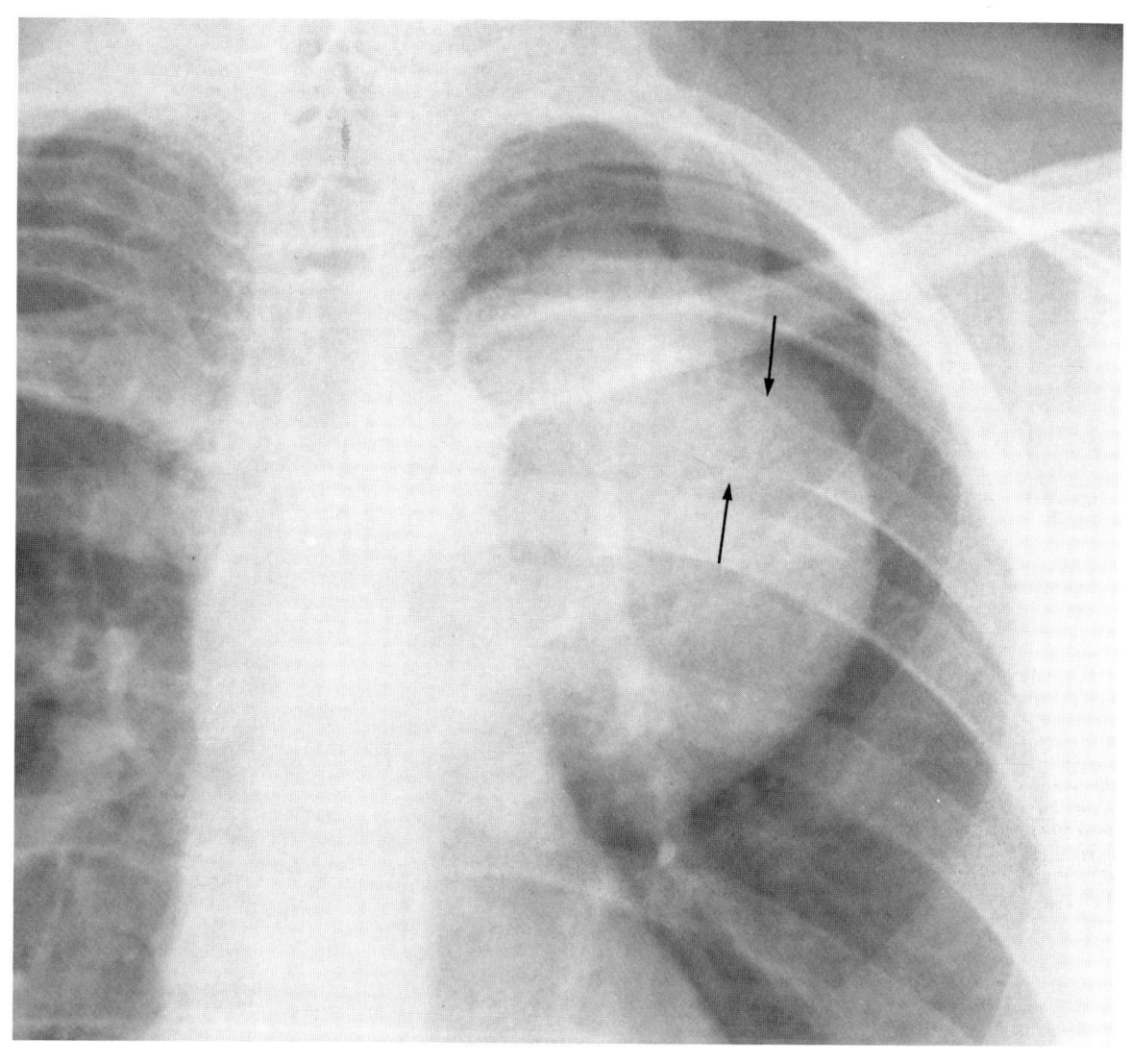

Figure 25 · Giant Cell Tumor of Rib / 99

Figure 26.—Giant cell tumor of the femur.

AFIP Case No. 1175158: **A,** anteroposterior, and **B,** lateral views.

DIAGNOSIS AND GRADE.—Giant cell tumor, femur; growth rate IC.

LIFE INFORMATION.—Male, 20 years; well three years after onset.

LOCATION.—The tumor, centered at the junction of the neck and intertrochanteric region of the femur, extends proximally to involve the epiphysis and reaching the subarticular cortex and distally to involve the intertrochanteric zone and lesser trochanter; a small soft tissue extension.

SIZE.—10 × 6 × 4 cm.

MINERALIZATION OF TUMOR.—None.

DESTRUCTION.—Geographic pattern; lobulated contour; total penetration of cortex medially.

PROLIFERATION.—Faint marginal sclerosis (**arrows**) and septation; slight expansion of the cortex at the base of the neck (**A, a**).

DIFFERENTIAL DIAGNOSIS	PROBABILITY
Giant cell tumor	.92
Chondromyxoid fibroma	.06
Fibrosarcoma	< .01
Osteoblastoma	< .01

COMMENT: A typical giant cell tumor in location and rate of growth.

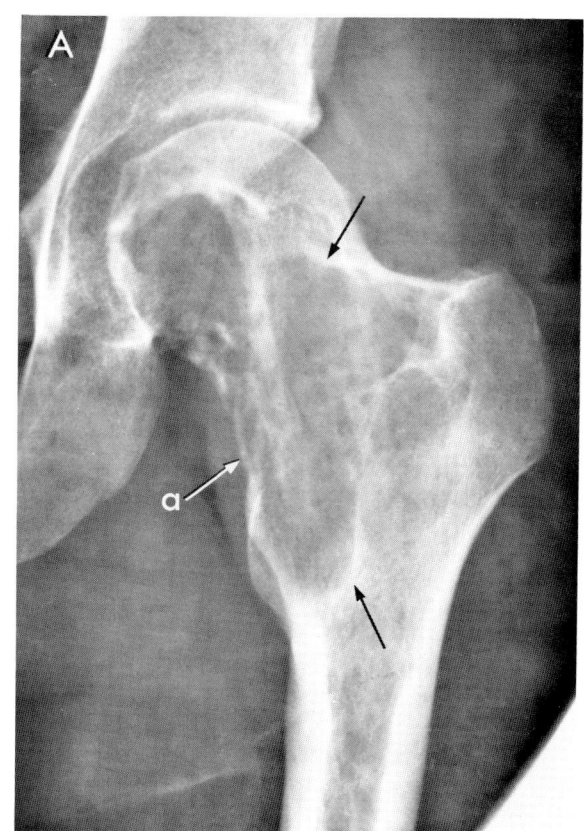
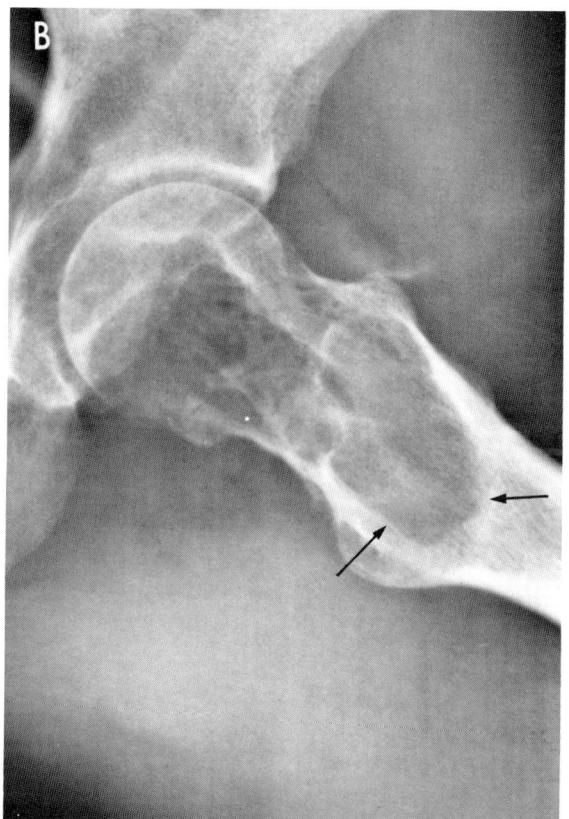

Figure 26 · Giant Cell Tumor of Femur / 101

Figure 27.—Giant cell tumors of the radius and humerus.

AFIP Case No. 910821: **A,** anteroposterior projection.

DIAGNOSIS AND GRADE.—Giant cell tumor, radius; growth rate IC.

LIFE INFORMATION.—Female, 22 years; survival unknown.

LOCATION.—The tumor, centered eccentrically in the distal third of the metaphysis, extends to the subchondral cortex and into the middle and proximal thirds of the metaphysis; small lateral extraosseous extension.

SIZE.—$3 \times 2 \times 1$ cm.

MINERALIZATION OF TUMOR.—None.

DESTRUCTION.—Essentially geographic; ragged contour; total loss of cortex laterally.

PROLIFERATION.—Probably none.

DIFFERENTIAL DIAGNOSIS	PROBABILITY
Giant cell tumor	.92
Fibrosarcoma	.06
Osteosarcoma	$< .01$

COMMENT: A remarkable looking tumor not typical of any histologic entity. The slow rate of growth is consistent with giant cell tumor. The computer zeros in on the diagnosis despite the bizarre appearance.

AFIP Case No. 1157309: **B,** anteroposterior projection.

DIAGNOSIS AND GRADE.—Giant cell tumor, humerus; growth rate IA.

LIFE INFORMATION.—Male, 37 years; last known to be well.

LOCATION.—The tumor, centered in the metaphysis of the medial epicondyle, extends into the epiphysis of the epicondyle and undermines the cortex.

SIZE.—$2 \times 2 \times 2$ cm.

MINERALIZATION OF TUMOR.—None.

DESTRUCTION.—Geographic pattern; regular contour.

PROLIFERATION.—Faint marginal sclerosis; no periosteal response.

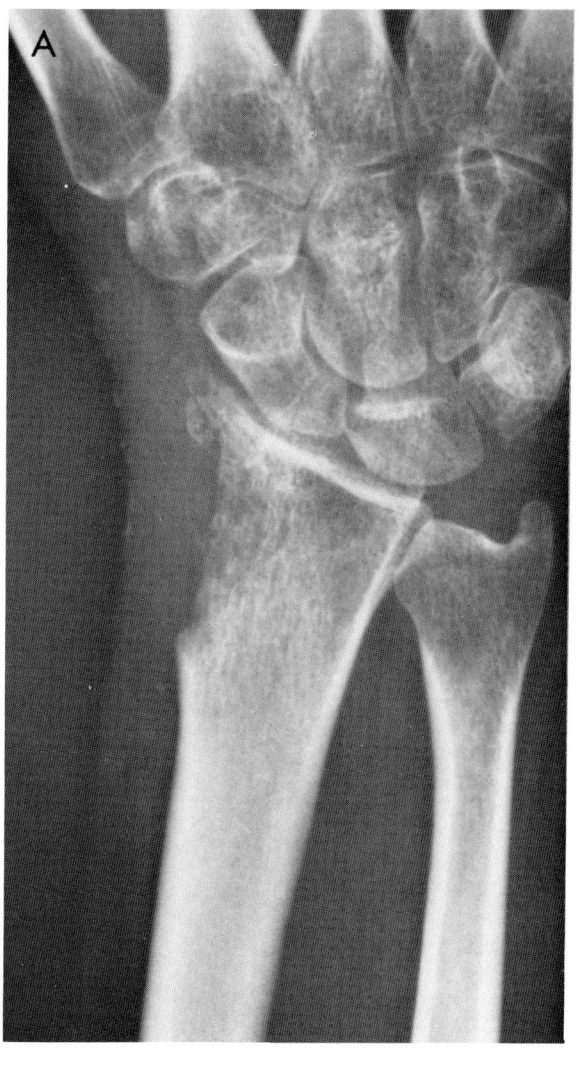
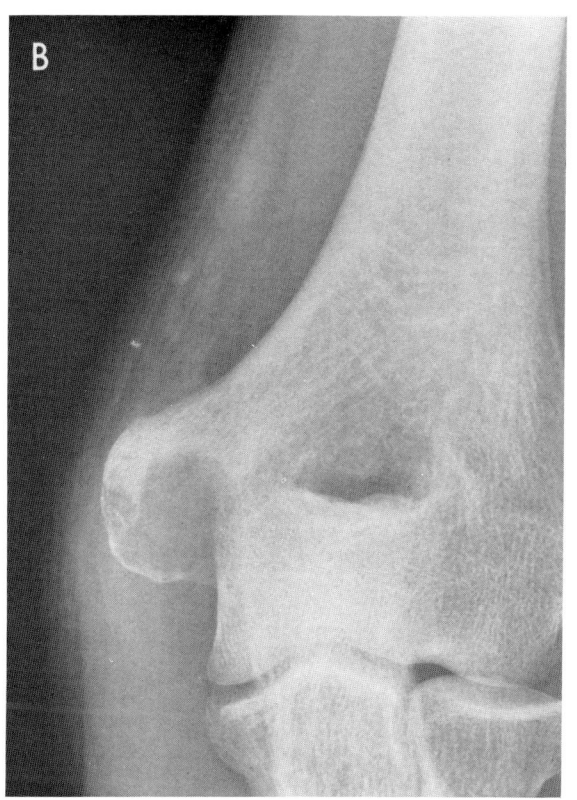

Differential Diagnosis	Probability
Giant cell tumor	.83
Cyst	.04
Osteoblastoma	.03
Benign cartilaginous tumor	.03
Chondrosarcoma	.02
Fibrosarcoma	.01
Chondromyxoid fibroma	< .01
Myeloma	< .01

COMMENT: A typical early giant cell tumor. Superficially it resembles a chondroblastoma, but it centers in the metaphysis, which is unheard of for chondroblastoma.

Figure 27 · Giant Cell Tumors of Radius & Humerus

Figure 28.—Giant cell tumor of the sacrum.

AFIP Case No. 1188553: **A,** anteroposterior, and **B,** lateral views.

DIAGNOSIS AND GRADE.—Giant cell tumor, sacrum; growth rate IC.

LIFE INFORMATION.—Female, 16 years; survival unknown.

LOCATION.—A large globular tumor centered at the anterior cortex of the fourth sacral segment with massive extraosseous extension (**arrows**); several vertebral bodies involved.

SIZE.—10 × 10 × 10 cm.

MINERALIZATION OF TUMOR.—None.

DESTRUCTION.—Centrally geographic; basically lobulated contour; marginal zones of questionable moth-eaten bone destruction (**A, a**).

PROLIFERATION.—An expanded cortex appears to have developed laterally, but has been overrun anteriorly and posteriorly; no conclusive evidence of marginal sclerosis.

DIFFERENTIAL DIAGNOSIS	PROBABILITY
Giant cell tumor	.42
Fibrosarcoma	.34
Chordoma	.21
Chondrosarcoma	.01
Cyst	< .01

COMMENT: Basically a tumor of relatively slow growth rate, fitting any of a number of entities. The age group is best for giant cell tumor, poor for chordoma. Also, the posterior extension and frank destruction of several vertebral bodies are unlikely behavior for chordoma.

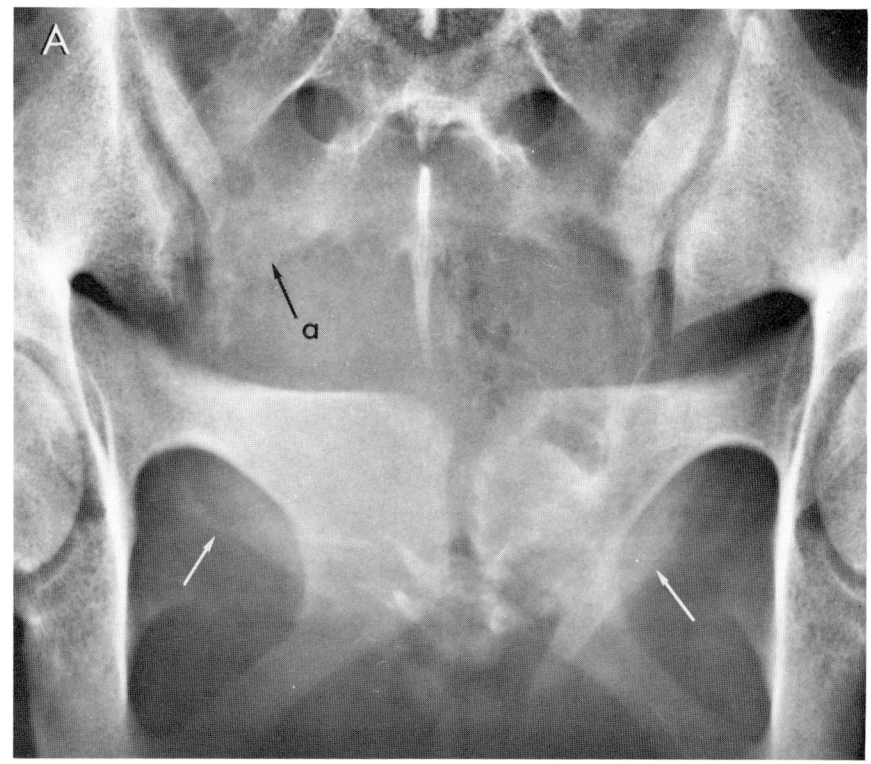
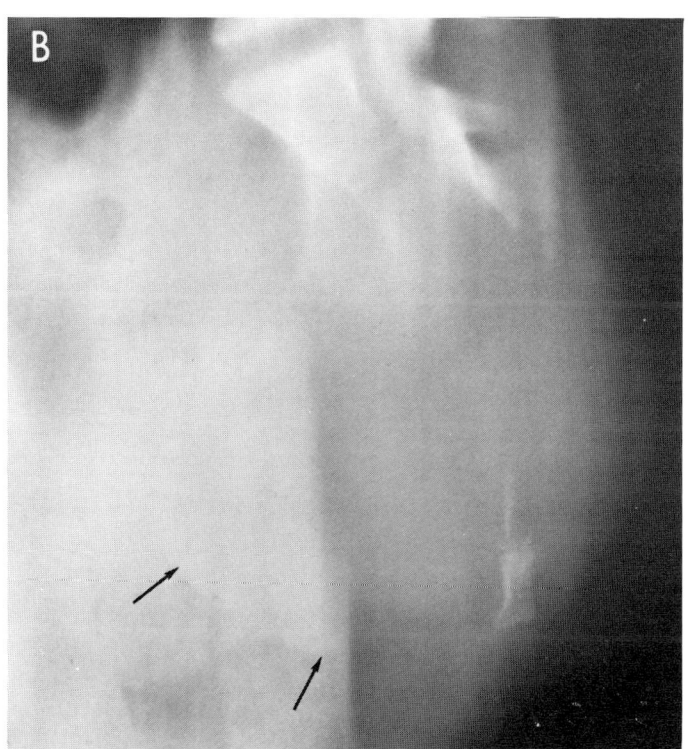

Figure 28 · Giant Cell Tumor of Sacrum / 105

Figure 29.—Giant cell tumor of the cervical spine.

AFIP Case No. 1109956: **A,** lateral, and **B,** anteroposterior views.

DIAGNOSIS AND GRADE.—Giant cell tumor, cervical spine; growth rate IC.
LIFE INFORMATION.—Female, age unknown; last known to be well.
LOCATION.—Total involvement of body and lateral processes of C6, with extension into C5 and C7.

SIZE.—5 × 4 × 2 cm.
MINERALIZATION OF TUMOR.—None.
DESTRUCTION.—Geographic; lobulated contour; compression fracture of the body of C6. Note prevertebral soft tissue swelling (**A, x**).
PROLIFERATION.—Ill-defined marginal sclerosis.

DIFFERENTIAL DIAGNOSIS	PROBABILITY
Cyst	.35
Giant cell tumor	.29
Osteoblastoma	.26
Chordoma	.06
Fibrosarcoma	.03

COMMENT: A typical giant cell tumor of the spine. The computer provides an excellent differential diagnosis for this case.

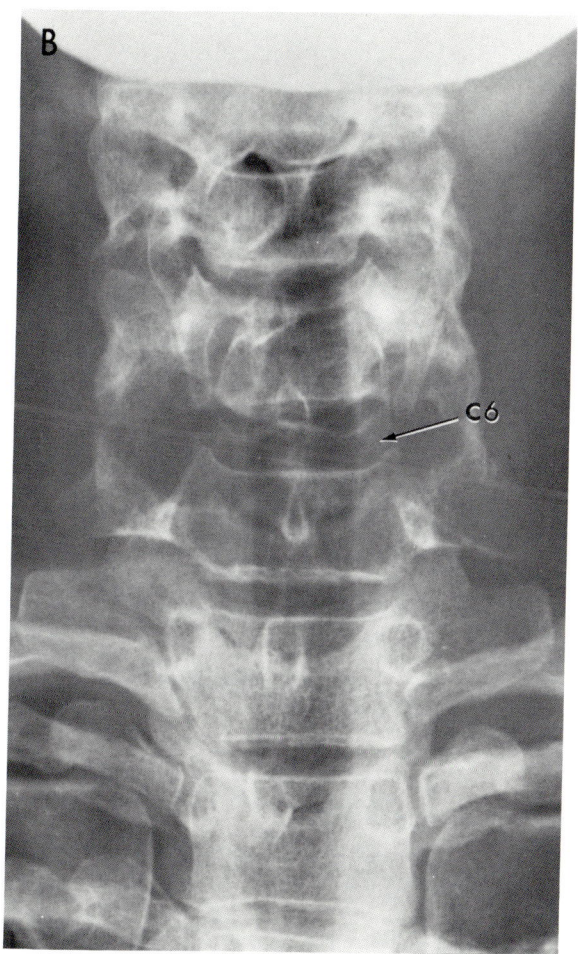
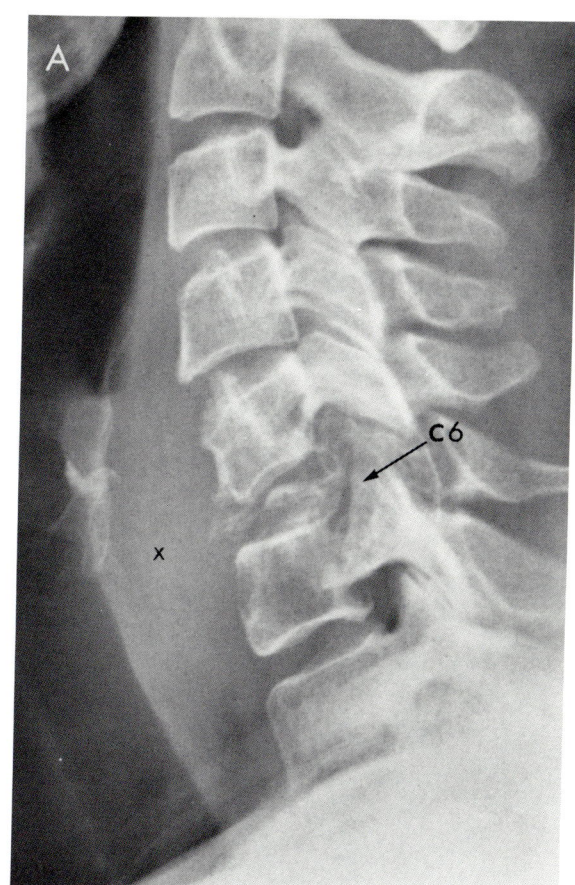

Figure 29 · Giant Cell Tumor of Cervical Spine / 107

Figure 30.—Giant cell tumor of the cervical spine.

AFIP Case No. 819218: **A**, lateral, and **B**, anteroposterior views.

DIAGNOSIS AND GRADE.—Giant cell tumor, cervical spine; growth rate IA.

LIFE INFORMATION.—Female, 16 years; survival unknown.

LOCATION.—The tumor centers in the lateral mass and extends into the body of C6 (**x**).

SIZE.—2 × 2 × 2 cm.

MINERALIZATION OF TUMOR.—None.

DESTRUCTION.—Geographic; essentially regular contour; partial penetration of the cortex laterally.

PROLIFERATION.—Faint zone of marginal sclerosis; slight expansion of lateral cortex (**B, arrow**).

DIFFERENTIAL DIAGNOSIS	PROBABILITY
Osteoblastoma	.78
Giant cell tumor	.11
Cyst	.09
Fibrosarcoma	< .01

COMMENT: A tumor of slow growth rate and so located that it probably would ultimately have penetrated the cortex.

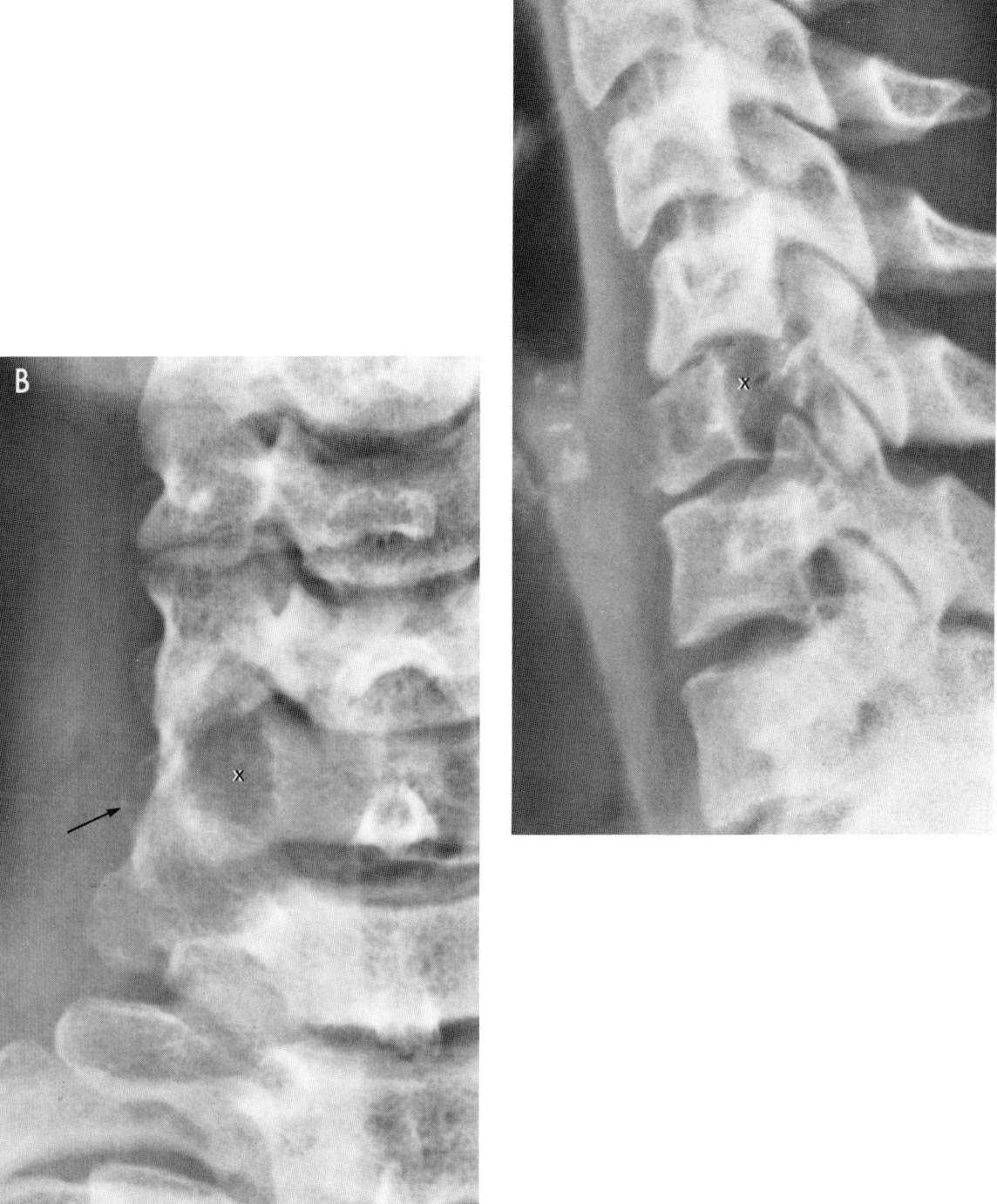

Figure 30 · Giant Cell Tumor of Cervical Spine / 109

Figure 31.—Giant cell tumor of the fibula.

AFIP Case No. 1129479: **A,** anteroposterior, and **B,** lateral views.

DIAGNOSIS AND GRADE.—Giant cell tumor, fibula; growth rate IC.

LIFE INFORMATION.—Female, 30 years; last known to be well.

LOCATION.—A lesion centered in the midmetaphysis at the proximal end of the fibula, extending down into the shaft and up into the epiphysis; no apparent soft tissue extension.

SIZE.—6 × 2 × 2 cm.

MINERALIZATION OF TUMOR.—None.

DESTRUCTION.—Centrally geographic. The transition zone between destroyed and intact bone is practically linear, but characterized by multiple moderate sized (up to 1 cm) oval foci of destruction of fairly uniform caliber, identified here as moth-eaten bone destruction, ragged contour. Total penetration of cortex. (See comment below.)

PROLIFERATION.—Several discontinuous areas of amorphous subperiosteal new bone (**arrows**).

DIFFERENTIAL DIAGNOSIS	PROBABILITY
Fibrosarcoma	.73
Giant cell tumor	.25
Osteosarcoma	< .01
Chondrosarcoma	< .01
Chondromyxoid fibroma	< .01

COMMENT: The principal problem concerns the distinction between this pattern of destruction—a combination of geographic and moth-eaten bone destruction—and the reticulate contour (Fig. 32) and permeated pattern of highly malignant tumors such as fibrosarcomas (Figs. 50 and 54). In the latter examples the central structure of cortex and medullary bone has been retained, showing principally a loss of density, while here there is total loss of structure within. Further, note the sharp zone of discontinuity at the junction of the tumor and shaft in this case and the fading discontinuity in the fibrosarcomas. The reticulate contour here is linear and finely lobulated, as seen usually in expanded lesions of the smaller bones. The combination of bone destruction illustrated here is principally seen in an early stage of growth.

The computer diagnosis strongly favored giant cell tumor until amorphous periostosis was considered in the differential diagnosis. Periostosis is so unusual in giant cell tumor that its presence greatly strengthened the probability of fibrosarcoma.

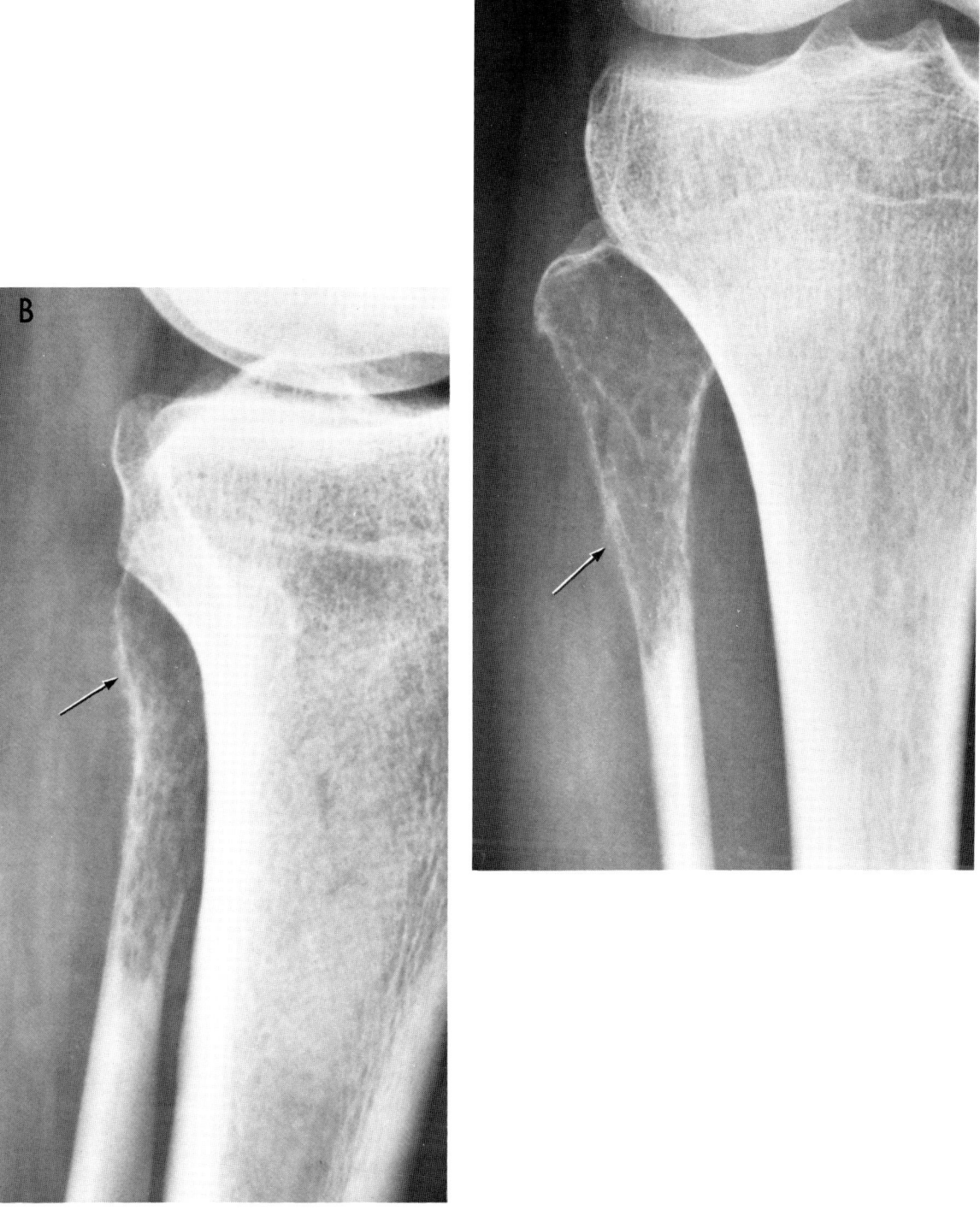

Figure 31 · Giant Cell Tumor of Fibula / 111

Figure 32.—Giant cell tumor of a metacarpal.

AFIP Case No. 1155465: Anteroposterior projection.

DIAGNOSIS AND GRADE.—Giant cell tumor, metacarpal; growth rate IA.

LIFE INFORMATION.—Male, 5 years; last known to be well.

LOCATION.—This round tumor, centered in the shaft of the fourth metacarpal, extends proximally to the proximal metaphysis and distally to the growth plate. Neither epiphysis is involved.

SIZE.—2 × 2 × 2 cm.

MINERALIZATION OF TUMOR.—None.

DESTRUCTION.—Geographic pattern; reticulate margin; incomplete penetration of cortex.

PROLIFERATION.—Symmetrically expanded shell; marginal sclerosis at ends of the tumor; fine septation.

DIFFERENTIAL DIAGNOSIS	PROBABILITY
Benign cartilaginous tumor	.55
Osteoblastoma	.38
Giant cell tumor	.04
Chondromyxoid fibroma	.01

COMMENT: The reticulate margin is similar in some respects to the pattern of destruction in the residual cortex of the giant cell tumor of the fibula seen in Figure 31. The location of the tumor in a metacarpal and its small size favor benign cartilaginous tumor over giant cell tumor.

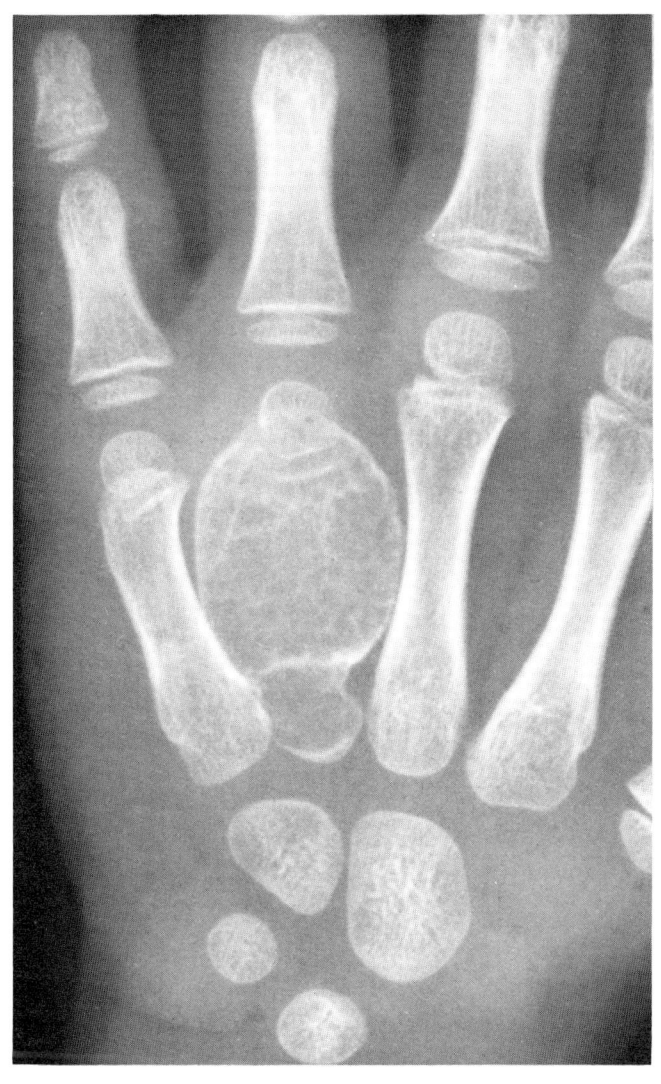

Figure 32 · Giant Cell Tumor of Metacarpal / 113

Figure 33.—Giant cell tumor of the os calcis.

AFIP Case No. 1148441: **A**, lateral, and **B**, sagittal views.

DIAGNOSIS AND GRADE.—Giant cell tumor, os calcis; growth rate IA.

LIFE INFORMATION.—Female, 8 years; well four years after onset.

LOCATION.—The tumor, centered eccentrically in the midbody of the os calcis, extends distally to the cartilage plate beneath the apophysis and anteriorly to within 1 cm of the anterior cortex.

SIZE.—5 × 3 × 3 cm.

MINERALIZATION OF TUMOR.—None.

DESTRUCTION.—Geographic; regular contour; largely reduction of cancellous bone.

PROLIFERATION.—Faint zone of marginal sclerosis (**arrows**); slight expansion of cortex laterally (**B, a**), with tumor completely encapsulated.

DIFFERENTIAL DIAGNOSIS	PROBABILITY
Cyst	.86
Chondromyxoid fibroma	.12
Giant cell tumor	< .01
Benign cartilaginous tumor	< .01
Fibrosarcoma	< .01

COMMENT: Were it not for the marginal sclerosis, this lesion might be missed. Note the location in the metaphysis in the presence of the unfused plate. In a child under 10, the elongated tumor with regular margin and sclerotic rim is far more typical of a cyst than of giant cell tumor.

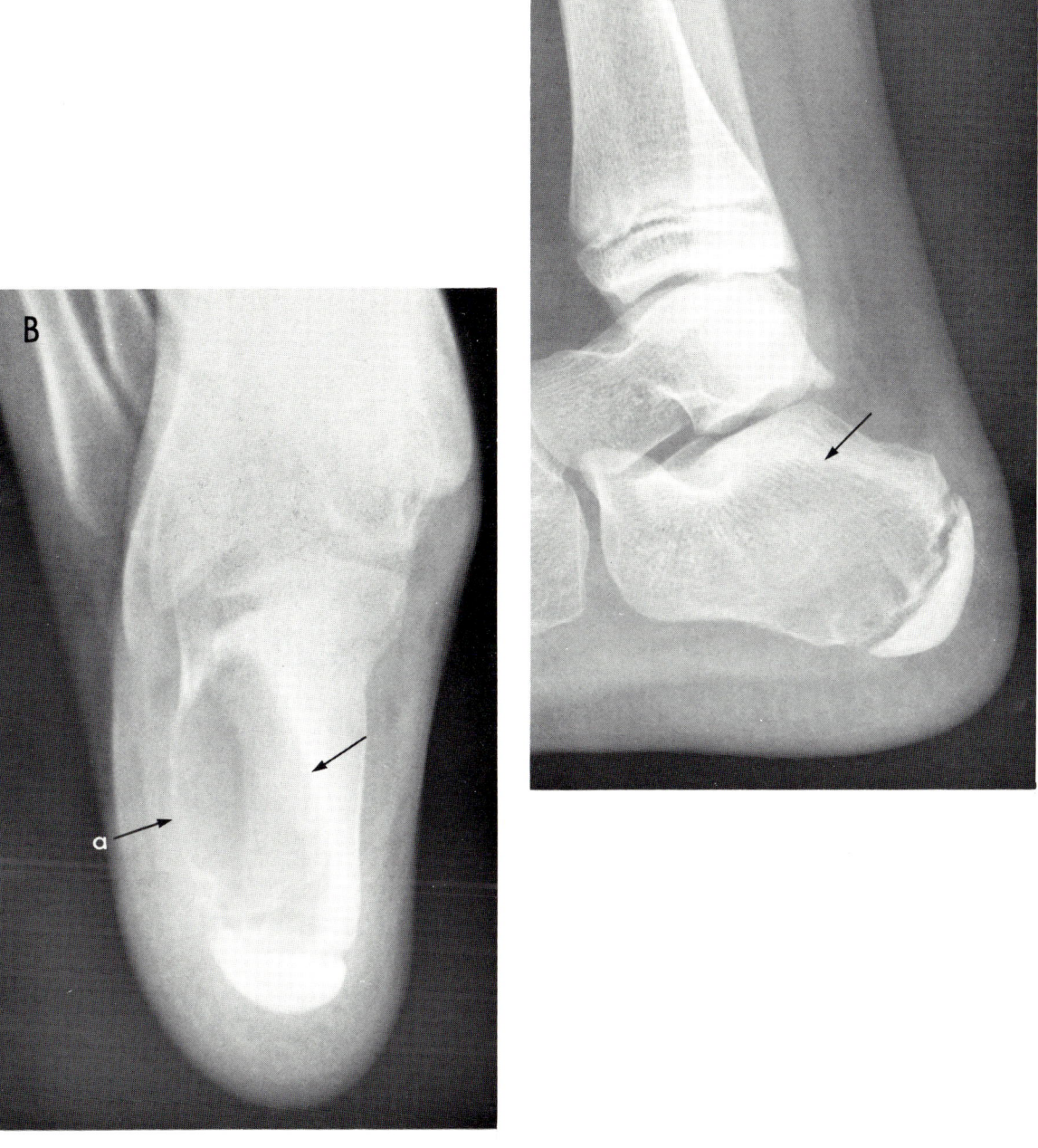

Figure 33 · Giant Cell Tumor of Os Calcis / 115

Figure 34.—Giant cell tumor of the pelvis.

AFIP Case No. 1151077: Anteroposterior projection.

DIAGNOSIS AND GRADE.—Giant cell tumor, pelvis; growth rate IC.
LIFE INFORMATION.—Male, 20 years; survival unknown.
LOCATION.—A large tumor centered in the medial acetabular area, involving ilium, ischium and subchondral cortex of the acetabulum; soft tissue extension medially into the pelvis (**arrow**).
SIZE.—9 × 7 × 5 cm.
MINERALIZATION OF TUMOR.—None.
DESTRUCTION.—Geographic; lobulated contour. Penetration of the cortex medially is postulated from presence of the extraosseous extension.
PROLIFERATION.—Faint marginal sclerosis: coarse, heavy septation; probably a slight expansion of cortex medially (**a**).

DIFFERENTIAL DIAGNOSIS	PROBABILITY
Chondromyxoid fibroma	.87
Cyst	.06
Myeloma	.03
Giant cell tumor	.02
Chondrosarcoma	< .01
Fibrosarcoma	< .01

COMMENT: Typical location and appearance of giant cell tumor of the pelvis. The computer apparently is not aware that this is not a typical location for chondromyxoid fibroma.

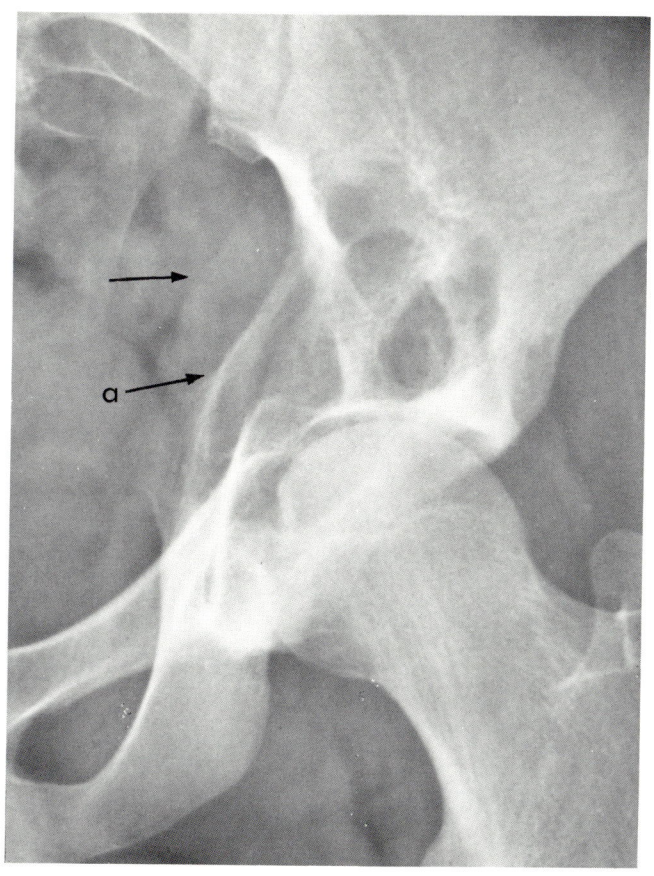

Figure 34 · Giant Cell Tumor of Pelvis / 117

Figure 35.—Cystic giant cell tumor of the pubis.

AFIP Case No. 1195256: Anteroposterior projection.

DIAGNOSIS AND GRADE.—Cystic giant cell tumor, pubis; growth rate IC.
LIFE INFORMATION.—Female, estimated age 5 years; last known to be well.
LOCATION.—A large tumor, centered in the pubic segment of the acetabulum, involves the entire pubic bone and parts of the ilium and ischium; large soft tissue extension (**arrows**).
SIZE.—8 × 8 cm.
MINERALIZATION OF TUMOR.—None.
DESTRUCTION.—Geographic; edge not seen; total loss of involved bone.
PROLIFERATION.—Several laminations of periosteal new bone medially (**a**); questionable marginal sclerosis.

DIFFERENTIAL DIAGNOSIS	PROBABILITY
Ewing's sarcoma	.74
Fibrosarcoma	.11
Chondrosarcoma	.05
Cyst	.04
Giant cell tumor	.04

COMMENT: Atypical for giant cell tumor. Absence of a definite sclerotic rim, septa, expanded cortex and presence of laminated periostosis led to the computer diagnosis of Ewing's sarcoma.

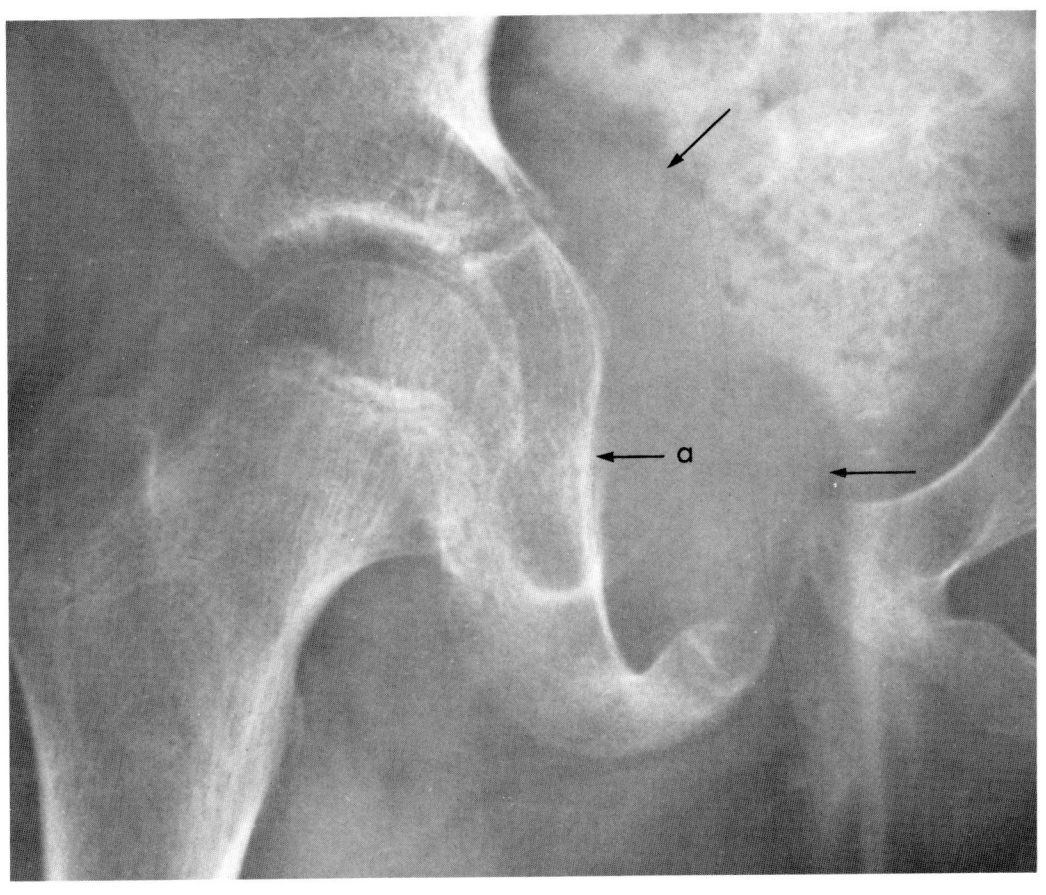

Figure 35 · Cystic Giant Cell Tumor of Pubis / 119

Figure 36.—Bone cyst of the radius.

AFIP Case No. 1022639: Anteroposterior projections—**A,** initial examination; **B,** three months later.

DIAGNOSIS AND GRADE.—Bone cyst, radius; growth rate IB.

LIFE INFORMATION.—Male, 7 years; well five years after onset.

LOCATION.—Oval lesion centered in middle third of the distal radial metaphysis, extending into the proximal and medial metaphyses but not reaching growth cartilage.

SIZE.—2.2 × 1.5 × 1.4 cm.

MINERALIZATION OF TUMOR.—None.

DESTRUCTION.—Geographic; regular contour; pathologic fracture (**arrows**).

PROLIFERATION.—First examination, none.

Three months later (**B**) the lesion, now 3.5 × 2.2 cm, extended to growth plate and into shaft. The cortex has been largely replaced by a newly expanded shell of periosteal new bone and the fracture has healed.

DIFFERENTIAL DIAGNOSIS	PROBABILITY
Cyst	.98
Chondromyxoid fibroma	< .01
Giant cell tumor	< .01

COMMENT: Note the shadow of the residual cortex inside the newly expanded shell (**B**). Growth rate is IB rather than IA because of absence of marginal sclerosis.

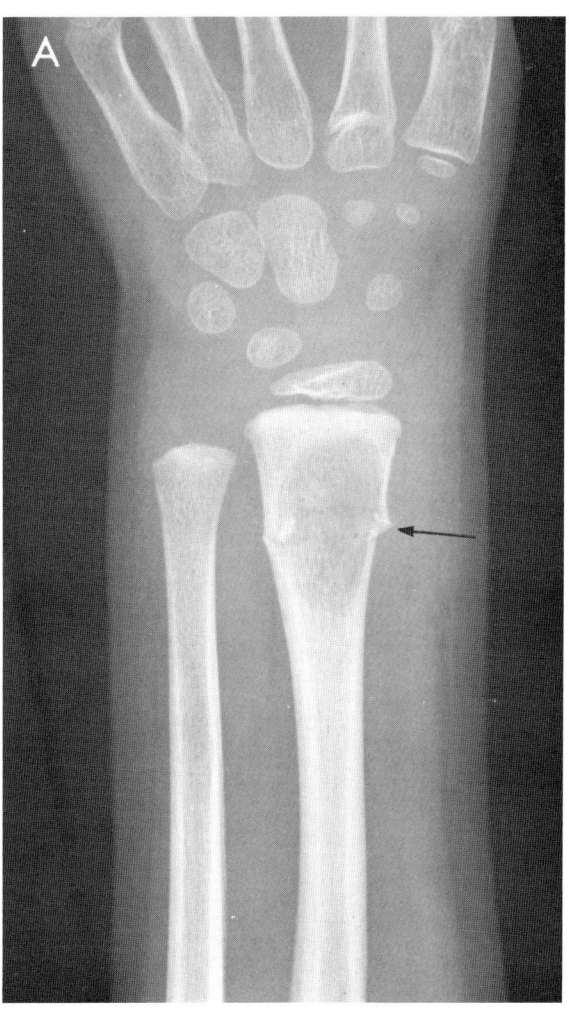
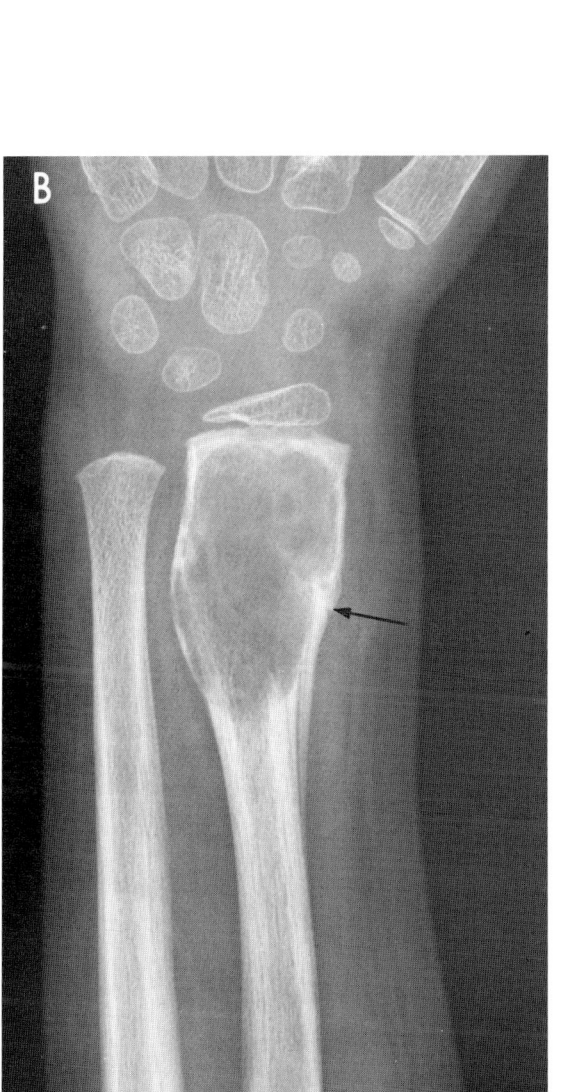

Figure 36 · Bone Cyst of Radius / 121

Figure 37.—Bone cysts of the humerus and ulna.

AFIP Case No. 1027619: **A,** anteroposterior projection.

DIAGNOSIS AND GRADE.—Cyst (unicameral), humerus; growth rate IB.
LIFE INFORMATION.—Male, estimated age 10 years; survival unknown.
LOCATION.—A circumscribed lesion centered in the middle third of the proximal metaphysis, extending proximally to the growth plate and distally to the origin of the shaft; no soft tissue extension.
SIZE.—6 × 3.5 cm.
MINERALIZATION OF TUMOR.—None.
DESTRUCTION.—Geographic; regular contour; pathologic fracture; thinning of cortex.
PROLIFERATION.—None.

DIFFERENTIAL DIAGNOSIS	PROBABILITY
Cyst	.95
Fibroxanthoma	.03
Benign cartilaginous tumor	.01
Fibrosarcoma	< .01
Chondromyxoid fibroma	< .01
Chondrosarcoma	< .01

COMMENT: At this stage, this lesion has the shape of a truncated cone (tear drop) typical of the juvenile unicameral cyst. The location is also typical. Growth rate is IB rather than IA because there is no marginal sclerosis. Note the fragment of bone in the cavity, a finding more suggestive of fluid content than of solid tissue.

AFIP Case No. 1087809: **B,** anteroposterior projection.

DIAGNOSIS AND GRADE.—Bone cyst, ulna; growth rate IA.
LIFE INFORMATION.—Male, 10 years; well at last contact.
LOCATION.—A lesion centered in the middle third of the proximal metaphysis extending into the remaining third; no soft tissue involvement.
SIZE.—3 × 2.5 × 2 cm.
MINERALIZATION OF TUMOR.—None.
DESTRUCTION.—Geographic; regular contour; thinning of cortex.
PROLIFERATION.—Broad zone of marginal sclerosis; about 6 mm of smoothly expanded cortex which completely encapsulates the tumor; faint septation.

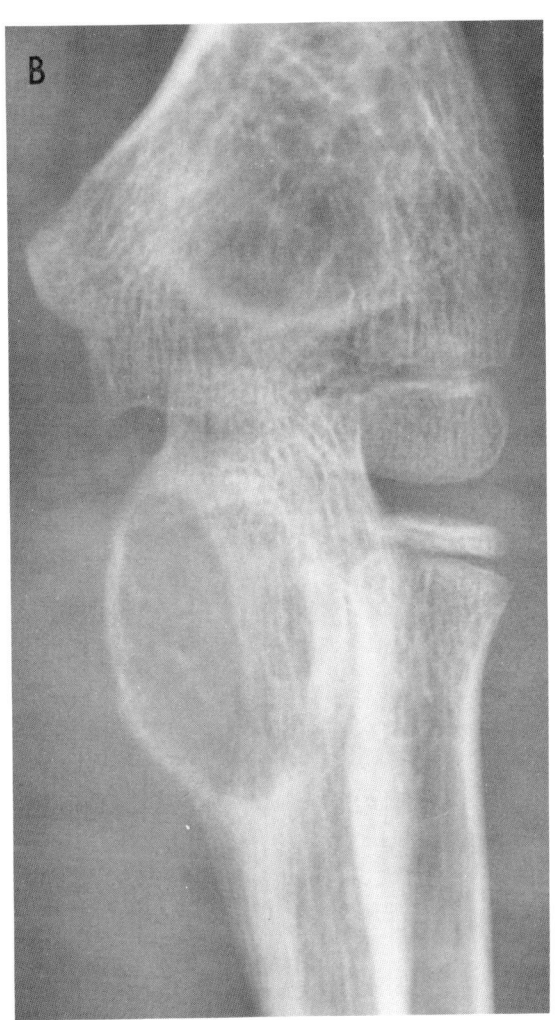
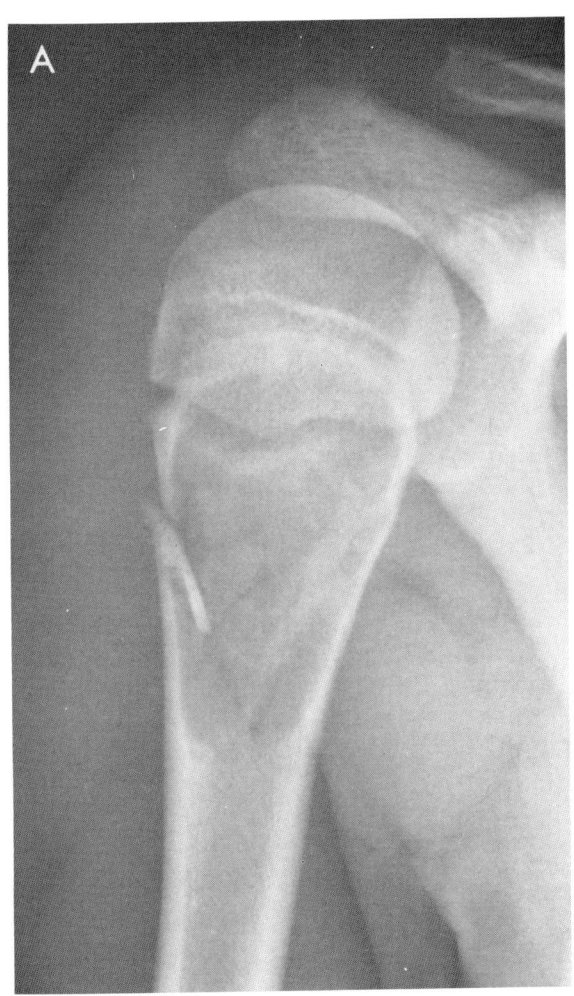

Differential Diagnosis	Probability
Cyst	.75
Chondromyxoid fibroma	.15
Fibroxanthoma	.08
Benign cartilaginous tumor	< .01

COMMENT: An expanding lesion which just reaches the subchondral cortex.

Figure 37 · Bone Cysts of Humerus and Ulna

Figure 38.—Bone cyst of the ilium.

AFIP Case No. 1194303: Anteroposterior views—**A,** initial study; **B,** four years later.

DIAGNOSIS AND GRADE.—Bone cyst, ilium; growth rate IC.

LIFE INFORMATION.—Female, 4 years; well four years after onset.

LOCATION.—Centered in the iliac wing, the lesion extends laterally to the crest and medially to within 1 cm of the sacroiliac joint.

SIZE.—6 × 4 cm on initial examination.

MINERALIZATION OF TUMOR.—Initially, some areas of cloudy matrix mineralization near the margins of the lesion (**A, x**).

DESTRUCTION.—Initially, geographic; ragged contour; penetration of cortex.

PROLIFERATION.—Initially, no definite proliferation.

Four years later, growth rate IB. The lesion has grown to 12 × 8 cm and involves the entire iliac wing. There is no evidence of matrix mineralization, and the lesion is encapsulated by a lobular septate shell.

DIFFERENTIAL DIAGNOSIS		PROBABILITY
Exam. 1	Cyst	.85
	Chondrosarcoma	.08
	Fibrosarcoma	.06
Exam. 2	Cyst	.65
	Chondromyxoid fibroma	.34
	Giant cell tumor	< .01
	Fibrosarcoma	< .01
	Chondrosarcoma	< .01

COMMENT: This lesion may provide insight into the development of cysts. It begins as a moderately aggressive bone cyst which has penetrated the cortex, diagnosed as of the aneurysmal variety by the contributor. Ultimately, though much enlarged, it appears to be multicompartmented and inactive.

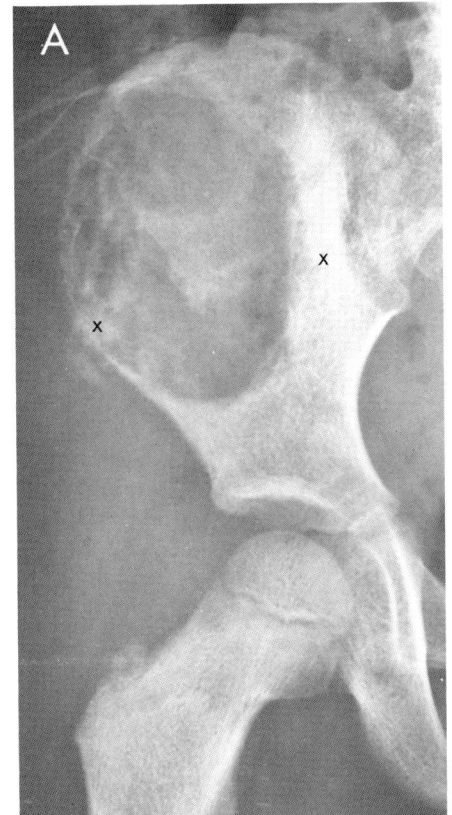
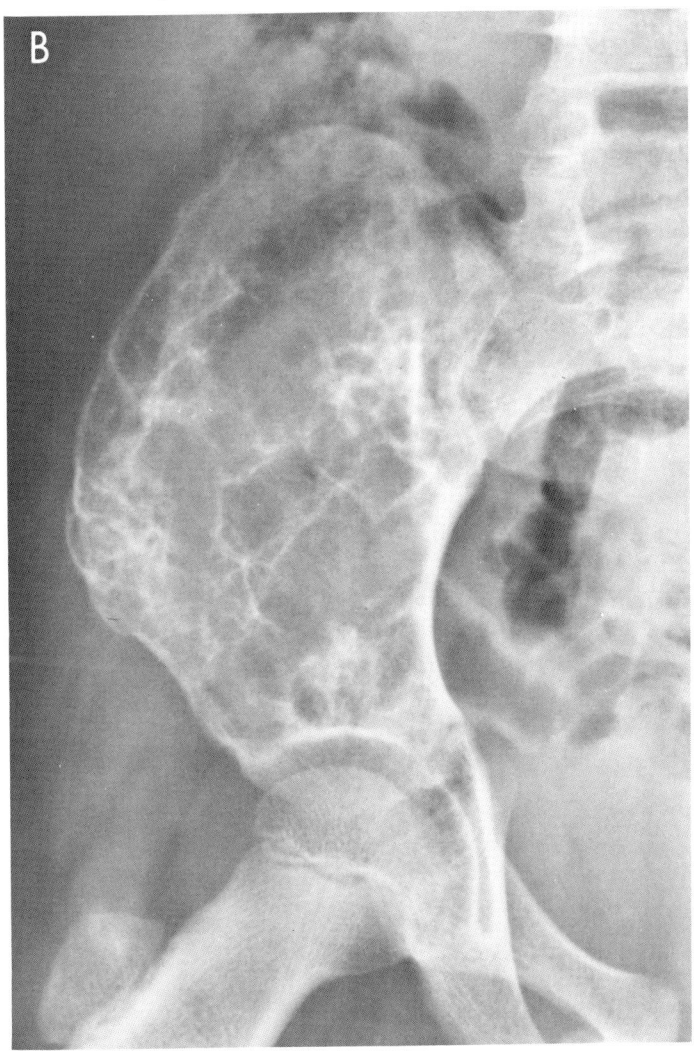

Figure 38 · Bone Cyst of Ilium

Figure 39.—Expanding bone cyst of the humerus.

AFIP Case No. 1193759: Series of anteroposterior exposures made at intervals over 25 months.

A, initial examination, showing pathologic fracture.
B, 5 months later, lesion has extended up and down the shaft.
C, immediately after curettage and installation of bone chips.
D, 6 months later, with recurrence.
For succeeding studies, see Figure 40.

DIAGNOSIS AND GRADE.—Cyst, expanding, humerus; growth rate IA.

LIFE INFORMATION.—Male, 5 years; well three years after onset.

LOCATION.—An elongated encapsulated lesion centered in the upper third of the shaft, confined to upper and middle thirds.

SIZE.—6 × 2 × 2 cm on initial examination.

MINERALIZATION OF TUMOR.—None.

DESTRUCTION.—Geographic; regular contour; internal buttresses at both ends.

PROLIFERATION.—Slightly expanded cortical shell in all examinations, with marginal sclerosis at ends of the lesion. After treatment a pronounced lobulated and septate pattern ultimately appears.

Subsequent course: Five months later (**B**) the cyst is substantially larger and the cortex is laterally expanded while the fracture has healed. There is no longer a sclerotic rim at the ends of the lesion, indicating an increase of growth rate to IB. Six months after curettage and installation of bone chips the lesion has recurred (**D**). Six months after re-treatment by bone grafting the lesion has extended farther along the shaft and the grafts are nearly resorbed (Fig. 40, *C*). Regrowth seems to be multifocal, with several discrete areas of destruction.

DIFFERENTIAL DIAGNOSIS	PROBABILITY
Cyst	.74
Fibroxanthoma	.13
Benign cartilaginous tumor	.10
Fibrosarcoma	.01
Chondrosarcoma	< .01
Chondromyxoid fibroma	< .01

(*Continued* in Figure 40.)

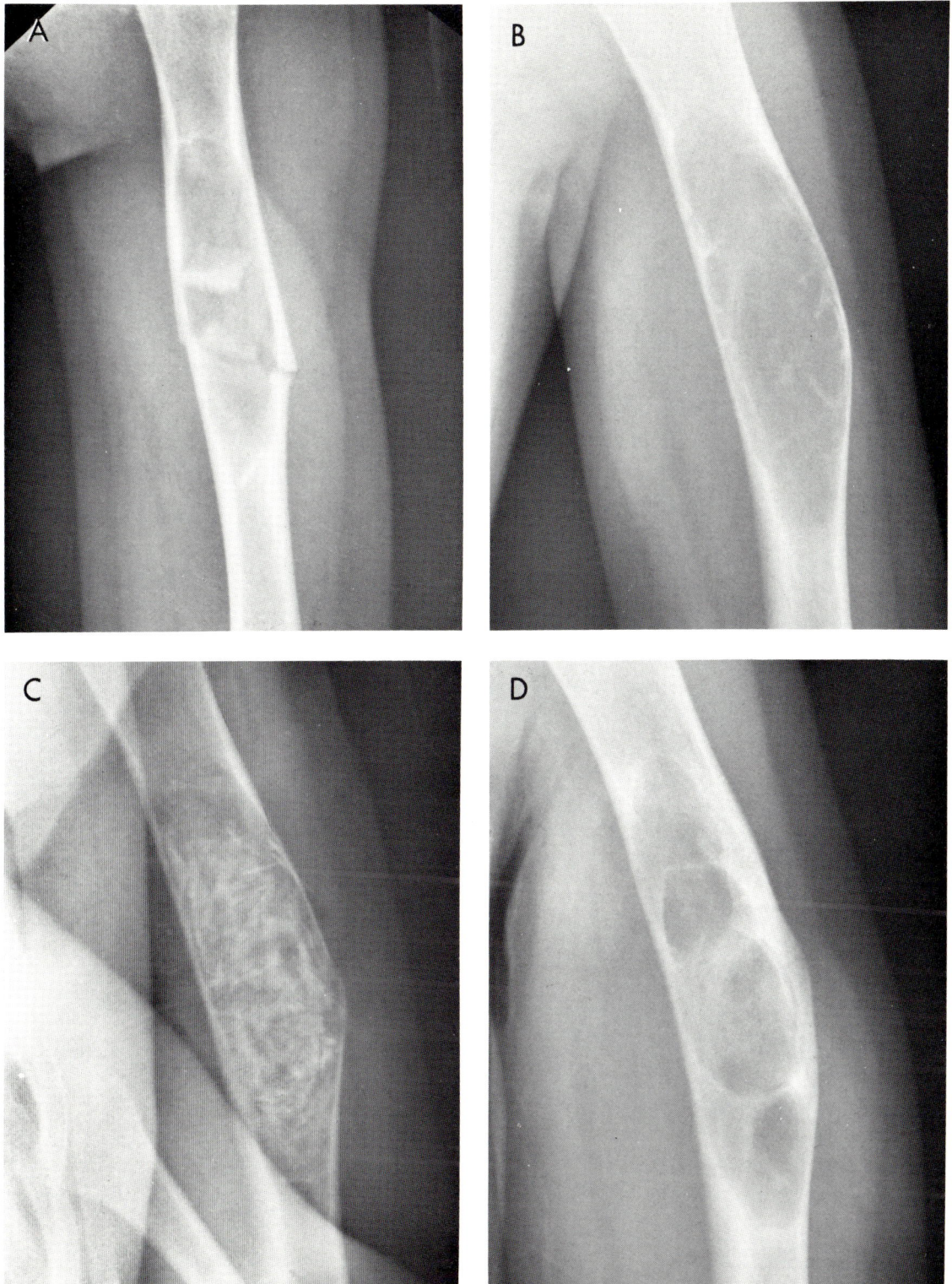

Figure 39 · Expanding Bone Cyst of Humerus

Figure 40.—Expanding bone cyst of the humerus (same case as in Figure 39).

A, immediately after second operation, 13 months after initial examination (Fig. 39, *A*). Note bone graft and bone chips.
B, 3 months later (16 months after initial study) the bone cysts are re-forming.
C, 3 months later (19 months after initial study) the bone graft has been resorbed and the cysts continue to grow.
D, Cystic humerus, removed 25 months after the patient was first examined.

COMMENT: This extraordinarily persistent cystic lesion appears to have had its origin in the shaft. At no time was it observed to lie within the metaphysis or near the growth plate. It expanded both lengthwise and laterally despite aggressive management. The histologic material was clearly that of a cyst, and the computer differential diagnosis is quite satisfactory.

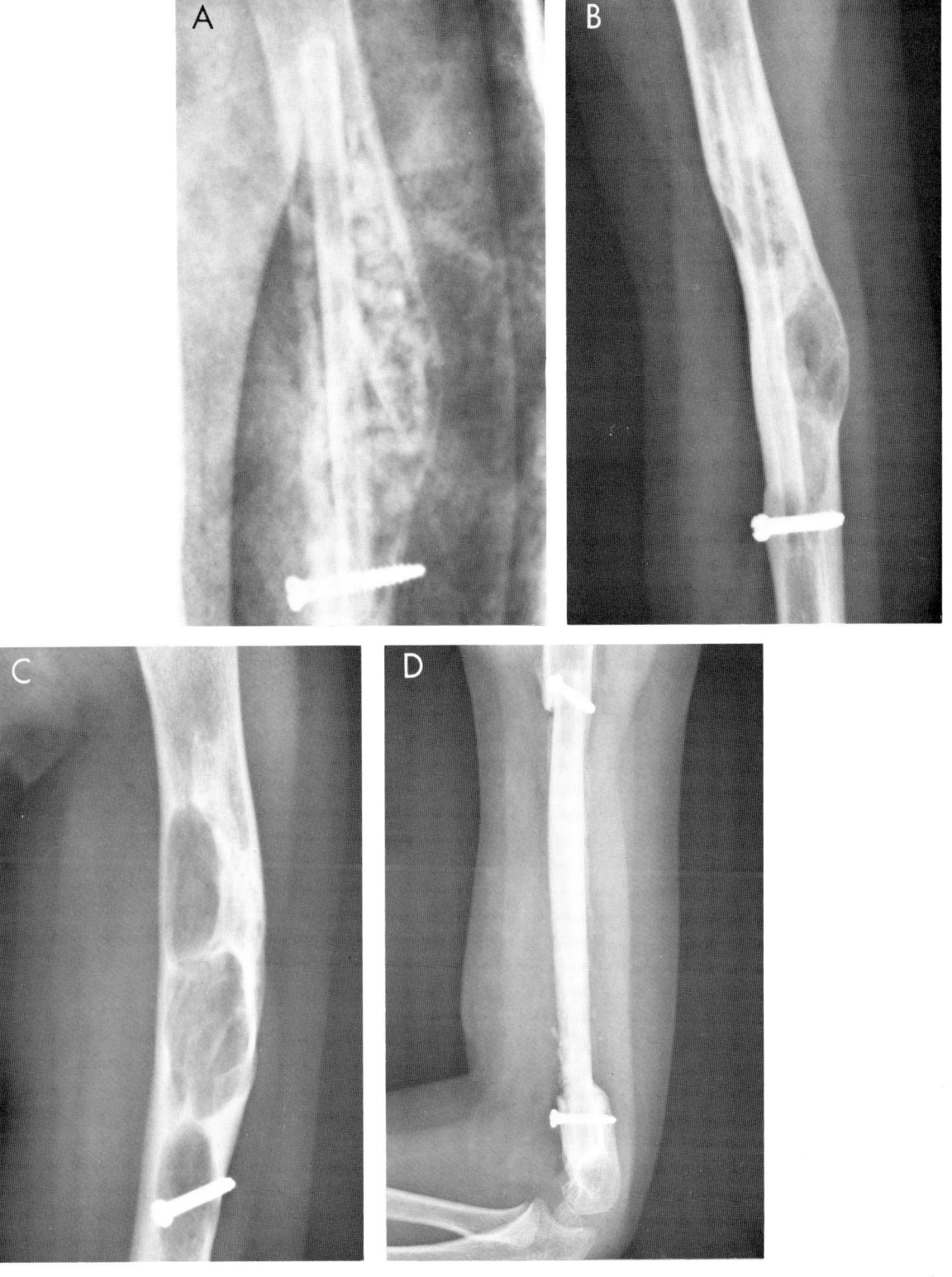

Figure 40 · Expanding Bone Cyst of Humerus

Figure 41.—Cystic giant cell tumor of the tibia.

AFIP Case No. 1111366: **A,** anteroposterior, and **B,** lateral views.

DIAGNOSIS AND GRADE.—Cystic giant cell tumor, tibia; growth rate IA.

LIFE INFORMATION.—Female, 17 years; last known to be well.

LOCATION.—An oval lesion (**arrows**) centered in the middle third of the proximal metaphysis, extending to involve the rest of the metaphysis and entering the epiphysis slightly, if at all; no involvement of the subarticular cortex or extraosseous extension.

SIZE.—7 × 3 × 4 cm

MINERALIZATION OF TUMOR.—None.

DESTRUCTION.—Geographic; essentially regular contour and slightly lobulated distal extension; incomplete lateral penetration of cortex. Most of the destruction that is visible is due to reduction of cancellous bone.

PROLIFERATION.—Faint marginal sclerosis; slight lateral expansion of cortex, which appears to encapsulate the tumor completely.

DIFFERENTIAL DIAGNOSIS	PROBABILITY
Cyst	.67
Chondromyxoid fibroma	.15
Giant cell tumor	.09
Fibrosarcoma	.03
Osteoblastoma	.03
Chondrosarcoma	< .01
Benign cartilaginous tumor	< .01

COMMENT: Lack of involvement of the epiphysis is unusual with giant cell tumor. The lesion more nearly resembles a cyst or chondromyxoid fibroma. Note the small lobulated lesion (**x**) at the distal margin of the large lesion, seen best in **B**. It seems quite separate and focally thins the cortex from within, as seen in **A**. This seems to be a separate benign lesion, less aggressive than the larger one. The heavier sclerotic rim around the small lesion may be explained as cancellous reinforcement of the weakened cortex.

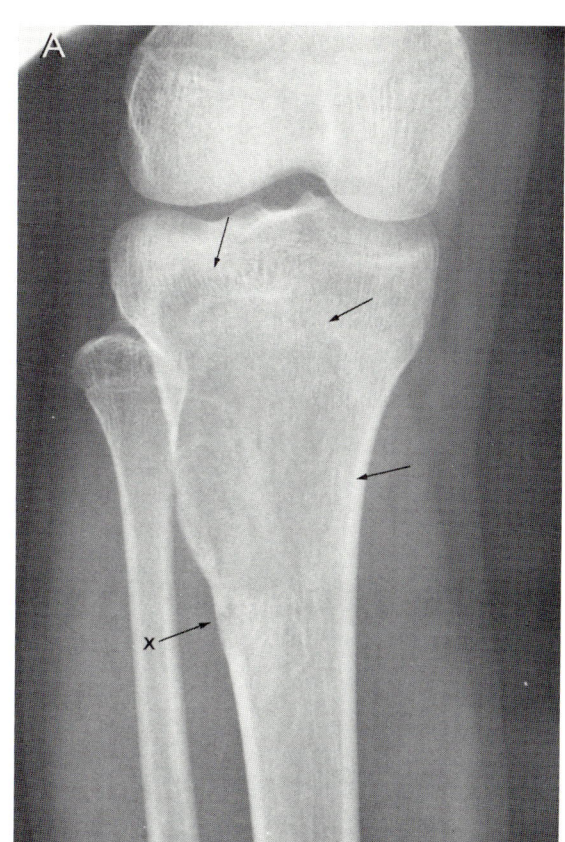
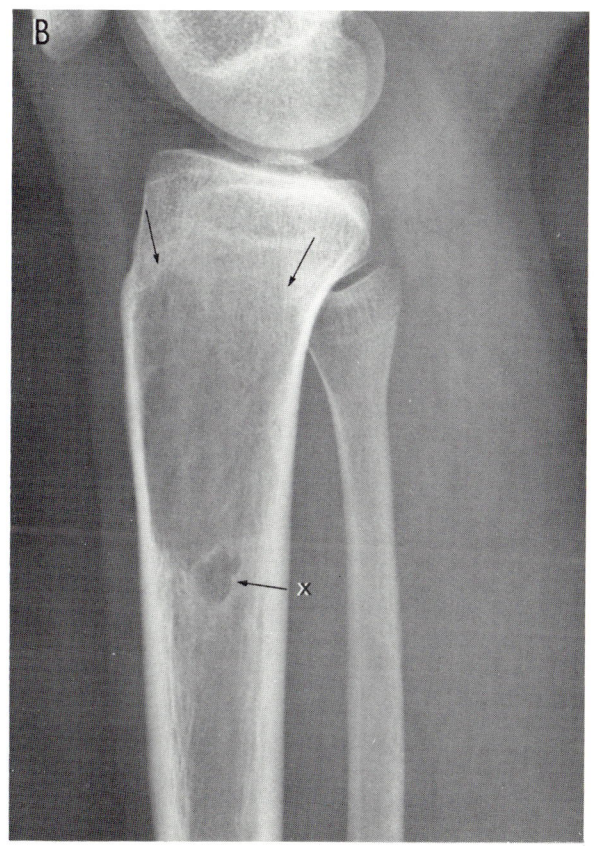

Figure 41 · Cystic Giant Cell Tumor of Tibia

Figure 42.—Bone cyst of the fibula.

AFIP Case No. 1165684: Anteroposterior projection.

DIAGNOSIS AND GRADE.—Bone cyst, fibula; growth rate IA.

LIFE INFORMATION.—Male, estimated 4 years; last known to be well.

LOCATION.—An elongated lesion centered in the mid-distal metaphysis of the fibula, extending to the growth cartilage and into the rest of the metaphysis.

SIZE.—3 × 1 × 2 cm.

MINERALIZATION OF TUMOR.—None.

DESTRUCTION.—Geographic; slightly lobulated contour; pathologic fracture; internal buttresses.

PROLIFERATION.—Faint marginal sclerosis; no conclusive evidence of expansion of cortex.

DIFFERENTIAL DIAGNOSIS	PROBABILITY
Cyst	.61
Osteoblastoma	.15
Benign cartilaginous tumor	.11
Chondromyxoid fibroma	.10
Giant cell tumor	.01
Osteosarcoma	< .01

COMMENT: This lesion is more probably a cyst than a nonossifying fibroma because the latter rarely reaches the growth plate. Note also that one of the fragments appears to lie free within the cyst cavity, a finding typical only of cysts.

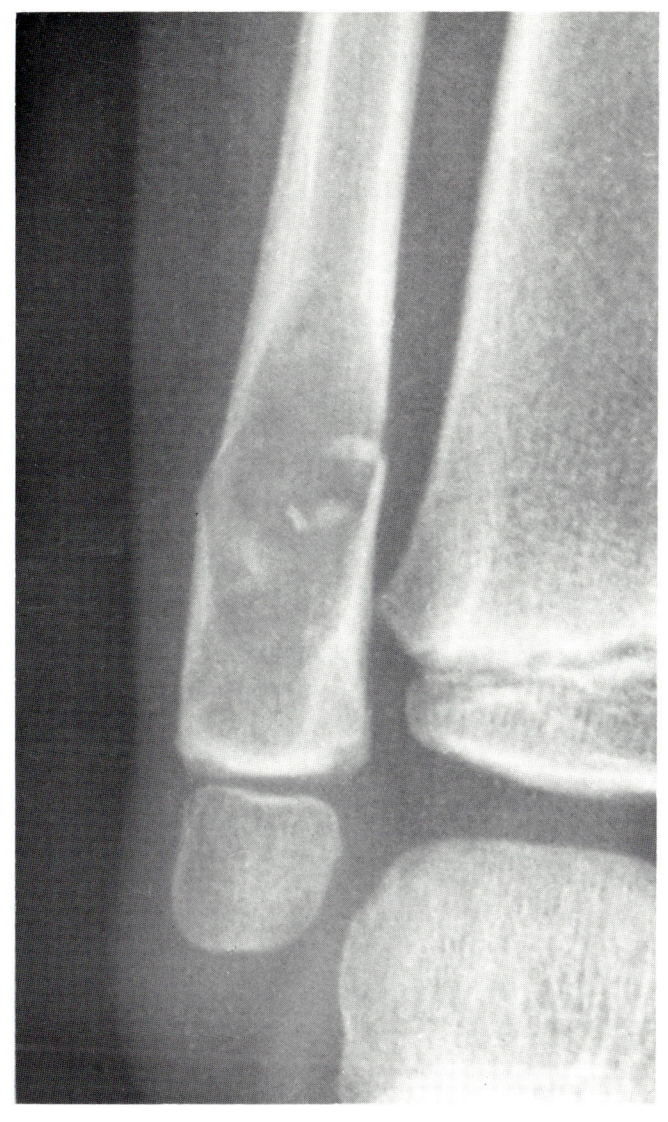

Figure 42 · Bone Cyst of Fibula / 133

Figure 43.—Bone cyst of the femur.

AFIP Case No. 1213808: Anteroposterior projection.

DIAGNOSIS AND GRADE.—Bone cyst, femur; growth rate IB.
LIFE INFORMATION.—Male, 21 years; last known to be well.
LOCATION.—The lesion, centered in the intertrochanteric region, extends down into the lesser trochanter and origin of the shaft and up to the base of the neck; no soft tissue extension.

SIZE.—7 × 5 cm.
MINERALIZATION OF TUMOR.—None.
DESTRUCTION.—Geographic; regular contour; pathologic fracture (**arrow**).
PROLIFERATION.—Smoothly symmetrical expansion of cortex into lesser trochanter and lateral cortex, estimated at 1 cm; definite marginal sclerosis; faint septation.

DIFFERENTIAL DIAGNOSIS	PROBABILITY
Cyst	.59
Fibroxanthoma	.24
Chondromyxoid fibroma	.09
Fibrosarcoma	.04
Villonodular synovitis	.01
Myeloma	< .01
Chondrosarcoma	< .01
Benign cartilaginous tumor	< .01

COMMENT: The smoothly symmetrical pattern of expansion is typical of a cyst. Note the unusual radiating pattern of septation.

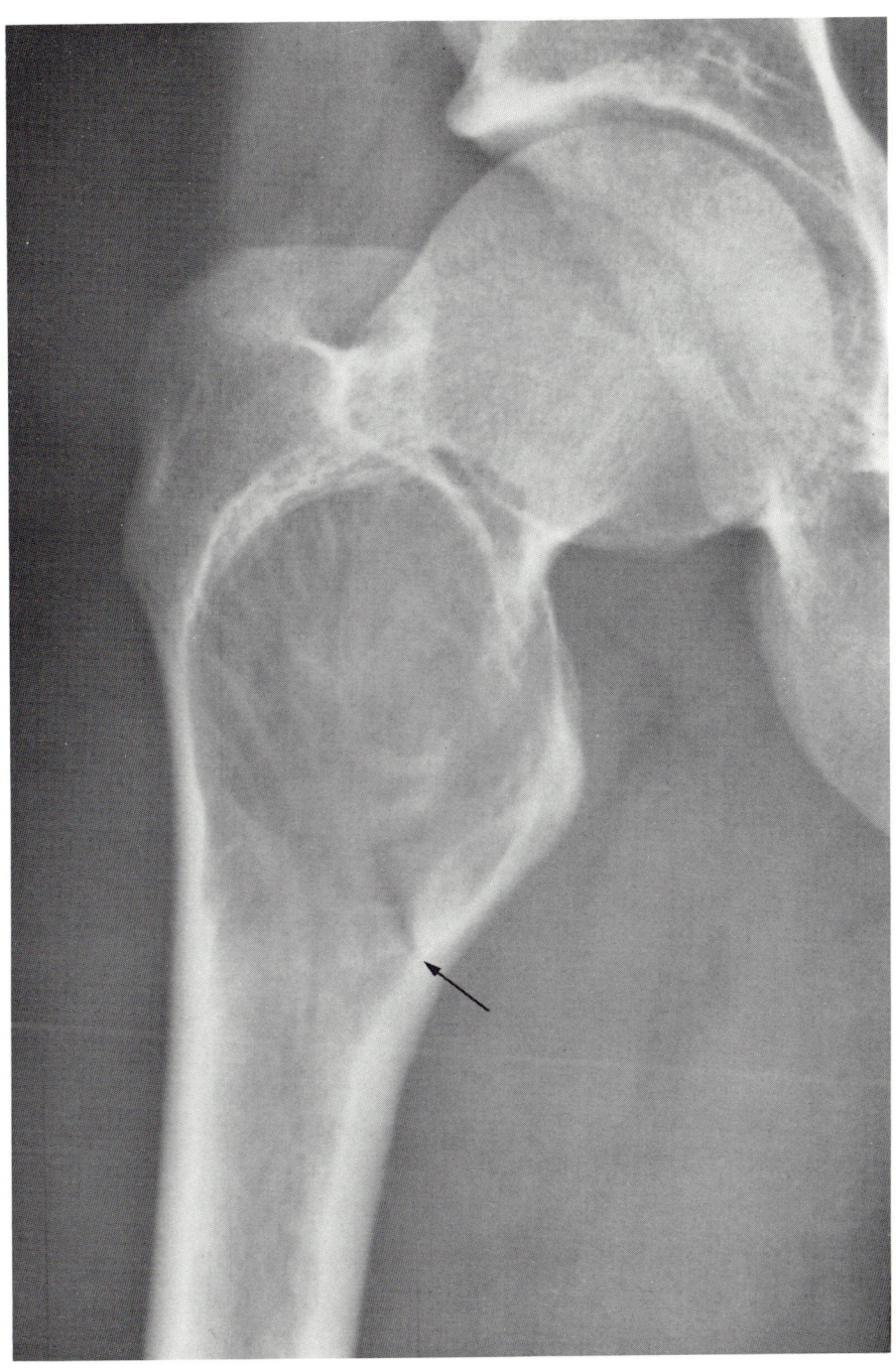

Figure 43 · Bone Cyst of Femur / 135

Figure 44.—Bone cysts of the clavicle and tibia.

AFIP Case No. 1120445: **A,** oblique projection.

DIAGNOSIS AND GRADE.—Bone cyst, clavicle; growth rate IA.

LIFE INFORMATION.—Female, 10 years; well three years after onset.

LOCATION.—A circumscribed lesion centered in the distal metaphysis of the clavicle, extending proximally into the shaft and terminating 1 cm short of the end of the bone; no soft tissue extension.

SIZE.—3 × 1 cm.

MINERALIZATION OF TUMOR.—None.

DESTRUCTION.—Geographic; lobulated contour; pathologic fracture through the lesion.

PROLIFERATION.—Faint marginal sclerosis; slightly expanded cortex which encapsulates the lesion.

DIFFERENTIAL DIAGNOSIS	PROBABILITY
Cyst	.59
Benign cartilaginous tumor	.40
Chondrosarcoma	< .01
Fibrosarcoma	< .01

COMMENT: A nonspecific appearance best fitting a diagnosis of cyst.

AFIP Case No. 1065938: **B,** anteroposterior projection.

DIAGNOSIS AND GRADE.—Bone cyst (cystic giant cell tumor), tibia; growth rate IA.

LIFE INFORMATION.—Male, 9 years; survival unknown.

LOCATION.—This lesion, centered eccentrically in the middle third of the proximal metaphysis, extends proximally, appearing to penetrate the growth plate with a small circumscribed extension into the epiphysis (**arrow**), and extends distally to a point just short of the shaft; no extraosseous extension.

SIZE.—5 × 3.5 cm.

MINERALIZATION OF TUMOR.—None.

DESTRUCTION.—Geographic; regular contour; incomplete penetration of medial cortex.

PROLIFERATION.—Dense marginal sclerosis; faint septation; small buttress with slight expansion of cortex.

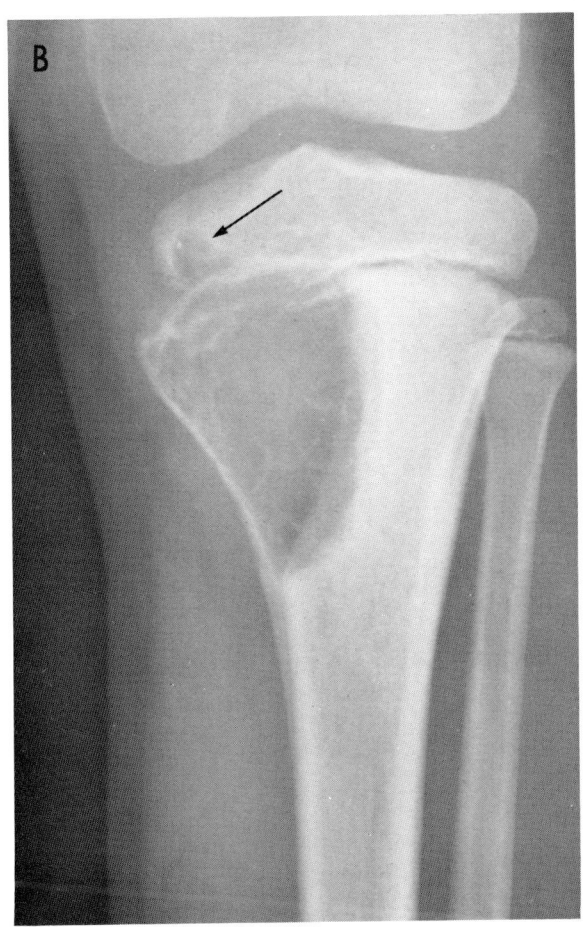
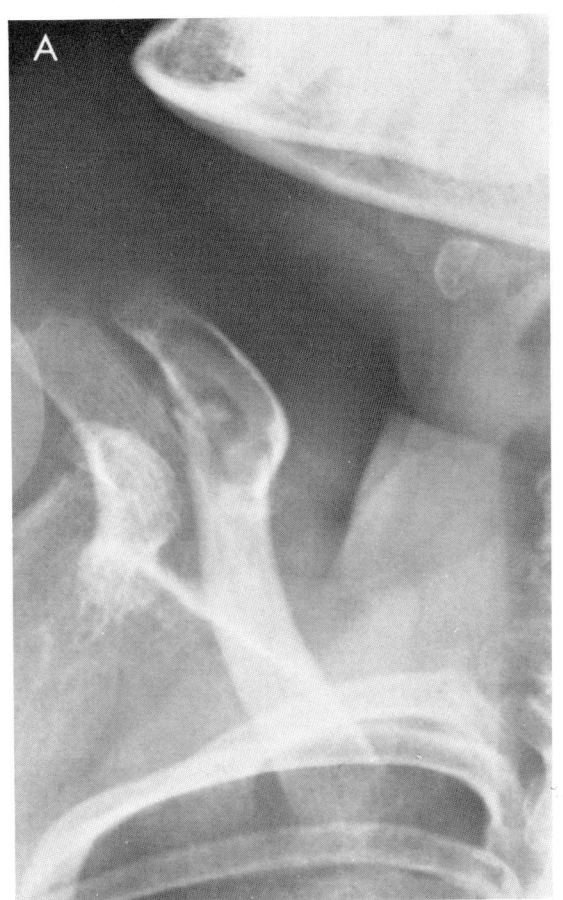

Differential Diagnosis	Probability
Giant cell tumor	.58
Cyst	.31
Chondromyxoid fibroma	.06
Osteoblastoma	.03

COMMENT: The lesion appears to have penetrated the growth cartilage and extended into the epiphysis without comparable extension into soft tissues. This may represent reflex absorption of bone adjacent to the tumor. The computer diagnosis of giant cell tumor is heavily in sympathy with the author's.

Figure 44 · Bone Cysts of Clavicle and Tibia

Figure 45.—Bone cysts of the ilium and femur.

AFIP Case No. 1126687: **A,** anteroposterior projection.

DIAGNOSIS AND GRADE.—Bone cyst, ilium; growth rate IA.
LIFE INFORMATION.—Male, 21 years; survival unknown.
LOCATION.—Large lesion centered in the ilium over the sacroiliac joint.

SIZE.—7 × 6 cm.
MINERALIZATION OF TUMOR.—None.
DESTRUCTION.—Geographic; lobulated contour.
PROLIFERATION.—Faint but definite marginal sclerosis; extensively septate pattern; large central zones of dense proliferative bone.

DIFFERENTIAL DIAGNOSIS	PROBABILITY
Chondromyxoid fibroma	.66
Cyst	.14
Myeloma	.12
Giant cell tumor	.05
Fibrosarcoma	.01
Chondrosarcoma	.01
Benign cartilaginous tumor	< .01

COMMENT: The lesion has a scarred inactive appearance. The eccentric location and lobulated contour are more strongly in favor of chondromyxoid fibroma than of cyst.

AFIP Case No. 1035921: **B,** lateral projection.

DIAGNOSIS AND GRADE.—Bone cyst, femur; growth rate IA.
LIFE INFORMATION.—Male, 9 years; survival unknown.
LOCATION.—A circumscribed lesion centered in the proximal metaphysis, extending distally to the origin of the shaft and proximally to within 1 cm of the growth plate. Both greater and lesser trochanters are involved. No extraosseous extension.

SIZE.—Estimated 5 × 3.5 cm.
MINERALIZATION OF TUMOR.—None.
DESTRUCTION.—Geographic; lobulated contour; incomplete penetration of cortex.
PROLIFERATION.—Distinct marginal sclerosis; moderate septate pattern; slight cortical expansion which completely encapsulates the lesion.

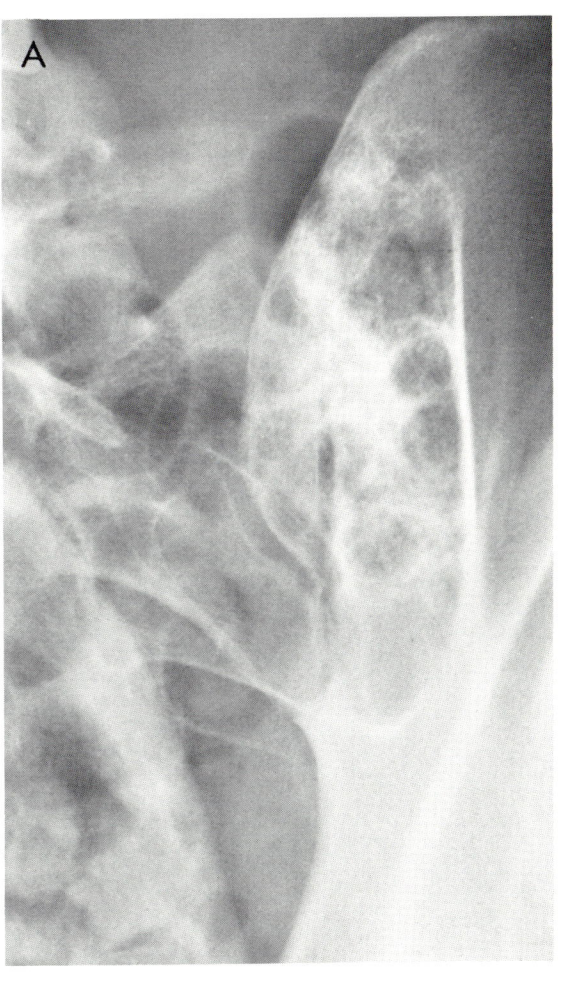
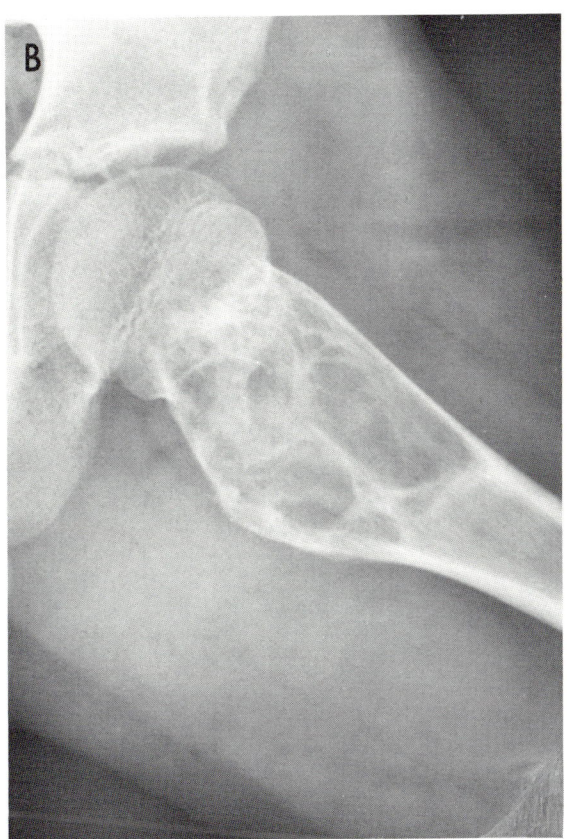

Differential Diagnosis	Probability
Chondromyxoid fibroma	.44
Fibroxanthoma	.31
Cyst	.21
Villonodular synovitis	.01
Myeloma	< .01
Fibrosarcoma	< .01
Benign cartilaginous tumor	< .01

COMMENT: This encapsulated, cystic appearing lesion demonstrates no real growth potential. The lobulated contour favors chondromyxoid fibroma more than a cyst.

Figure 45 · Bone Cysts of Ilium and Femur

Figure 46.—Simple bone cyst of the pelvis.

AFIP Case No. 978219: Anteroposterior projection.

DIAGNOSIS AND GRADE.—Bone cyst (simple), pelvis; growth rate IA.
LIFE INFORMATION.—Male, 41 years; survival unknown.
LOCATION.—A large lesion centrally located in the ilium, with major marginal contact with the crest.
SIZE.—12 × 11 cm.
MINERALIZATION OF TUMOR.—None.
DESTRUCTION.—Geographic; lobulated contour; incomplete penetration of cortex.
PROLIFERATION.—Distinct marginal sclerosis: multiple septation with loculated pattern.

DIFFERENTIAL DIAGNOSIS	PROBABILITY
Chondrosarcoma	.30
Fibrosarcoma	.28
Myeloma	.27
Giant cell tumor	.08
Chondromyxoid fibroma	.04
Cyst	< .01

COMMENT: A picture very similar to that of Figure 38, *B,* possibly with the same kind of origin. The greater age here and absence of expanded cortex make for a quite different differential diagnosis, however.

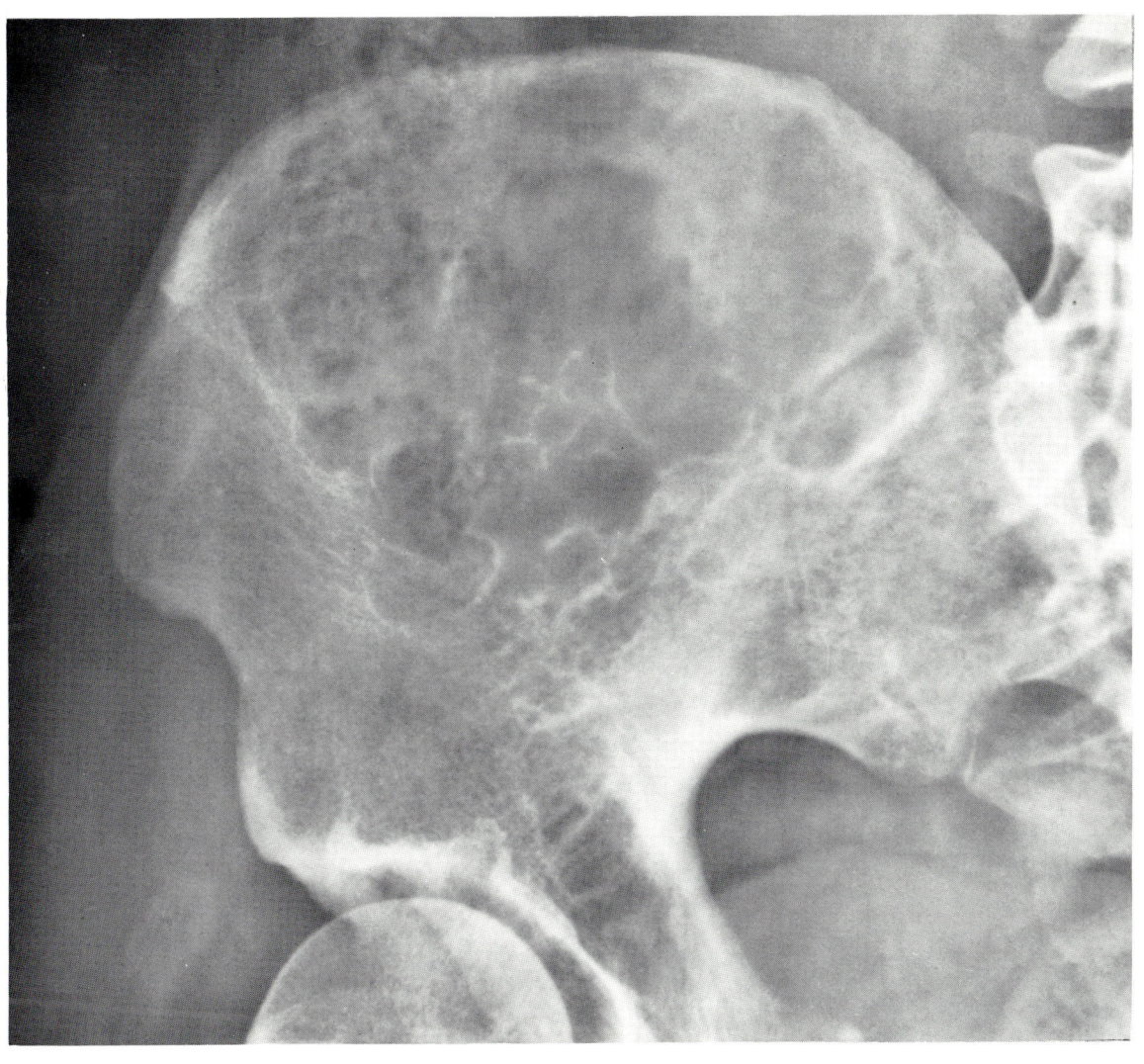

Figure 46 · Bone Cyst of Pelvis / 141

Figure 47.—Bone cyst of the radius.

AFIP Case No. 1129433: Anteroposterior projection.

DIAGNOSIS AND GRADE.—Bone cyst, radius; growth rate IC.

LIFE INFORMATION.—Male, 23 years; last known to be well.

LOCATION.—An elongated lesion apparently centered on the medial cortex of the distal radius, occupying a narrow strip of the metaphysis; soft tissue extension.

SIZE.—5 × 1 × 1 cm.

MINERALIZATION OF TUMOR.—None.

DESTRUCTION.—Geographic; regular contour; total penetration of cortex.

PROLIFERATION.—Dense marginal sclerosis, tiny buttress; a few septa. There is no apparent encapsulation of the tumor by bone, but encapsulation by periosteum is suspected based on the sharp encapsulation elsewhere.

DIFFERENTIAL DIAGNOSIS	PROBABILITY
Fibroxanthoma	.99
Benign cartilaginous tumor	< .01
Fibrosarcoma	< .01

COMMENT: An unusual lesion, of low growth potential. A fibrous lesion would be the first choice. Interestingly, the cortex beneath the lesion appears to have been expanded inward or held in position by a long-standing tumor while the rest of the bone grew around it. The decision scheme does not allow for the possibility of a cyst in this location.

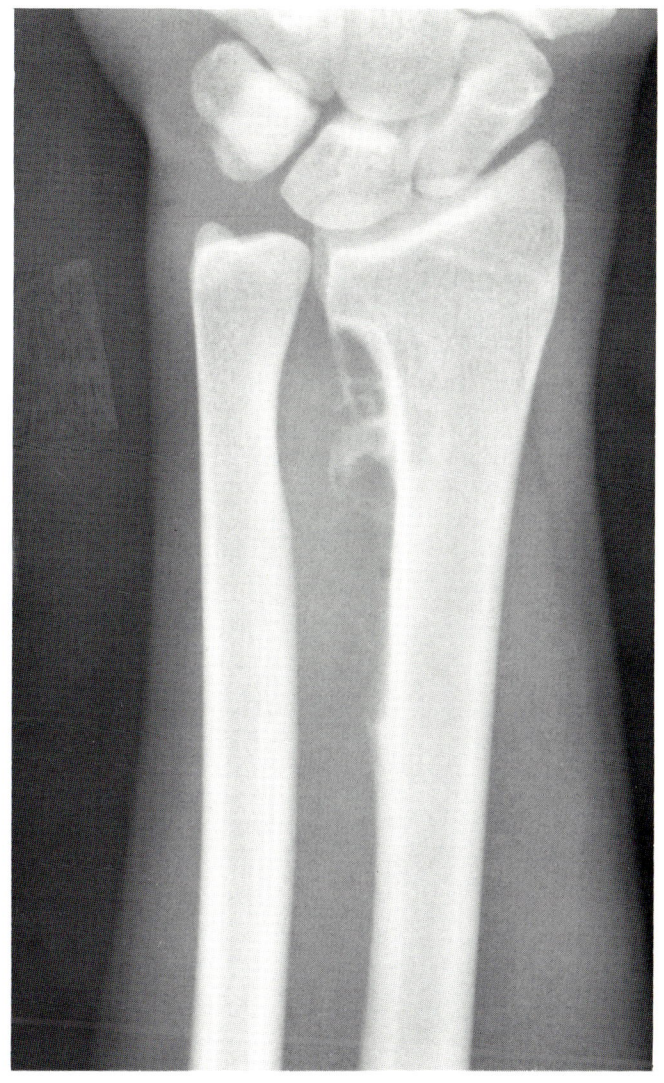

Figure 47 · Bone Cyst of Radius / 143

PART 3

Fibrous Tumors

Figure 48.—Fibrosarcoma of the frontal bone.

AFIP Case No. 1152297: Posteroanterior projection.

DIAGNOSIS AND GRADE.—Fibrosarcoma, frontal bone; growth rate IC.
LIFE INFORMATION.—Female, 38 years; survival unknown.
LOCATION.—A circumscribed lesion in the lateral frontal sinus.

SIZE.—Estimated 4 × 4 cm.
MINERALIZATION OF TUMOR.—A slight cloudy matrix mineralization is scattered throughout the tumor (**x**).
DESTRUCTION.—Geographic; regular contour; total penetration of orbital roof (**arrows**).
PROLIFERATION.—Slight marginal sclerosis.

DIFFERENTIAL DIAGNOSIS	PROBABILITY
Fibrosarcoma	.96
Chondrosarcoma	.03

COMMENT: It is interesting that there should be cloudy matrix mineralization in this fibrosarcoma. Fibromas in the skull are frequently of ground-glass density due to multiple tiny trabeculae within the neoplasm. The finding in this case may be a reflection of the same kind of density within a fibrous lesion of more aggressive potential.

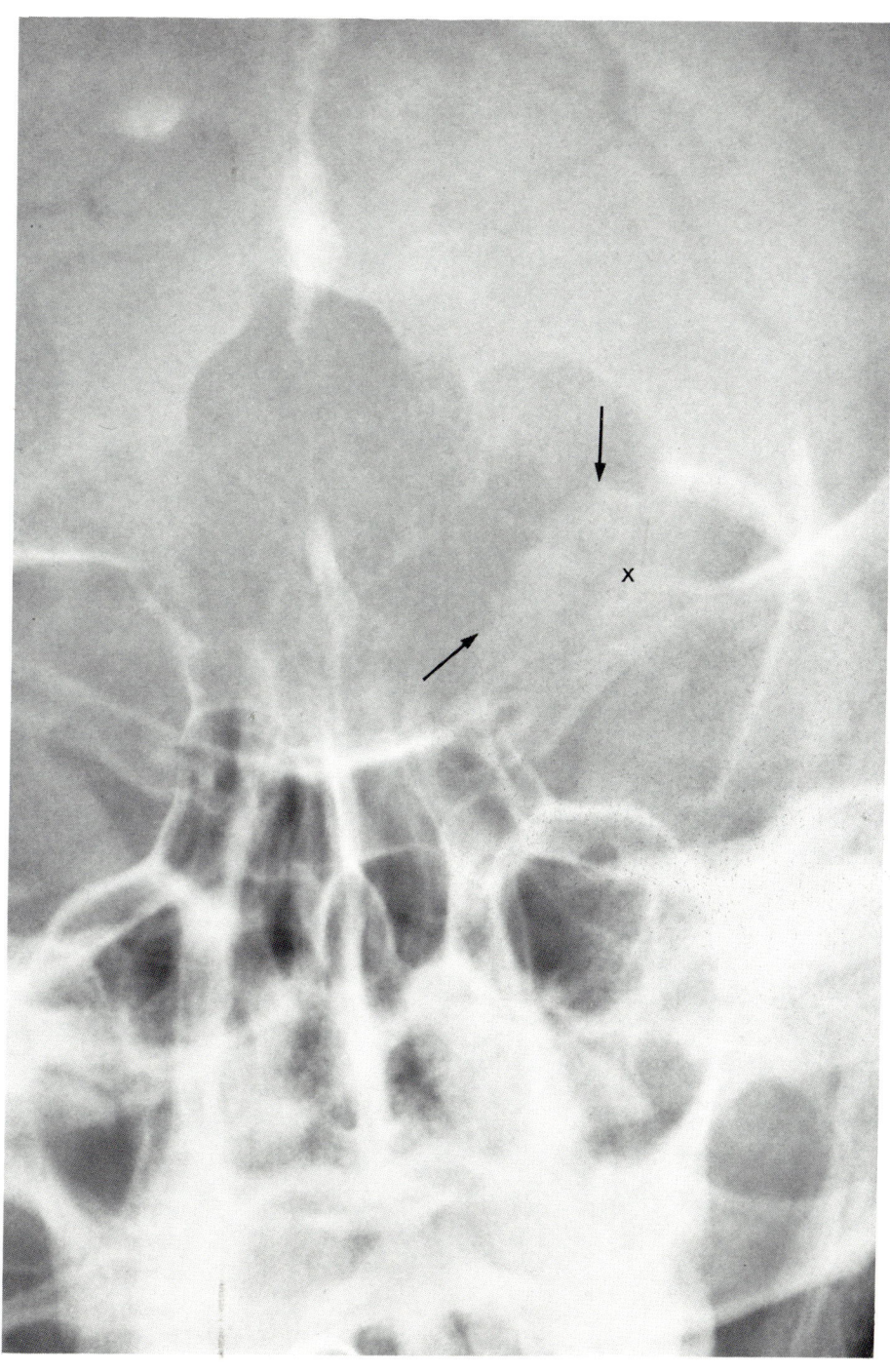

Figure 48 · Fibrosarcoma of Frontal Bone / 147

Figure 49.—Fibrosarcoma of the os calcis.

AFIP Case No. 1081826: **A,** lateral, and **B,** sagittal projections.

DIAGNOSIS AND GRADE.—Fibrosarcoma, os calcis; growth rate IA.
LIFE INFORMATION.—Male, 40 years; alive five years after onset.
LOCATION.—A circumscribed tumor involving most of the os calcis, without extraosseous extension.
SIZE.—7 × 3 × 4 cm.
MINERALIZATION OF TUMOR.—None.
DESTRUCTION.—Geographic; lobulated contour; extensive loss of cancellous bone.
PROLIFERATION.—Scant marginal sclerosis; slight septation; about 7 mm expansion of cortex laterally, with amorphous periosteal response (**B, arrow**).

DIFFERENTIAL DIAGNOSIS	PROBABILITY
Fibrosarcoma	.82
Cyst	.08
Giant cell tumor	.03
Chondrosarcoma	.03
Chondromyxoid fibroma	.02
Benign cartilaginous tumor	< .01

COMMENT: This slowly growing tumor was diagnosed variously by consulting pathologists as malignant spindle cell tumor, probably malignant (neuro-) fibroma, fibrosarcoma, and poorly differentiated chondroid tumor.

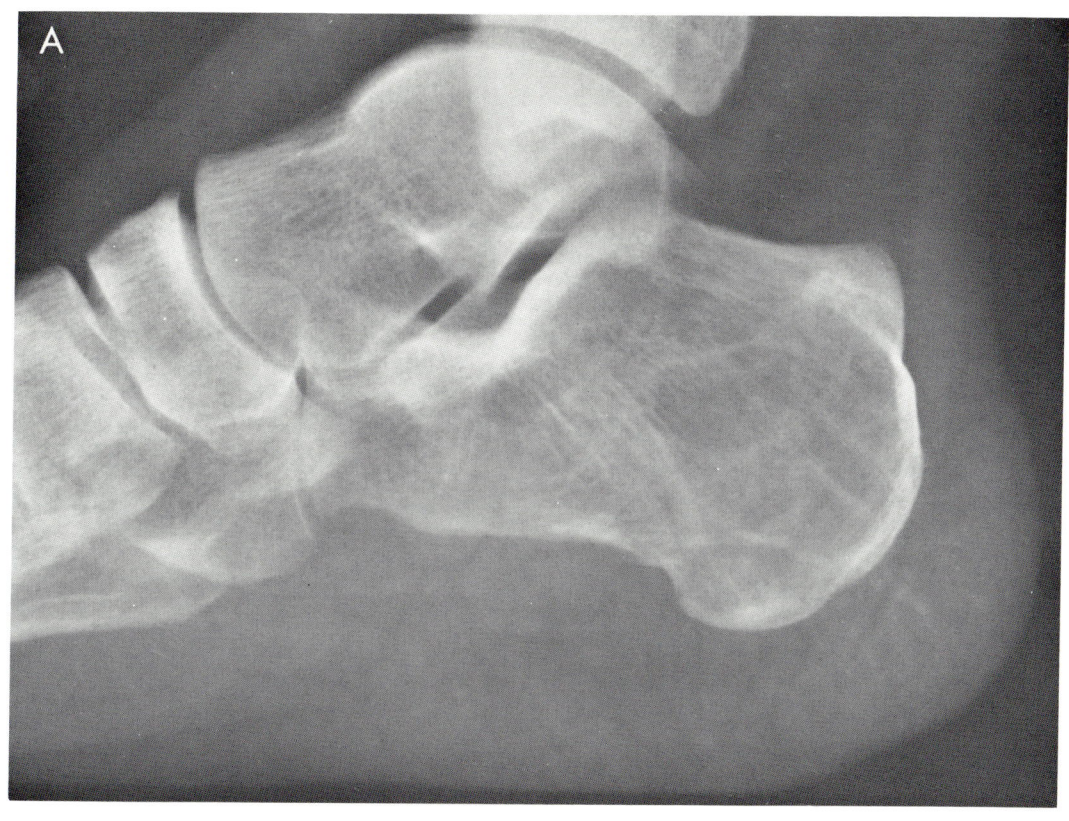
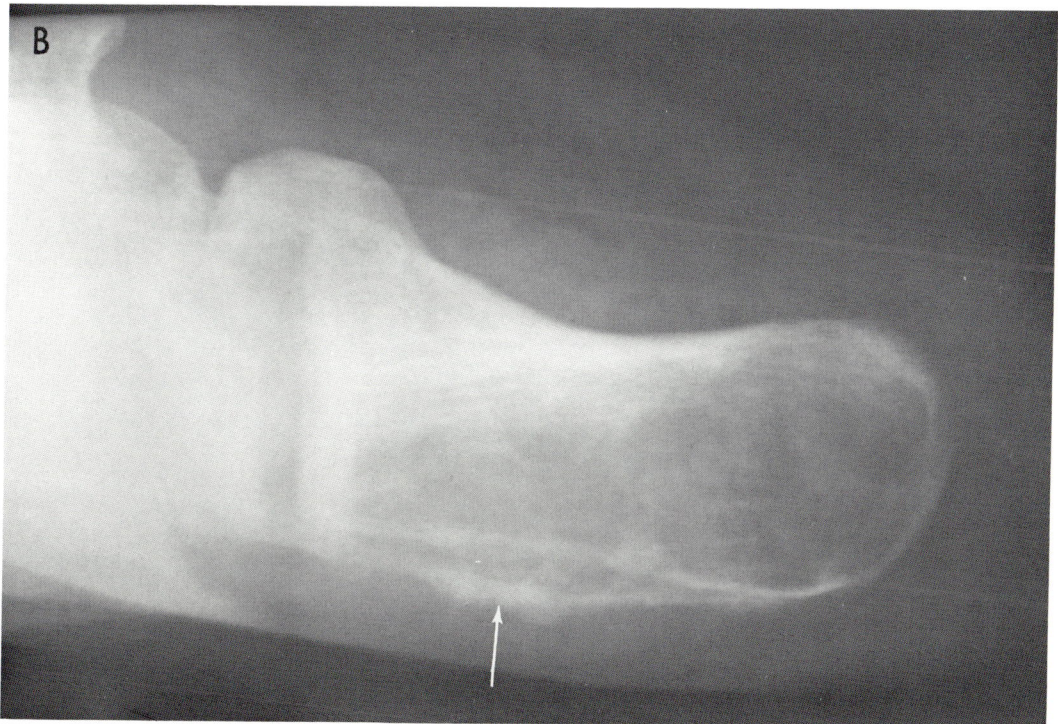

Figure 49 · Fibrosarcoma of Os Calcis / 149

Figure 50.—Fibrosarcomas of the fibula and scapula.

AFIP Case No. 1061467: **A,** lateral, and **B,** anteroposterior views.

DIAGNOSIS AND GRADE.—Fibrosarcoma, fibula; growth rate IC.
LIFE INFORMATION.—Male 69 years; survived 29 months.
LOCATION.—A tumor centrally located in the distal fibular metaphysis, extending up into the distal shaft; substantial extraosseous component.

SIZE.—11 × 5 × 4 cm.
MINERALIZATION OF TUMOR.—None.
DESTRUCTION.—Geographic; lobulated contour; total penetration of cortex.
PROLIFERATION.—Extensive septate, honeycomb pattern of proliferative response, with slight expansion of the cortex near upper edge of tumor.

DIFFERENTIAL DIAGNOSIS	PROBABILITY
Fibrosarcoma	.79
Chondrosarcoma	.19
Osteosarcoma	< .01
Reticulum cell sarcoma	< .01

COMMENT: The honeycomb pattern is seen most often in angiomas and angiomyomas. The computer provided a surprisingly good differential diagnosis. Angiomyomas are mentioned only in the rare categories. This tumor resembles the Ewing sarcoma in Figure 143.

AFIP Case No. 907257: **C,** anteroposterior view.

DIAGNOSIS AND GRADE.—Fibrosarcoma, scapula; growth rate IC.
LIFE INFORMATION.—Female, 11 years; last known to be well.
LOCATION.—An apparently circumscribed lesion involving the glenoid and neck of the scapula.

SIZE.—5 × 5 cm.
MINERALIZATION OF TUMOR.—None.
DESTRUCTION.—Principally geographic; with ragged contour.
PROLIFERATION.—Reactive sclerosis in the edge of the destroyed area, with rather nondescript spiculation (**arrow**) extending into the soft tissues, possibly an early effort at sunburst.

DIFFERENTIAL DIAGNOSIS	PROBABILITY
Fibrosarcoma	.74
Chondrosarcoma	.25
Ewing's sarcoma	< .01

COMMENT: Spiculation is rare in fibrosarcoma. The radiologic pattern better fits a fibroblastic type of osteosarcoma.

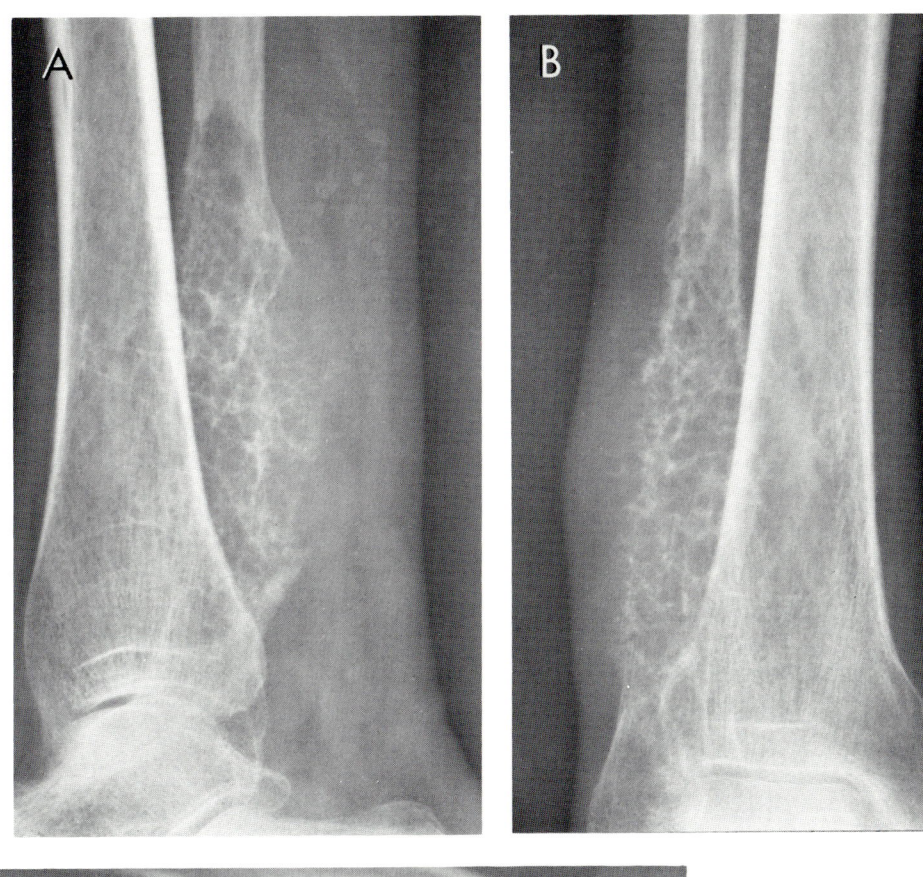
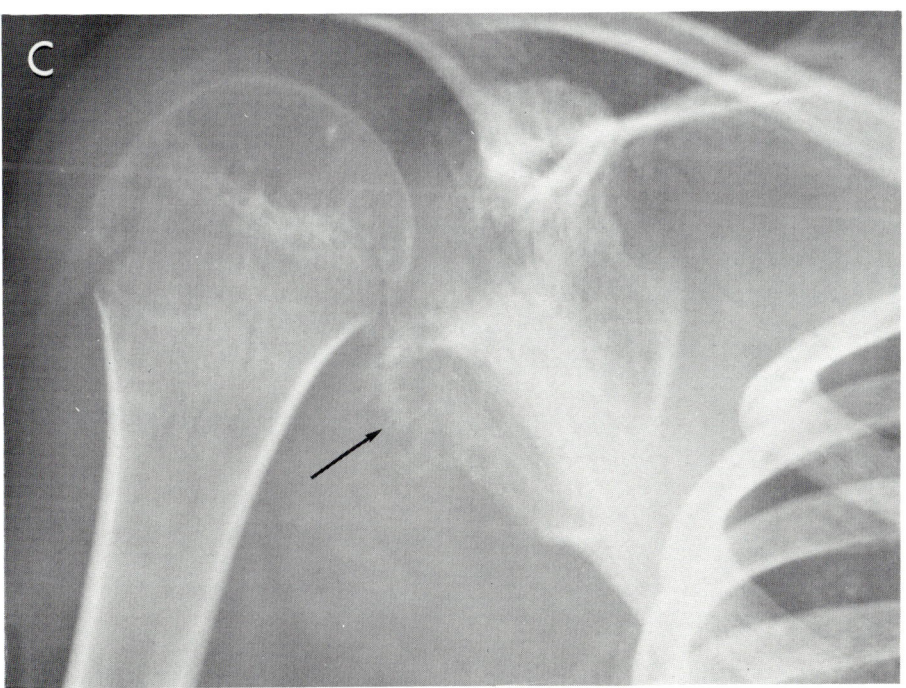

Figure 50 · Fibrosarcomas of Fibula and Scapula / 151

Figure 51.—Fibrosarcomas of the tibia.

AFIP Case No. 1035222: **A,** lateral projection.

DIAGNOSIS AND GRADE.—Fibrosarcoma, tibia; growth rate IC.

LIFE INFORMATION.—Male, 69 years; survived three years.

LOCATION.—A circumscribed lesion (**arrows**) located eccentrically in the central third of the proximal tibial metaphysis. The 90° projection (not shown) revealed a definite extraosseous component.

SIZE.—3 × 2.5 cm.

MINERALIZATION OF TUMOR.—None.

DESTRUCTION.—Geographic; lobulated contour.

PROLIFERATION.—Very slight marginal sclerosis.

DIFFERENTIAL DIAGNOSIS	PROBABILITY
Fibrosarcoma	.79
Chondrosarcoma	.10
Osteosarcoma	.09
Reticulum cell sarcoma	.01

COMMENT: A rather indolent appearing tumor which behaved otherwise.

AFIP Case No. 1128996: **B,** anteroposterior projection.

DIAGNOSIS AND GRADE.—Fibrosarcoma, tibia; growth rate III.

LIFE INFORMATION.—Male, 21 years; died three years after onset.

LOCATION.—A diffuse lesion centered eccentrically in the midproximal metaphysis, extending into the epiphysis, with moderate extraosseous component.

SIZE.—8 × 6 cm.

MINERALIZATION OF TUMOR.—None.

DESTRUCTION.—Permeated pattern.

PROLIFERATION.—Slight mottled increased density in intramedullary spongy bone (**arrows**).

DIFFERENTIAL DIAGNOSIS	PROBABILITY
Fibrosarcoma	.52
Ewing's sarcoma	.17
Osteosarcoma	.16
Reticulum cell sarcoma	.12
Chondrosarcoma	< .01

COMMENT: Fibrosarcoma typically induces little proliferative response. Note that the cortex gradually loses normal density (**a**) as the center of the tumor is approached—typical of permeated bone destruction.

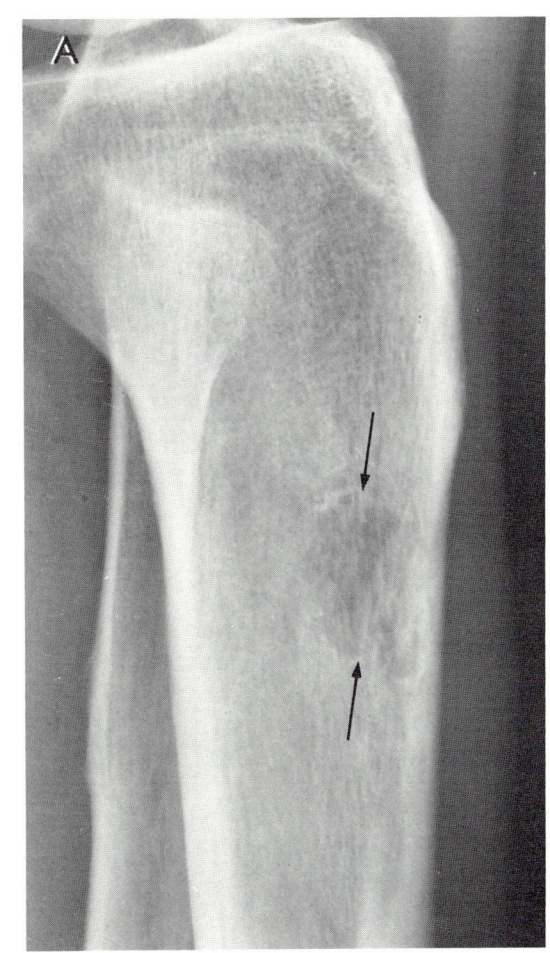
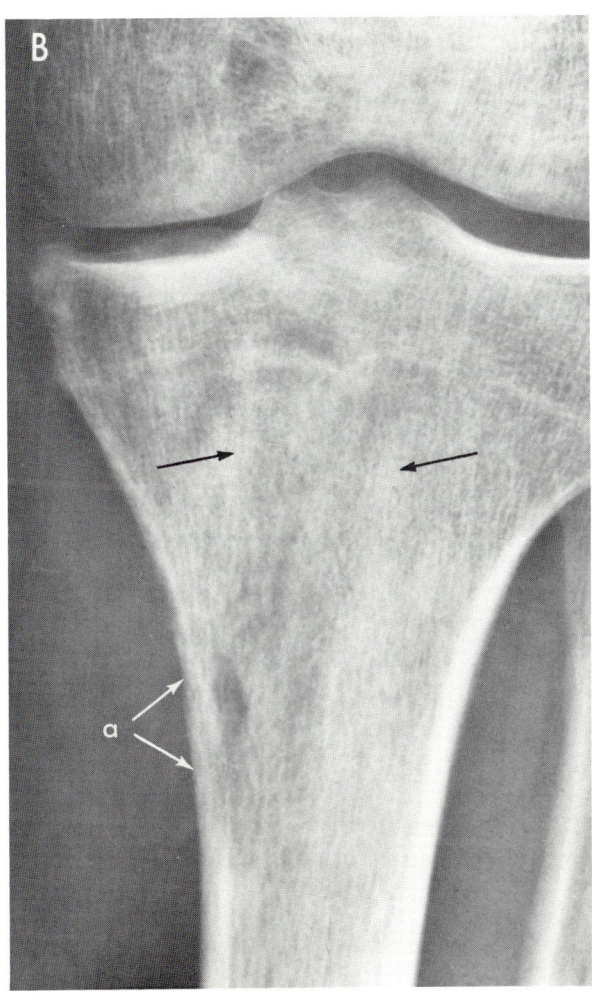

Figure 51 · Fibrosarcomas of Tibia

Figure 52.—Fibrosarcoma of the tibia.

AFIP Case No. 1106260: **A,** anteroposterior, and **B,** lateral views.

DIAGNOSIS AND GRADE.—Fibrosarcoma, tibia; growth rate IA.

LIFE INFORMATION.—Male, 41 years; dead 18 months after onset.

LOCATION.—A circumscribed lesion centered eccentrically in the proximal tibia, involving epiphysis and proximal third of metaphysis; no extraosseous extension.

SIZE.—5 × 4 × 3 cm.

MINERALIZATION OF TUMOR.—None.

DESTRUCTION.—Geographic pattern, lobulated contour.

PROLIFERATION.—Marginal sclerosis (**arrows**), slight septation.

DIFFERENTIAL DIAGNOSIS	PROBABILITY
Fibrosarcoma	.47
Villonodular synovitis	.35
Giant cell tumor	.09
Chondromyxoid fibroma	.06
Chondrosarcoma	< .01

COMMENT: This view, obtained after biopsy, shows no evidence that the cortex has been broached by the tumor. The patient probably had pulmonary metastases on initial examination.

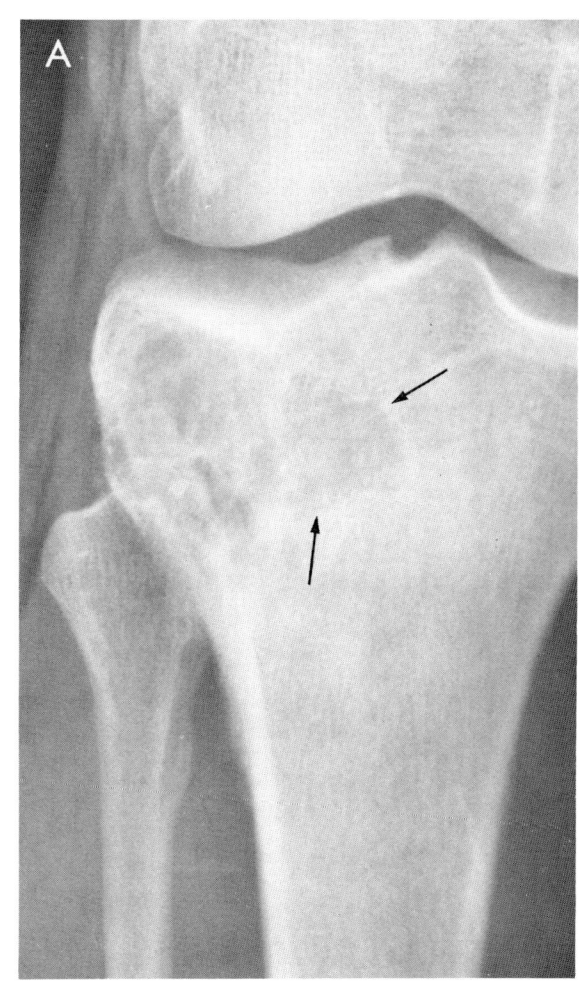
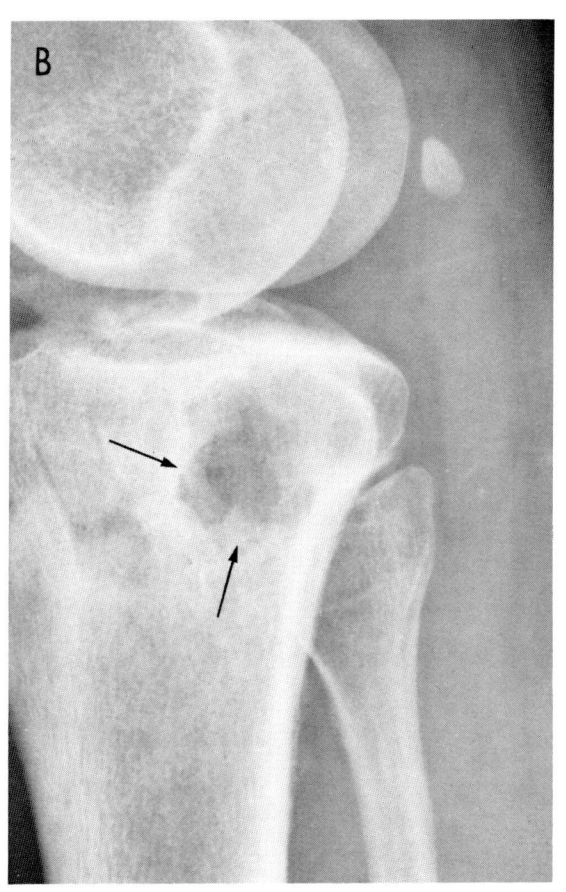

Figure 52 · Fibrosarcoma of Tibia / 155

Figure 53.—Fibrosarcoma of the femur.

AFIP Case No. 949448: **A,** anteroposterior, and **B,** lateral views, initial examination; **C** and **D,** 29 months later.

DIAGNOSIS AND GRADE.—Fibrosarcoma, femur; growth rate IC.

LIFE INFORMATION.—Male, 30 years; survived six years.

LOCATION.—Initially, a circumscribed lesion in the distal femoral metaphysis, extending slightly into the epiphysis; no invasion of soft tissues.

SIZE.—8 × 3 × 5 cm on initial examination.

MINERALIZATION OF TUMOR.—None.

DESTRUCTION.—Geographic; lobulated contour. Initially, partial penetration of cortex and evidence suggesting pathologic fracture, (**B, arrow**).

PROLIFERATION.—Initially, dense marginal sclerosis; slight expansion of cortex and septation.

Twenty-nine months later (**C** and **D**) the lesion, now 9 × 8 × 7 cm, involves practically the entire metaphysis and epiphysis including the subarticular cortex. There are large extraosseous extensions of tumor and total penetration of cortex. Marginal sclerosis and septation are more pronounced. The expanded shell no longer encapsulates the tumor.

	DIFFERENTIAL DIAGNOSIS	PROBABILITY
Exam. 1	Chondromyxoid fibroma	.35
	Fibrosarcoma	.28
	Giant cell tumor	.15
	Cyst	.14
	Villonodular synovitis	.04
	Chondrosarcoma	.01
Exam. 2	Giant cell tumor	.99
	Fibrosarcoma	< .01
	Chondromyxoid fibroma	< .01

COMMENT: An excellent example of a slowly growing fibrosarcoma. Preoperative diagnosis was giant cell tumor; postoperative and initial pathologic diagnoses were benign nonosteogenic fibroma. Fibrosarcoma was not diagnosed until the tumor recurred. Evidently the computer favors a lesion more benign than fibrosarcoma.

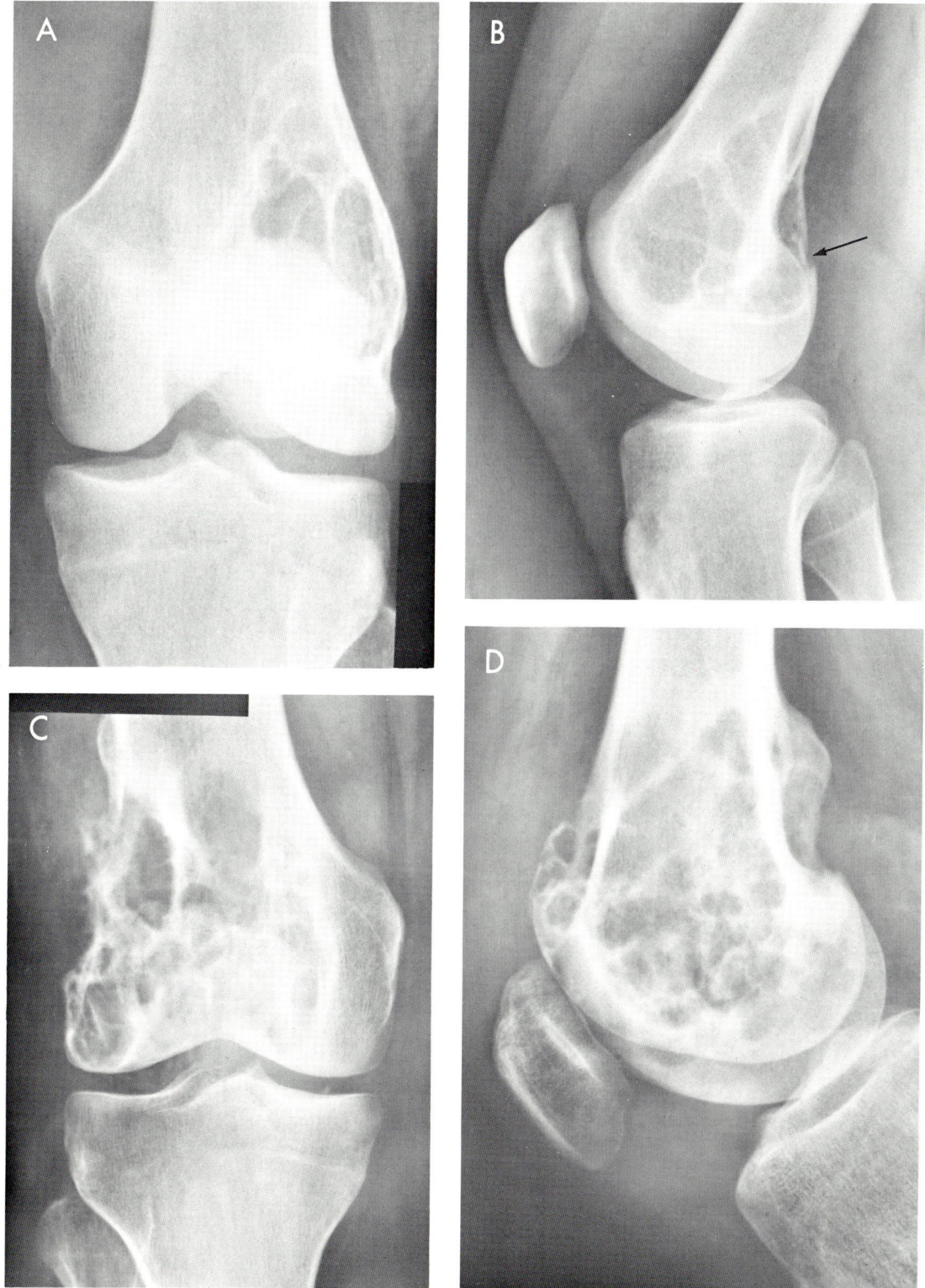

Figure 53 · Fibrosarcoma of Femur / 157

Figure 54.—Fibrosarcoma of the fibula.

AFIP Case No. 1096840: **A,** anteroposterior, and **B,** oblique views.

DIAGNOSIS AND GRADE.—Fibrosarcoma, fibula; growth rate III.

LIFE INFORMATION.—Male, 18 years; survived 10 months.

LOCATION.—A diffuse tumor involving the proximal metaphysis; large extraosseous component.

SIZE.—7 × 5 × 5 cm.

MINERALIZATION OF BONE.—None.

DESTRUCTION.—Permeative; total penetration of the cortex; pathologic fracture (**a**).

PROLIFERATION.—Irregular, amorphous subperiosteal response (**b**).

DIFFERENTIAL DIAGNOSIS	PROBABILITY
Osteosarcoma	.52
Fibrosarcoma	.24
Reticulum cell sarcoma	.14
Ewing's sarcoma	.08
Chondrosarcoma	< .01

COMMENT: A highly malignant-appearing tumor, which behaves accordingly. A quite satisfactory computer differential diagnosis.

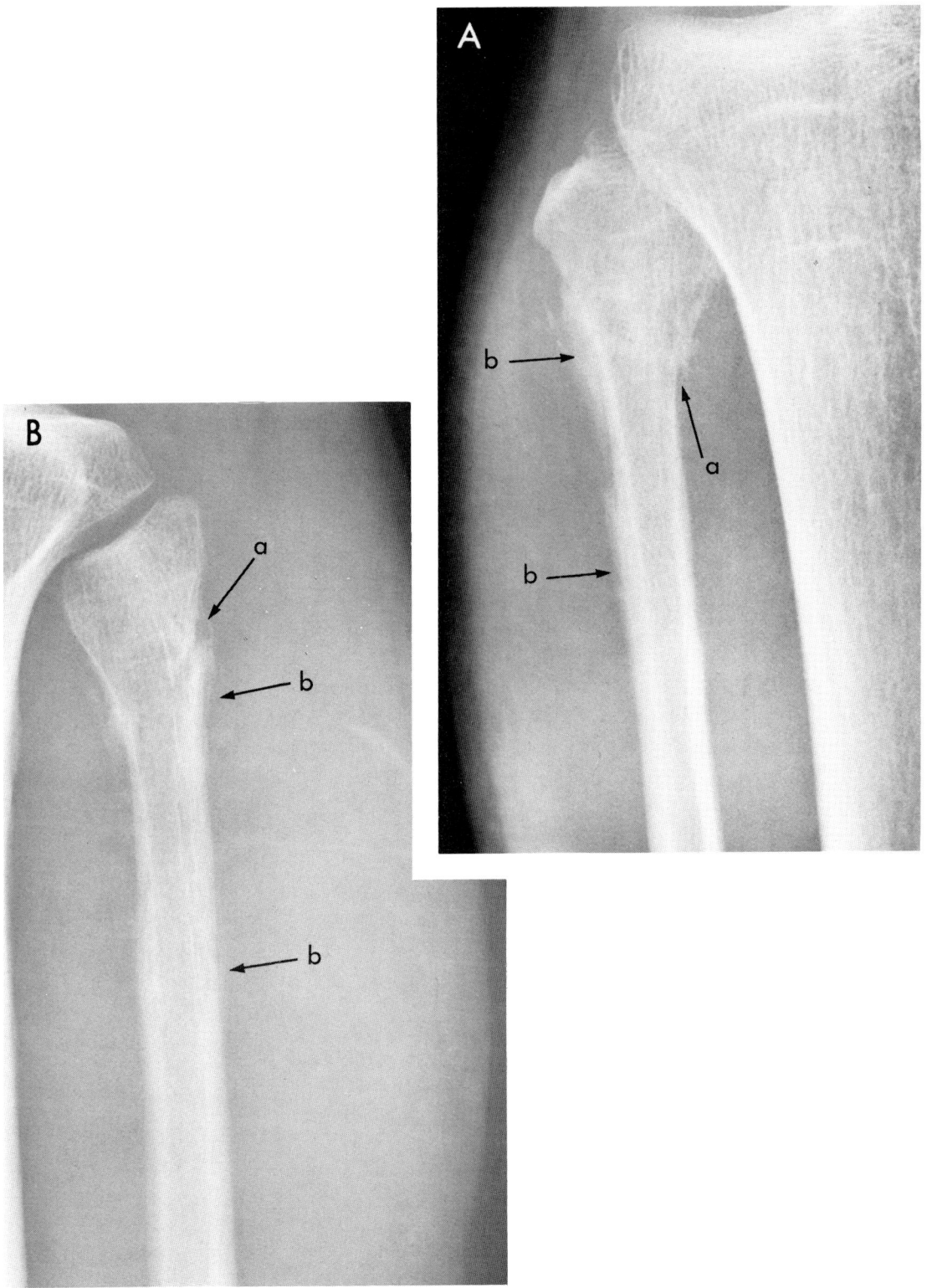

Figure 54 · Fibrosarcoma of Fibula

Figure 55.—Fibrosarcoma of the pubis.

AFIP Case No. 1081268: Anteroposterior projection.

DIAGNOSIS AND GRADE.—Fibrosarcoma, pubis; growth rate IC.

LIFE INFORMATION.—Male, 53 years; survival unknown.

LOCATION.—A seemingly circumscribed lesion of the pubis, with huge extraosseous extension in the pelvis.

SIZE.—15 × 7 cm.

MINERALIZATION OF TUMOR.—Many clouds in the extraosseous component (**x**); crescentic patterns of tumor matrix mineralization at the edge of the tumor.

DESTRUCTION.—Geographic (**y**); regular contour; pathologic fracture (**b**).

PROLIFERATION.—Sclerosis at the lower margin of the tumor (**a**), with some amorphous periosteal response.

DIFFERENTIAL DIAGNOSIS	PROBABILITY
Chondrosarcoma	.85
Fibrosarcoma	.14

COMMENT: Clouds and crescentic marginal patterns of tumor bone may be found in tumors having a predominantly fibrosarcomatous stroma. Some pathologists believe this is evidence for osteosarcoma, but there is evidence that such a tumor with matrix mineralization behaves like a fibrosarcoma, not an osteosarcoma. The patient's age, large tumor size and matrix mineralization motivate the computer strongly in the direction of chondrosarcoma.

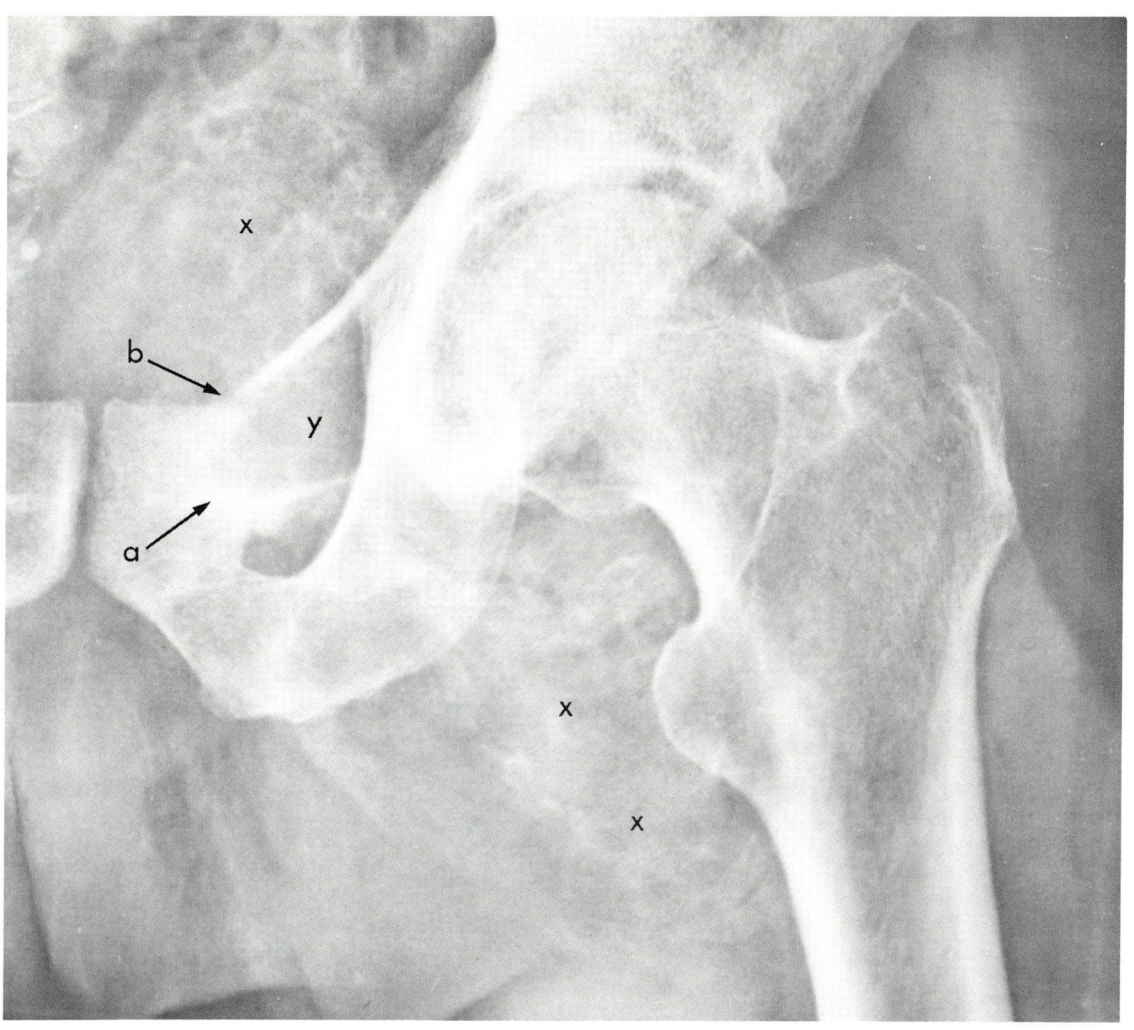

Figure 55 · Fibrosarcoma of Pubis / 161

Figure 56.—Fibrosarcoma arising in an old enchondroma in the tibia.

AFIP Case No. 1063737: **A,** anteroposterior, and **B,** lateral views.

DIAGNOSIS AND GRADE.—Fibrosarcoma arising in an old calcified enchondroma, tibia; growth rate IB.

LIFE INFORMATION.—Female, 65 years; first symptom, pathologic fracture; survived three years following diagnosis.

LOCATION.—A circumscribed lesion in the proximal half of the tibia.

SIZE.—6 × 3 × 2 cm.

MINERALIZATION OF TUMOR.—There is a dense clump of flocculent calcification in the center of the lesion.

DESTRUCTION.—Geographic; ragged contour; pathologic fracture.

PROLIFERATION.—None.

DIFFERENTIAL DIAGNOSIS	PROBABILITY
Chondrosarcoma	.84
Fibrosarcoma	.08
Benign cartilaginous tumor	.06

COMMENT: In view of the central flocculent calcification, chondrosarcoma might seem the best diagnosis. However, it is not unusual to find fibrosarcomatous and chondrosarcomatous elements in the same tumor. Treatment and prognosis are essentially the same with either cell type.

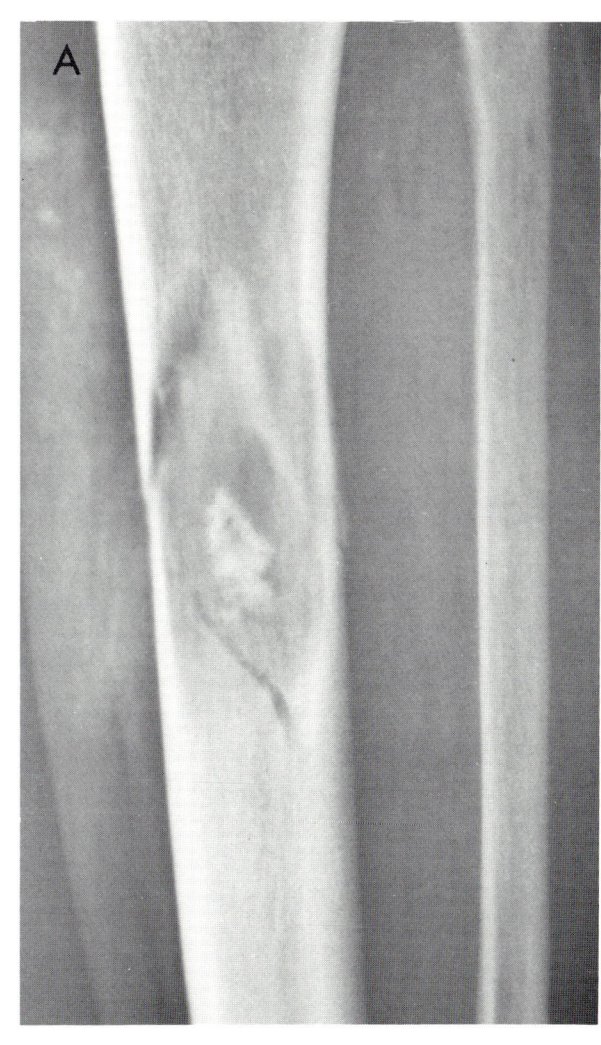
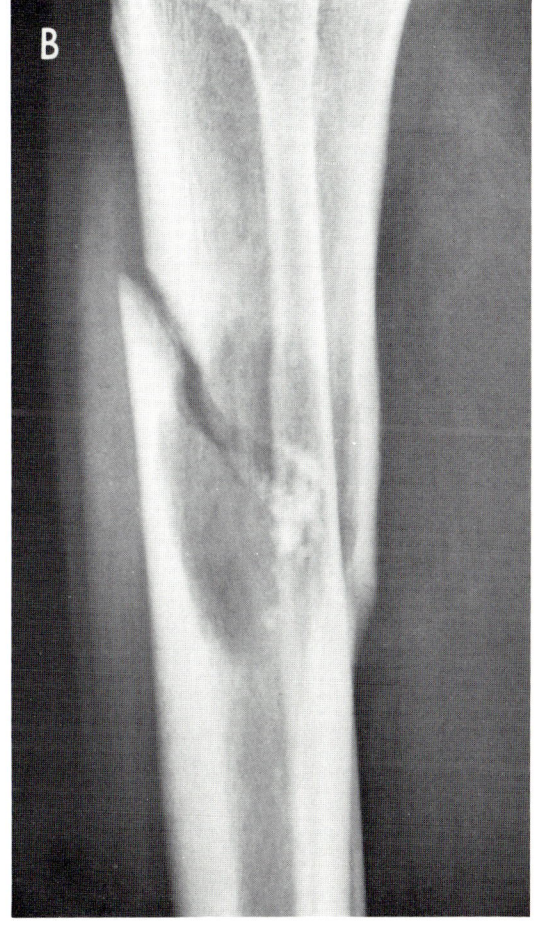

Figure 56 · Fibrosarcoma in Enchondroma of Tibia / 163

Figure 57.—Fibrosarcoma of the femur.

AFIP Case No. 1065289: **A,** anteroposterior, and **B,** lateral views.

DIAGNOSIS AND GRADE.—Fibrosarcoma, femur; growth rate III.

LIFE INFORMATION.—Female, 77 years; died of other causes 3½ years after onset.

LOCATION.—An extensive tumor centered at the junction of the distal shaft in the metaphysis of the femur, extending throughout the metaphysis and epiphysis and up into the shaft; scant extraosseous component.

SIZE.—$16 \times 6 \times 5$ cm.

MINERALIZATION OF TUMOR.—None.

DESTRUCTION.—Permeative pattern; pathologic fracture; extensive loss of cancellous bone.

PROLIFERATION.—Amorphous periosteal response; callus at fracture site.

DIFFERENTIAL DIAGNOSIS	PROBABILITY
Reticulum cell	.98
Fibrosarcoma	.01

COMMENT: The irregular, amorphous periosteal response (**A, arrows**) is frequently seen with both fibrosarcoma and reticulum cell sarcoma and in any kind of tumor following radiation therapy.

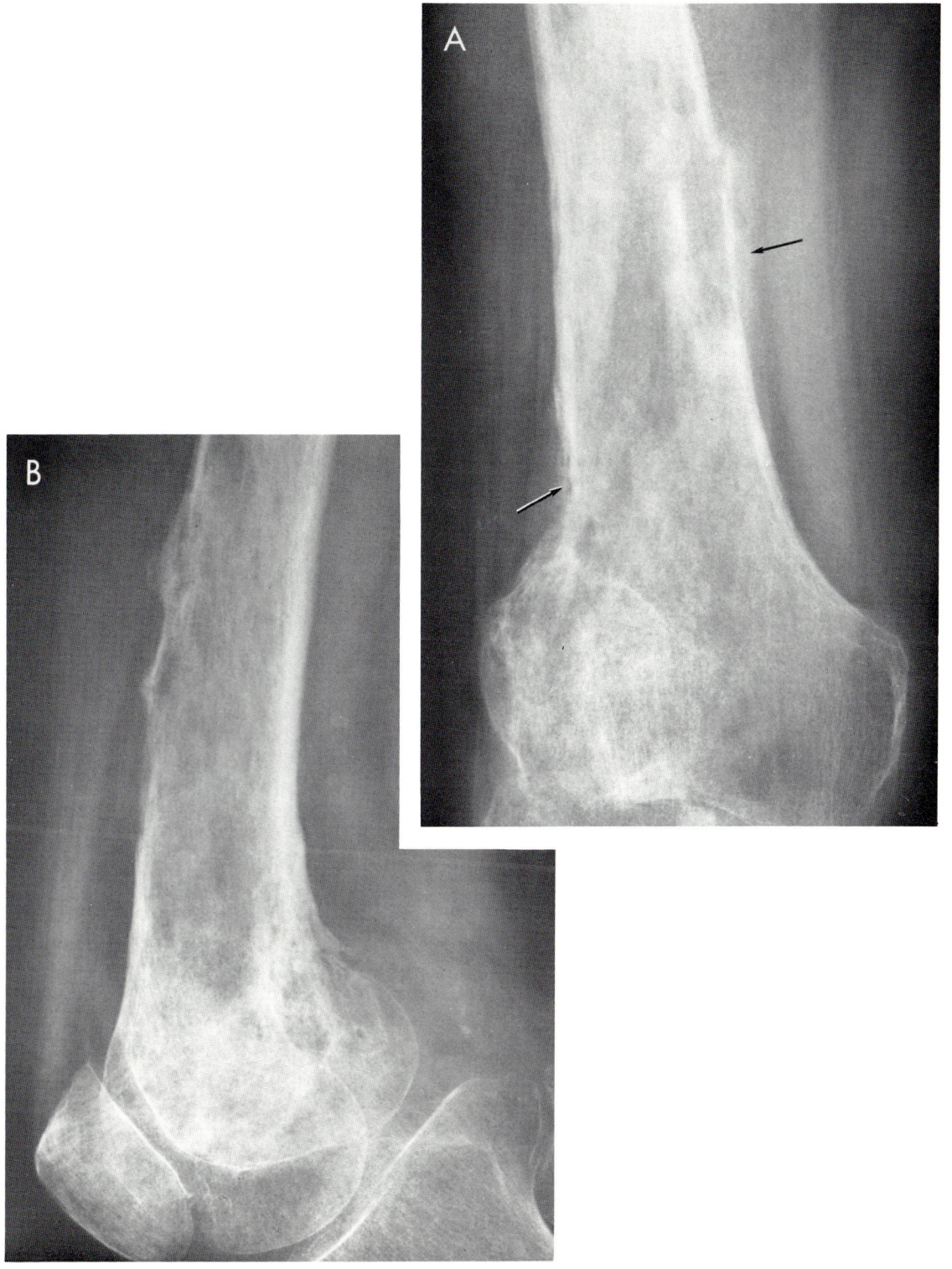

Figure 57 · Fibrosarcoma of Femur / 165

Figure 58.—Fibrosarcomas of the tibia and fibula.

AFIP Case No. 1028513: **A,** anteroposterior, and **B,** lateral views.

DIAGNOSIS AND GRADE.—Fibrosarcoma, tibia; growth rate IC.
LIFE INFORMATION.—Male, 18 years; survival unknown.
LOCATION.—A circumscribed lesion centered in the anterior cortex of the tibial shaft; large extraosseous component (**B, x**).
SIZE.—3 × 2 × 2 cm.
MINERALIZATION OF TUMOR.—None.
DESTRUCTION.—Geographic; saucerized erosion (**B, b**); lobulated contour; incomplete penetration of cortex, the inner surface of which is intact.
PROLIFERATION.—Distinct marginal sclerosis, slight expansion (**A, a**); slight septation.

DIFFERENTIAL DIAGNOSIS	PROBABILITY
Benign cartilaginous tumor	.99
Fibrosarcoma	< .01
Chondrosarcoma	< .01

COMMENT: Another of the slowly growing fibrosarcomas.

AFIP Case No. 1165869: **C,** anteroposterior, and **D,** lateral views.

DIAGNOSIS AND GRADE.—Fibrosarcoma, fibula; growth rate III.
LIFE INFORMATION.—Male, 18 years; survived 14 months.
LOCATION.—A diffuse tumor involving the proximal metaphysis and shaft. The growth plate seems to have been penetrated at one margin (**C, a**). Note small extraosseous extension (**C, arrows**).
SIZE.—6 × 5 × 5 cm.
MINERALIZATION OF TUMOR.—None.
DESTRUCTION.—Permeative pattern (**x**).
PROLIFERATION.—Two very delicate Codman triangles (**b**).

DIFFERENTIAL DIAGNOSIS	PROBABILITY
Ewing's sarcoma	.79
Osteosarcoma	.20
Reticulum cell sarcoma	< .01
Fibrosarcoma	< .01

COMMENT: A rapidly growing highly malignant tumor. The density and structure of cancellous bone are practically unchanged. The probability for fibrosarcoma in this case is low, and the Codman triangles make it even less likely.

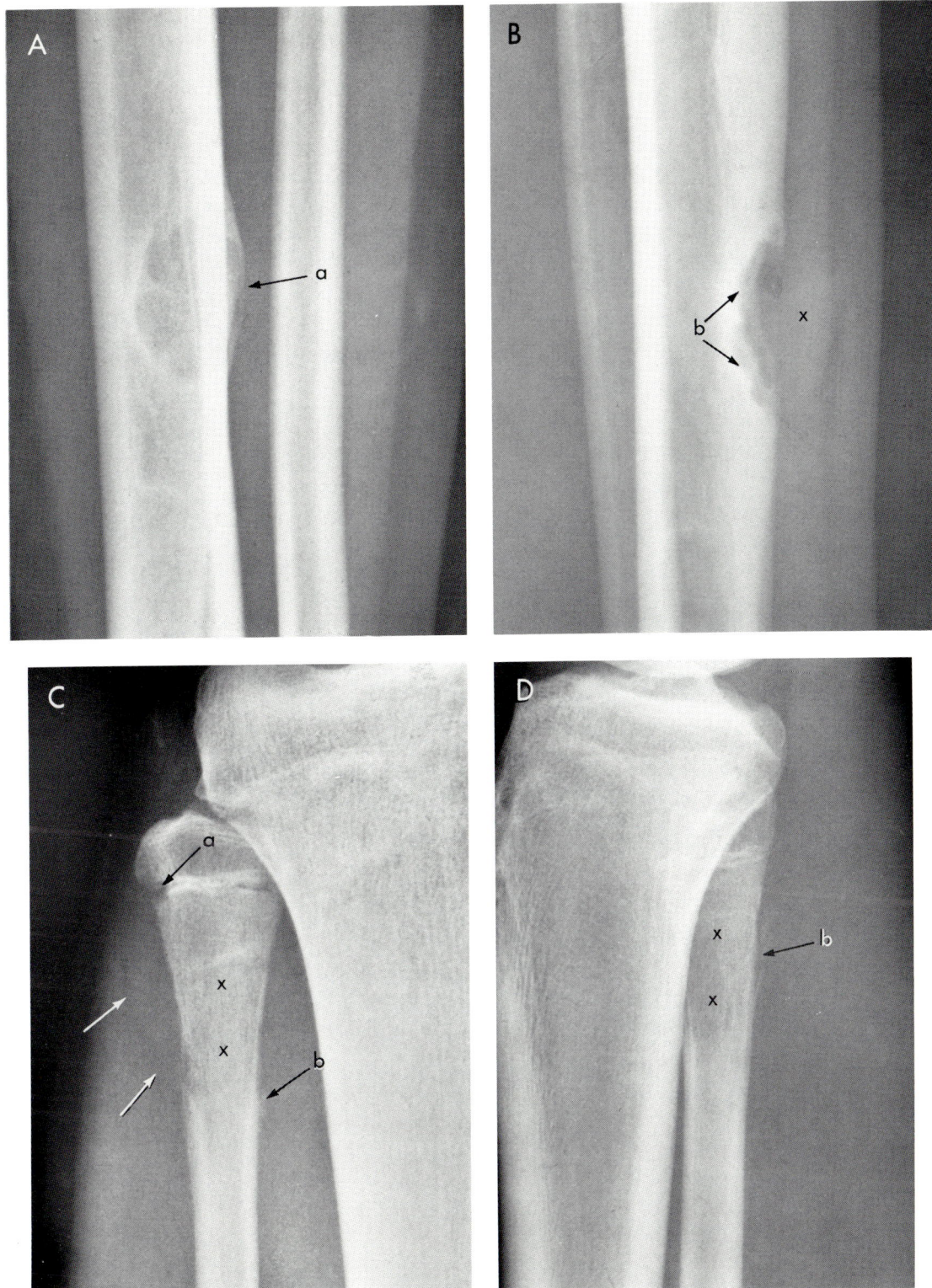

Figure 58 · Fibrosarcomas of Tibia & Fibula / 167

Figure 59.—Chondromyxoid fibromas of the radius and femur.

AFIP Case No. 1002914: **A,** posteroanterior projection.

>   DIAGNOSIS AND GRADE.—Chondromyxoid fibroma, distal radius; growth rate IC.
>   LIFE INFORMATION.—Male, 4 years; last known to be well.
>   LOCATION.—A sharply circumscribed eccentrically centered lesion of the distal metaphysis.
>   SIZE.—3 × 1.5 × 1 cm.
>   MINERALIZATION OF TUMOR.—None.
>   DESTRUCTION.—Geographic; reticulate contour.
>   PROLIFERATION.—Dense sclerotic rim; buttress (**arrow**).
>
> | DIFFERENTIAL DIAGNOSIS | PROBABILITY |
> |---|---|
> | Chondromyxoid fibroma | .99 |
> | Giant cell tumor | < .01 |
>
>   COMMENT: There is slightly more dense marginal proliferation and buttress formation than usual in giant cell tumor or simple cyst.

AFIP Case No. 1009537: **B,** lateral projection.

>   DIAGNOSIS AND GRADE.—Chondromyxoid fibroma, femur; growth rate IA.
>   LIFE INFORMATION.—Female, 10 years; well 10 years later.
>   LOCATION.—A large sharply circumscribed lesion involving the intertrochanteric region and proximal shaft.
>   SIZE.—6 × 4 cm.
>   MINERALIZATION OF TUMOR.—None.
>   DESTRUCTION.—Geographic; lobulated contour; incomplete penetration of cortex in this projection.
>   PROLIFERATION.—Heavy, coarse marginal sclerosis; septation; slightly expanded cortex with amorphous periosteal response (**arrows**).
>
> | DIFFERENTIAL DIAGNOSIS | PROBABILITY |
> |---|---|
> | Chondromyxoid fibroma | .87 |
> | Chondrosarcoma | .06 |
> | Benign cartilaginous tumor | .05 |
> | Fibrosarcoma | .01 |
>
>   COMMENT: Again, the heavy proliferative response that characterizes many of these lesions.

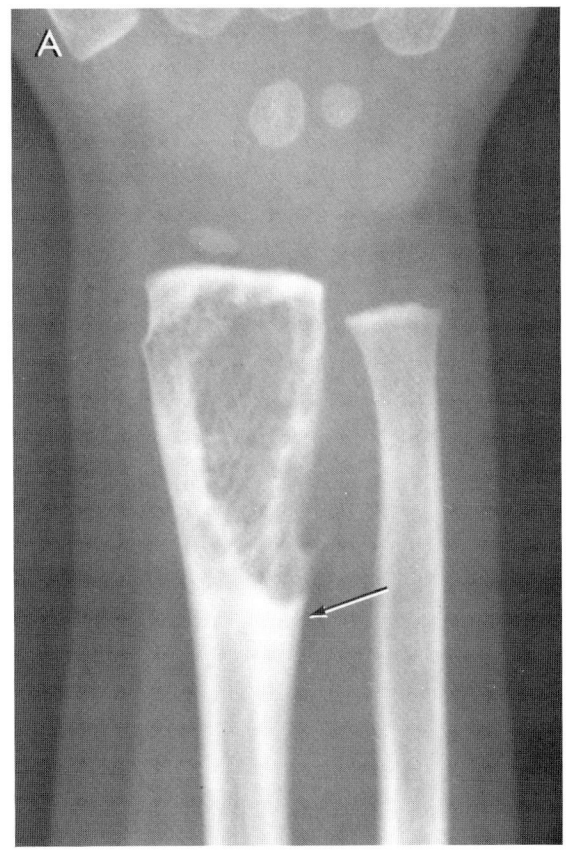
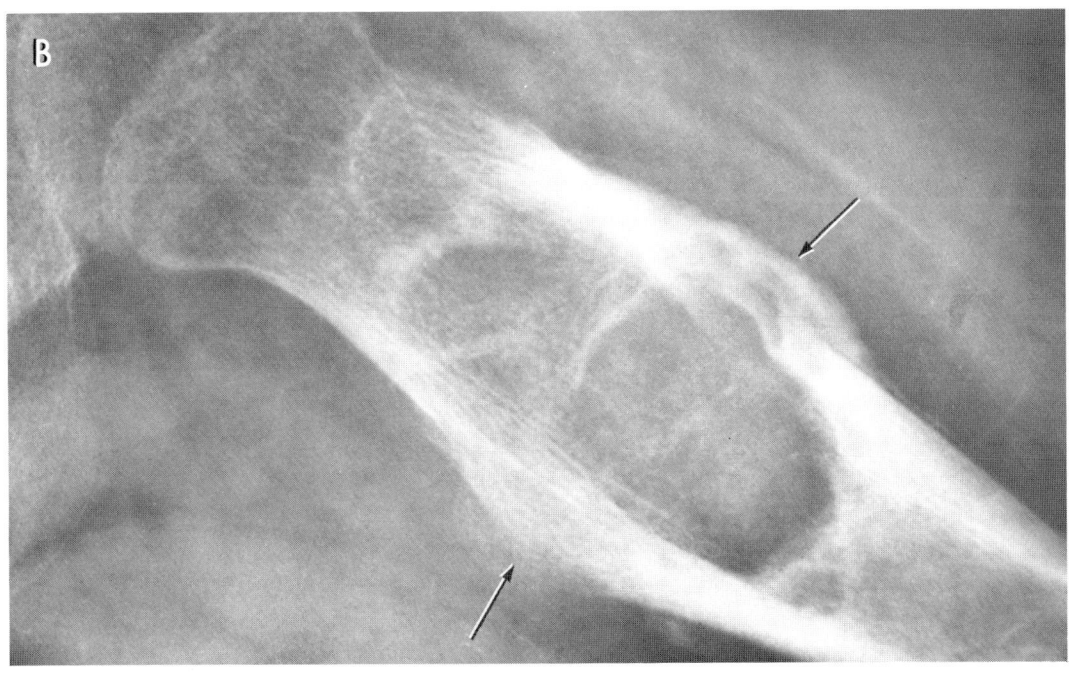

Figure 59 · Chondromyxoid Fibromas / 169

Figure 60.—Chondromyxoid fibroma of the pelvis.

AFIP Case No. 933894: Anteroposterior projection.

DIAGNOSIS AND GRADE.—Chondromyxoid fibroma, pelvis; growth rate IA.
LIFE INFORMATION.—Male, 18 years; well eight years after onset.
LOCATION.—A large, circumscribed lesion in the center of the ilium.

SIZE.—10 × 7 cm.
MINERALIZATION OF TUMOR.—None.
DESTRUCTION.—Geographic; regular contour.
PROLIFERATION.—Faintly sclerotic rim (**a**); delicate septate pattern (**b**).

DIFFERENTIAL DIAGNOSIS	PROBABILITY
Chondromyxoid fibroma	.61
Chondrosarcoma	.34
Fibrosarcoma	.03
Ewing's sarcoma	< .01

COMMENT: This closely resembles the bone cyst in Figure 38.

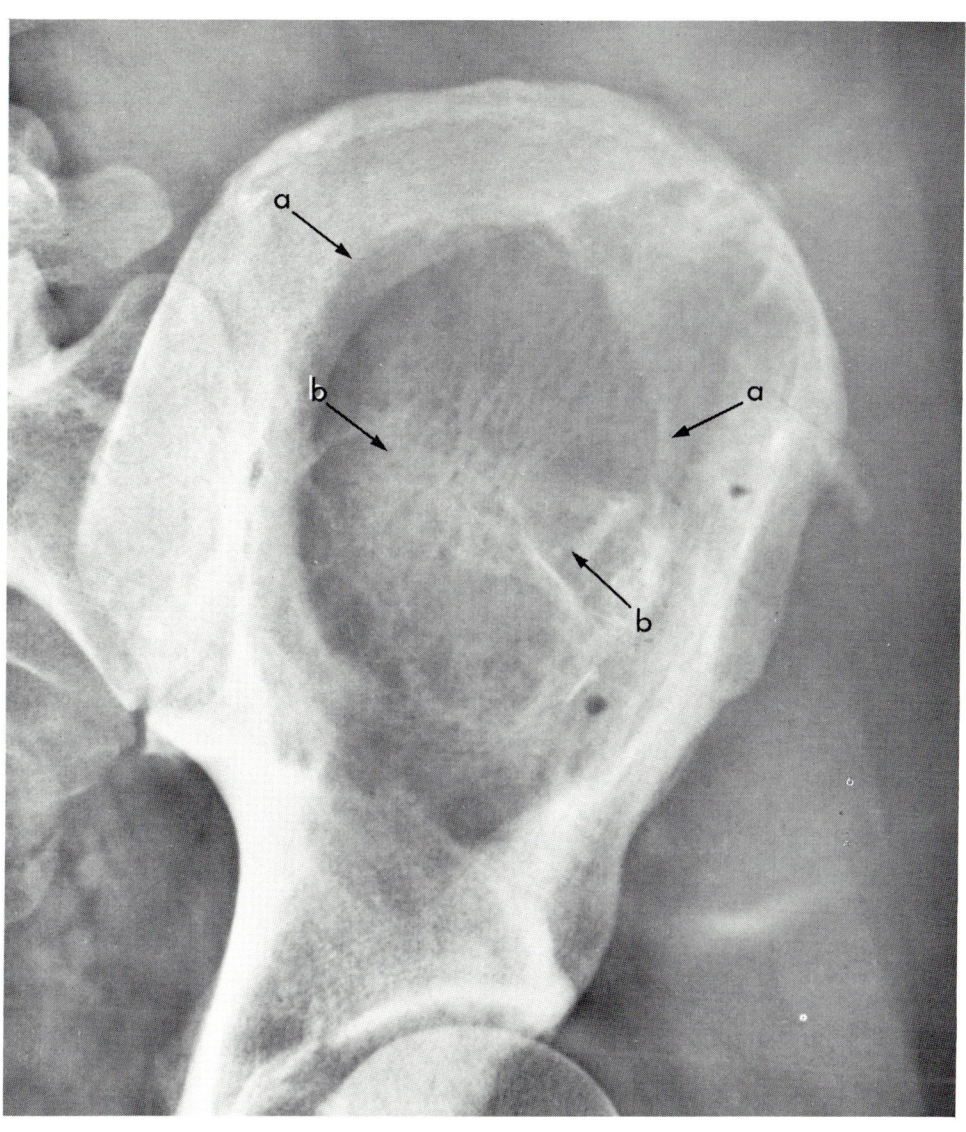

Figure 60 · Chondromyxoid Fibroma of Pelvis / 171

Figure 61.—Chondromyxoid fibroma of the fibula.

AFIP Case No. 932830: Anteroposterior projection.

DIAGNOSIS AND GRADE.—Chondromyxoid fibroma, fibula; growth rate IC.
LIFE INFORMATION.—Male, 15 years; survival unknown.
LOCATION.—A sharply circumscribed lesion at the junction of the proximal metaphysis and shaft.
SIZE.—6 × 4 cm.
MINERALIZATION OF TUMOR.—None.
DESTRUCTION.—Geographic; lobulated contour; total penetration of cortex (**arrow**).
PROLIFERATION.—Heavy sclerotic rim; multiple buttresses; expanded cortex laterally which does not totally encapsulate the tumor; moderate septation.

DIFFERENTIAL DIAGNOSIS	PROBABILITY
Chondromyxoid fibroma	.60
Fibroxanthoma	.31
Cyst	.07
Fibrosarcoma	< .01

COMMENT: This tumor has the same coarse, heavy proliferative change as seen in Figure 65.

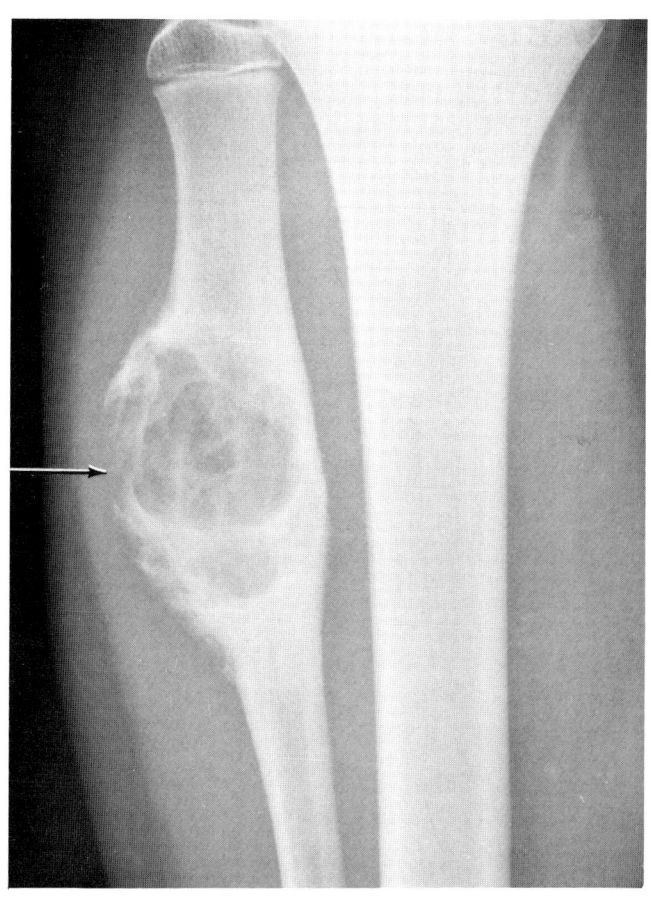

Figure 61 · Chondromyxoid Fibroma of Fibula / 173

Figure 62.—Chondromyxoid fibroma of the ulna.

AFIP Case No. 1189541: Lateral projection.

Diagnosis and Grade.—Chondromyxoid fibroma, ulna; growth rate IB.
Life Information.—Male, 23 years; survival unknown.
Location.—A sharply circumscribed lesion centered at the junction of the proximal metaphysis and shaft.
Size.—3.5 × 2.5 cm.
Mineralization of Tumor.—None.
Destruction.—Geographic; regular contour; pathologic fracture (**arrow**).
Proliferation.—Very slight expansion of cortex.

Differential Diagnosis	Probability
Chondromyxoid fibroma	.52
Fibroxanthoma	.31
Cyst	.13
Osteoblastoma	.02
Giant cell tumor	< .01
Fibrosarcoma	< .01
Benign cartilaginous tumor	< .01
Chondrosarcoma	< .01

COMMENT: This sharply delineated lesion with pathologic fracture is graded IB because no sclerotic rim has developed.

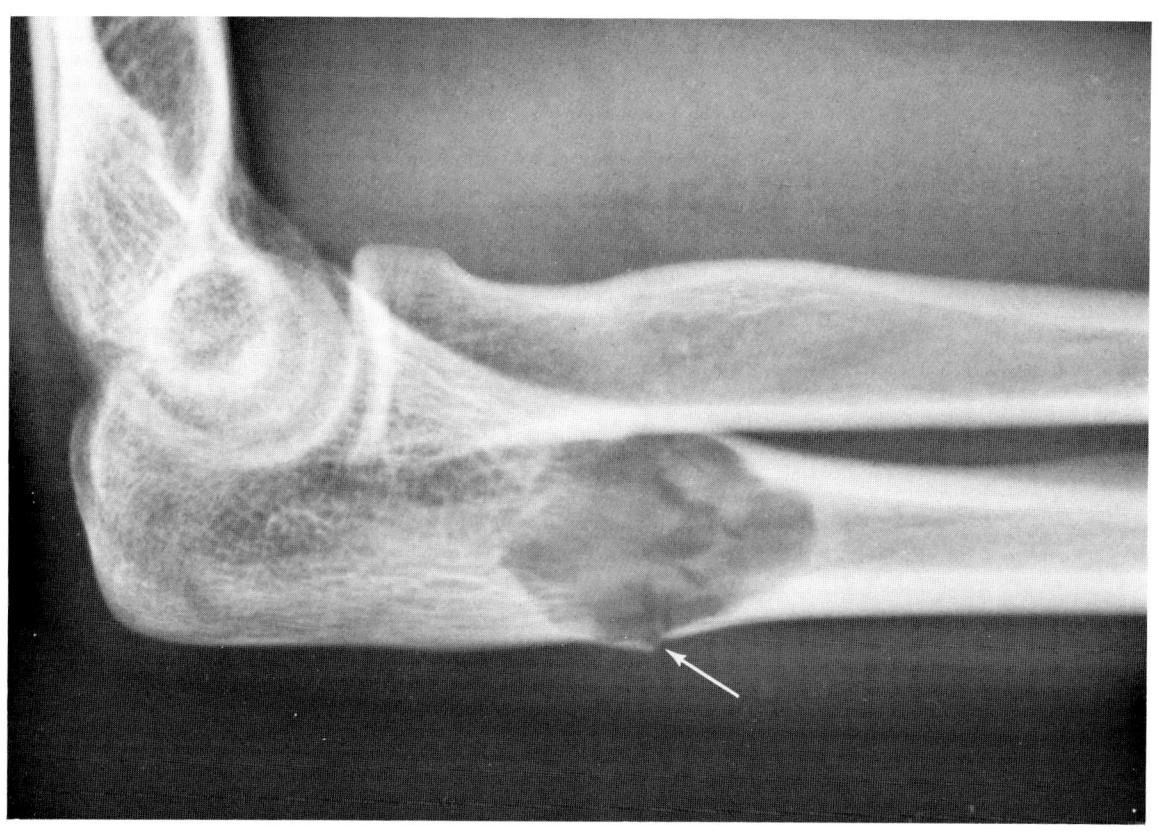

Figure 62 · Chondromyxoid Fibroma of Ulna / 175

Figure 63.—Chondromyxoid fibromas of the pelvis and tibia.

AFIP Case No. 1080586: **A,** anteroposterior projection.

DIAGNOSIS AND GRADE.—Chondromyxoid fibroma, pelvis; growth rate IA.
LIFE INFORMATION.—Female, 33 years; well seven years later.
LOCATION.—A sharply circumscribed lesion in the medial half of the ilium.

SIZE.—8 × 5 cm.
MINERALIZATION.—None.
DESTRUCTION.—Geographic; lobulated (hint of moth-eaten) contour.
PROLIFERATION.—Dense sclerotic new bone around the lesion medially (**arrow**); delicate sclerotic rim laterally; faint septation.

DIFFERENTIAL DIAGNOSIS	PROBABILITY
Chondromyxoid fibroma	.53
Chondrosarcoma	.42
Benign cartilaginous tumor	.06
Fibrosarcoma	< .01

COMMENT: A nondescript quiescent lesion.

AFIP Case No. 1004844: **B,** anteroposterior, and **C,** lateral views.

DIAGNOSIS AND GRADE.—Chondromyxoid fibroma, tibia; growth rate IA.
LIFE INFORMATION.—Female, 48 years; well five years later.
LOCATION.—A sharply circumscribed lesion centered in the proximal metaphysis, extending slightly into the epiphysis but not involving the subchondral cortex.

SIZE.—7 × 6 × 5 cm.
MINERALIZATION OF TUMOR.—None.
DESTRUCTION.—Geographic; moth-eaten contour; incomplete penetration of cortex. (See comment.)
PROLIFERATION.—Moderately heavy; slight cortical expansion laterally (**B, a**); heavy septation (**B, b**).

DIFFERENTIAL DIAGNOSIS	PROBABILITY
Chondromyxoid fibroma	.38
Giant cell tumor	.35
Fibrosarcoma	.20
Chondrosarcoma	.04
Benign cartilaginous tumor	< .01

COMMENT: A coarse, heavy proliferative response. The finely serrated lobular contour is seen principally in cartilaginous tumors.

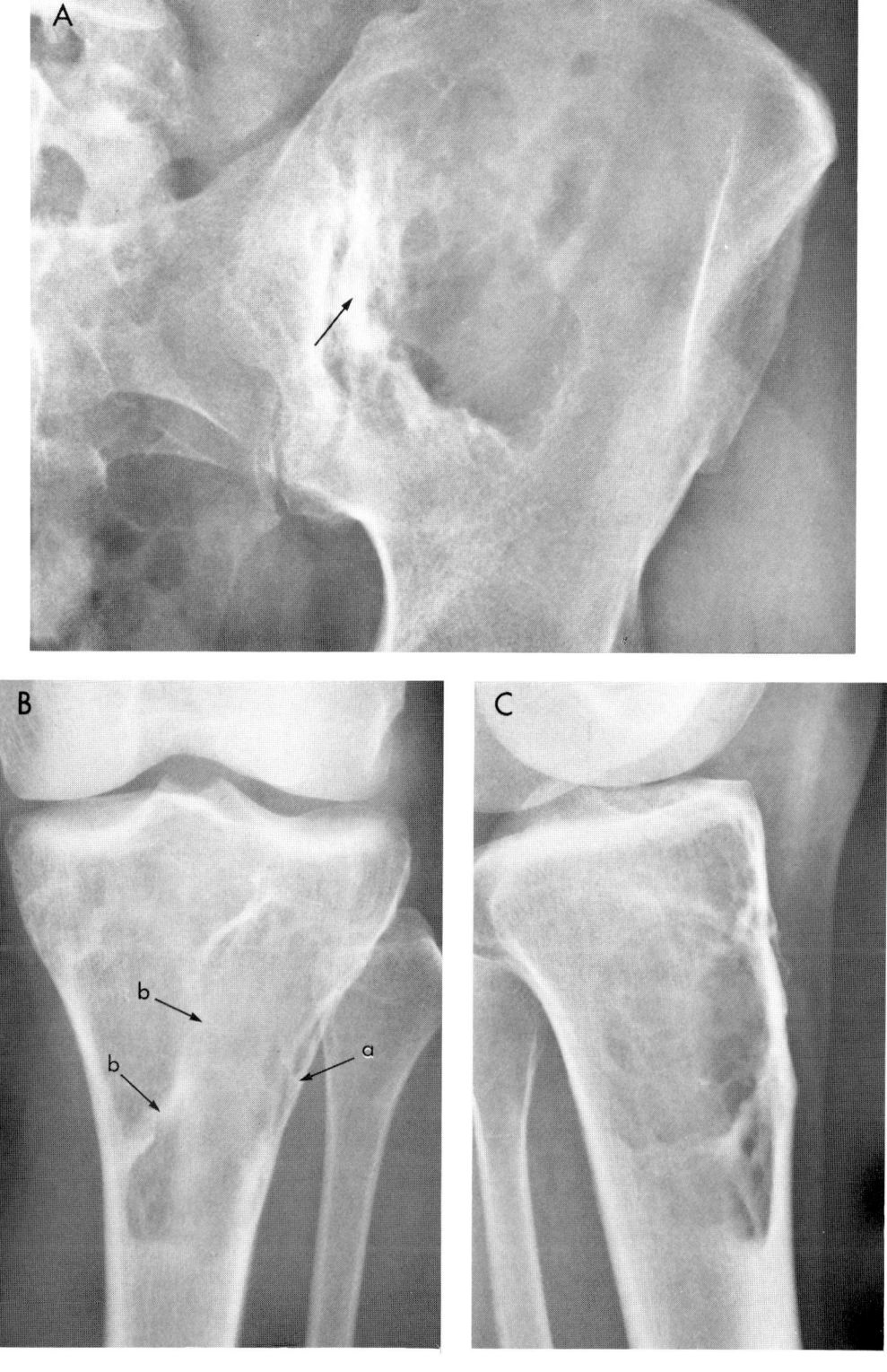

Figure 63 · Chondromyxoid Fibromas / 177

Figure 64.—Chondromyxoid fibroma of the fibula.

AFIP Case No. 1207088: anteroposterior projection.

DIAGNOSIS AND GRADE.—Chondromyxoid fibroma, fibula; growth rate IA.
LIFE INFORMATION.—Male, 9 years; survival unknown.
LOCATION.—A sharply circumscribed lesion confined to the lower metaphysis.
SIZE.—6 × 2 cm.
MINERALIZATION OF TUMOR.—None.
DESTRUCTION.—Geographic; regular contour.
PROLIFERATION.—Sclerotic rim; two small buttresses (**a**); slightly expanded shell (**b**) which encapsulates the tumor; faint septation (**c**).

DIFFERENTIAL DIAGNOSIS	PROBABILITY
Cyst	.61
Chondromyxoid fibroma	.37
Giant cell tumor	< .01
Osteoblastoma	< .01

COMMENT: This lesion resembles a nonossifying fibroma, but the absence of an uninvolved zone between the edge of the lesion and the growth plate is a mark against this diagnosis.

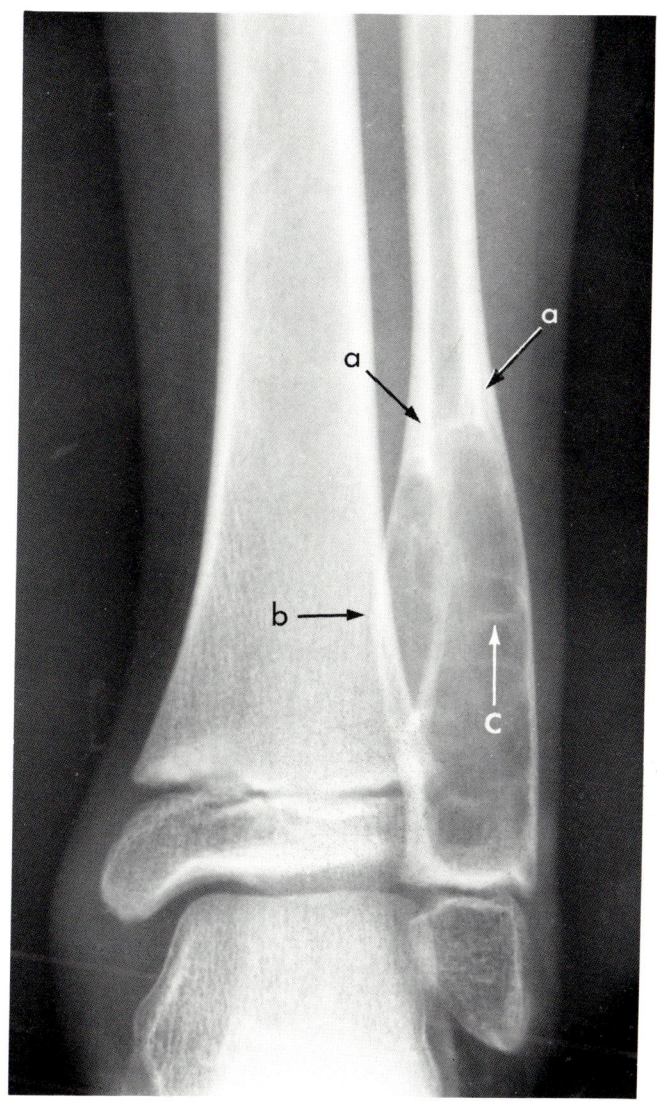

Figure 64 · Chondromyxoid Fibroma of Fibula / 179

Figure 65.—Chondromyxoid fibroma of the tibia.

AFIP Case No. 795574: **A,** anteroposterior, and **B,** lateral views.

DIAGNOSIS AND GRADE.—Chondromyxoid fibroma, tibia; growth rate IC.
LIFE INFORMATION.—Male, 23 years; well 10 years later.
LOCATION.—A sharply circumscribed lesion centered eccentrically in the midproximal metaphysis, extending into the epiphysis.
SIZE.—9 × 8 × 6 cm.
MINERALIZATION OF TUMOR.—None.
DESTRUCTION.—Geographic; lobulated contour; total penetration of the cortex (**B, a**); expanded shell (**B, b**).
PROLIFERATION.—Dense heavy marginal sclerosis (**B, c**); heavy coarse septation (**d**); expanded shell posteriorly which does not completely encapsulate the tumor.

DIFFERENTIAL DIAGNOSIS	PROBABILITY
Giant cell tumor	.82
Chondromyxoid fibroma	.11
Villonodular synovitis	.03
Cyst	.01
Fibrosarcoma	< .01
Osteoblastoma	< .01

COMMENT: The preoperative diagnosis was giant cell tumor, but the sclerotic rim and septa are too coarse and heavy, and the tumor does not extend as close to the subarticular cortex as giant cell tumor usually does.

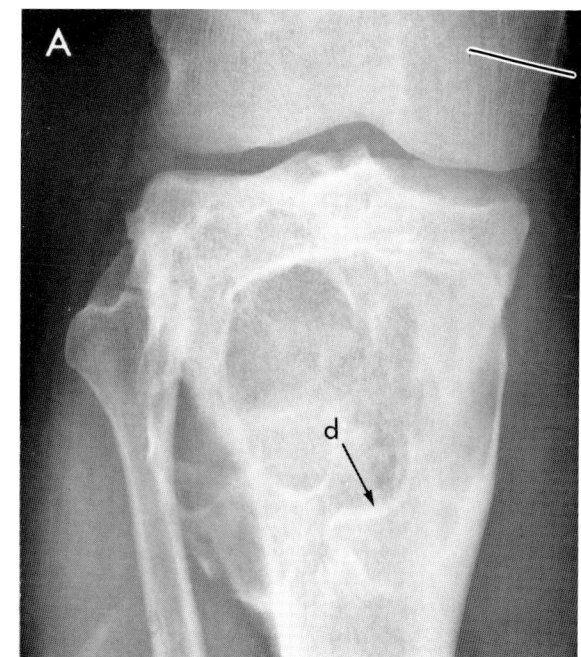
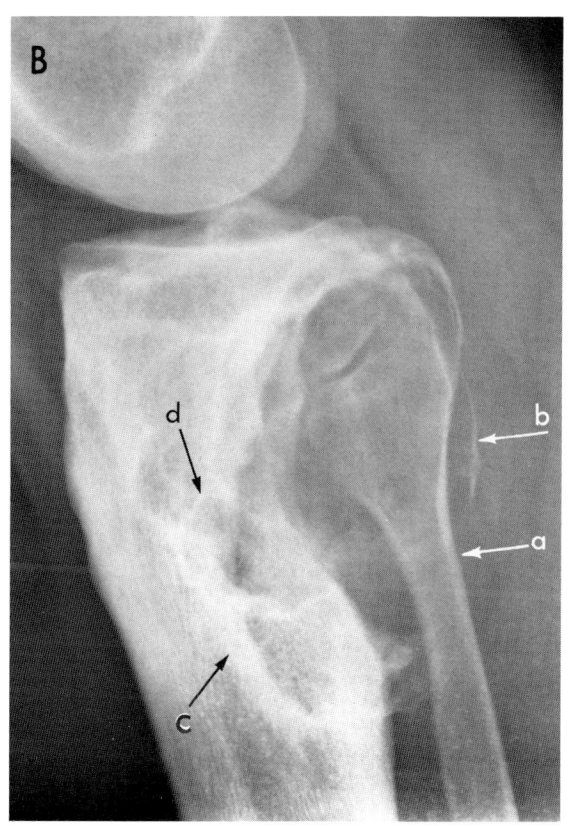

Figure 65 · Chondromyxoid Fibroma of Tibia / 181

Figure 66.—Chondromyxoid fibromas of the os calcis and rib.

AFIP Case No. 972983: **A,** lateral projection.

   DIAGNOSIS AND GRADE.—Chondromyxoid fibroma, os calcis; growth rate IA.
   LIFE INFORMATION.—Male, 25 years; survival unknown.
   LOCATION.—A sharply circumscribed lesion of the os calcis.

SIZE.—3.5 × 3 cm.
MINERALIZATION OF TUMOR.—None.
DESTRUCTION.—Geographic; principally reduction of medullary spongy bone; regular contour.
PROLIFERATION.—Thin sclerotic rim.

DIFFERENTIAL DIAGNOSIS	PROBABILITY
Giant cell tumor	.54
Fibrosarcoma	.24
Cyst	.12
Chondromyxoid fibroma	.06
Benign cartilaginous tumor	.01
Myeloma	.01
Chondrosarcoma	< .01

   COMMENT: This could be any of several kinds of lesions. The thin rim of marginal sclerosis (**arrows**) sets off what otherwise might be an invisible lesion.

AFIP Case No. 1035794: **B,** anteroposterior oblique projection.

   DIAGNOSIS AND GRADE.—Chondromyxoid fibroma, rib; growth rate IA.
   LIFE INFORMATION.—Female, 47 years; last known to be well.
   LOCATION.—Tiny circumscribed lesion in the center of the eleventh rib (**arrow**).

SIZE.—1 × 1 cm.
MINERALIZATION OF TUMOR.—None.
DESTRUCTION.—Geographic; slightly lobulated contour.
PROLIFERATION.—Pronounced zone of marginal sclerosis.

DIFFERENTIAL DIAGNOSIS	PROBABILITY
Myeloma	.60
Benign cartilaginous tumor	.36
Chondrosarcoma	.01
Fibroxanthoma	.01
Fibrosarcoma	< .01
Chondromyxoid fibroma	< .01

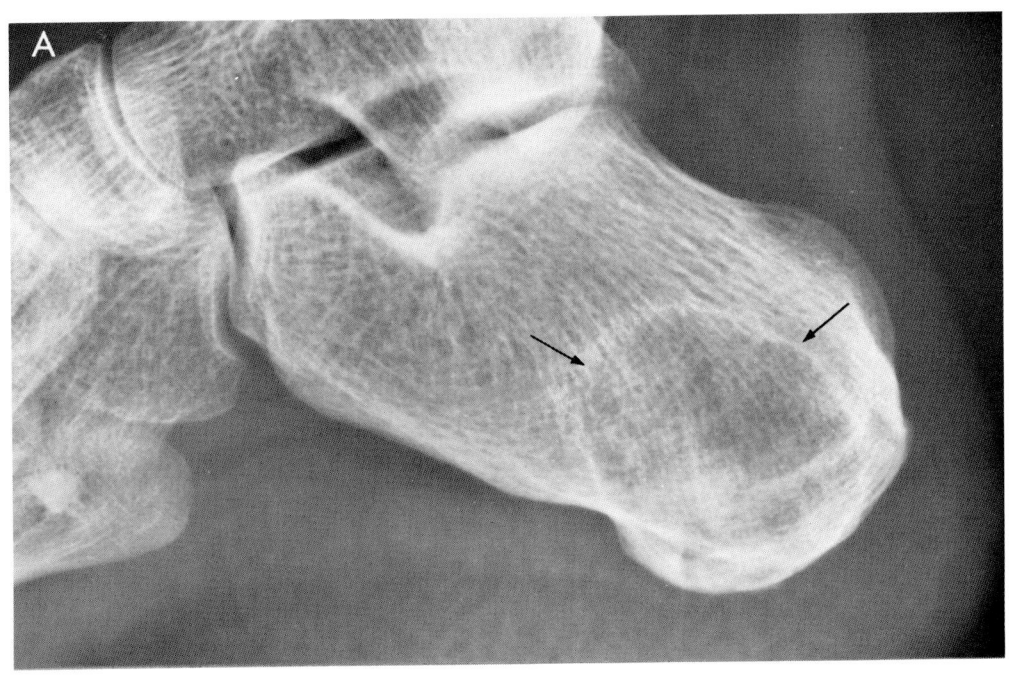

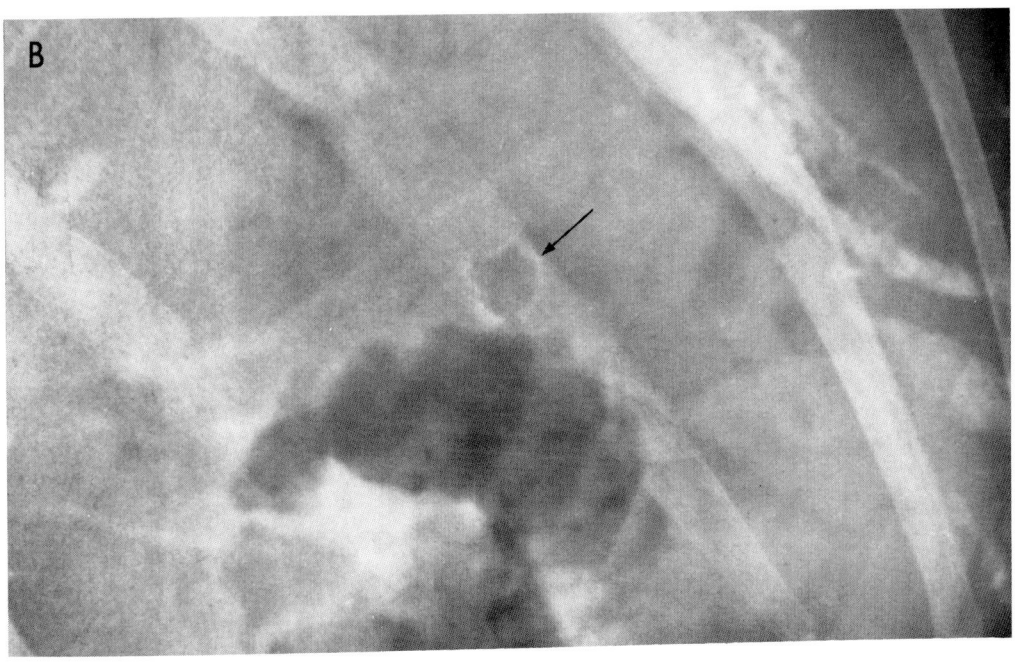

COMMENT: The best radiologic diagnosis is benign fibrous lesion. The computer evidently does not know that a myelomatous lesion this small is rarely lobulated.

Figure 67.—Fibroxanthomas of the tibia.

AFIP Case No. 1167299: **A,** anteroposterior, and **B,** lateral views.

DIAGNOSIS AND GRADE.—Fibroxanthoma, tibia; growth rate IC.

LIFE INFORMATION.—Male, 15 years; survival unknown.

LOCATION.—A partially circumscribed lesion arising in the medial cortex of the proximal tibial metaphysis.

SIZE.—2 × 1.5 × 1 cm.

MINERALIZATION OF TUMOR.—None.

DESTRUCTION.—Deeply excavated cortex of geographic pattern; lobulated contour (**B, arrows**).

PROLIFERATION.—Narrow zone of marginal sclerosis.

DIFFERENTIAL DIAGNOSIS	PROBABILITY
Fibroxanthoma	.99
Benign cartilaginous tumor	< .01

COMMENT: An atypical fibroxanthoma because there is no covering cortex.

AFIP Case No. 1207290: **C,** anteroposterior, and **D,** lateral views.

DIAGNOSIS AND GRADE.—Fibroxanthoma, tibia; growth rate IC.

LIFE INFORMATION.—Male, 5 years; survival unknown.

LOCATION.—A circumscribed lesion in the lateral cortex of the distal tibial metaphysis; extraosseous component.

SIZE.—1 cm × 6 × 4 mm.

MINERALIZATION OF TUMOR.—None.

DESTRUCTION.—Geographic; total penetration of cortex (**D, arrow**); regular contour.

PROLIFERATION.—Faint reduction of cancellous bone (**C, x**). Two wedge-shaped segments of subperiosteal new bone (**D, a**) partially encapsulate the lesion. In **C**, a faint zone of marginal sclerosis may reflect the periosteal response.

DIFFERENTIAL DIAGNOSIS	PROBABILITY
Fibroxanthoma	.99
Fibrosarcoma	< .01

COMMENT: This case is unusual in that the periosteal reaction seems fresh and active, most of the lesion is on the surface, and there is no fracture to account for the peculiar periosteal response without which the lesion might be missed.

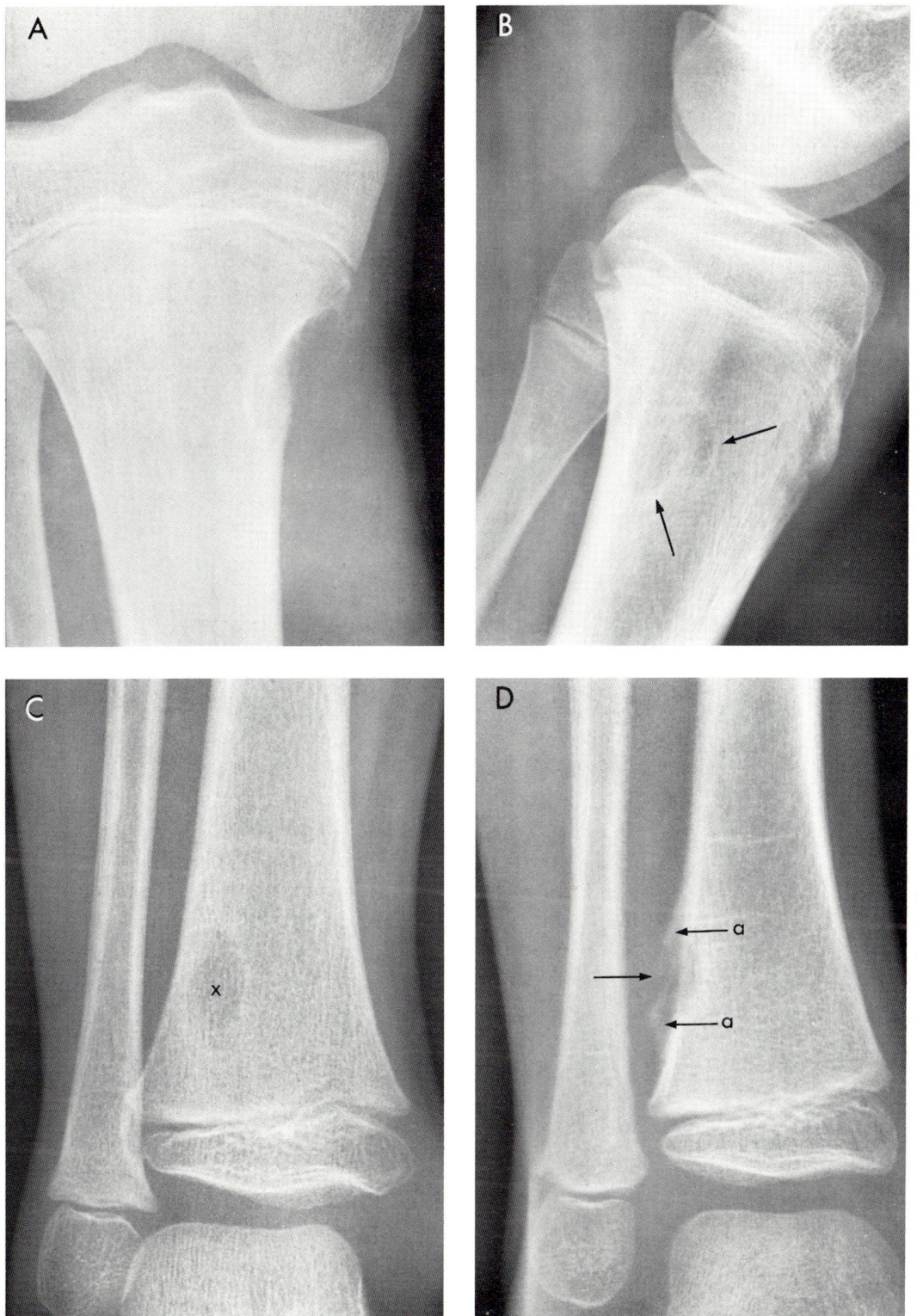

Figure 67 · Fibroxanthomas of Tibia / 185

Figure 68.—Fibroxanthomas of the femur and tibia.

AFIP Case No. 1164168: **A,** lateral projection.

DIAGNOSIS AND GRADE.—Fibroxanthoma, femur; growth rate IA.
LIFE INFORMATION.—Female, 18 years; last known to be well.
LOCATION.—An elongated circumscribed lesion occupying the posterior cortex of the distal femoral shaft and metaphysis.
SIZE.—11 × 3 × 3 cm.
MINERALIZATION OF TUMOR.—None.
DESTRUCTION.—Geographic; lobulated contour.
PROLIFERATION.—Distal half of the lesion surrounded by a thin shell of expanded cortex and thin sclerotic rim; slight septation; proximal half enveloped in dense heavy reparative bone.

DIFFERENTIAL DIAGNOSIS	PROBABILITY
Fibroxanthoma	.96
Chondromyxoid fibroma	.03
Fibrosarcoma	< .01

COMMENT: The proximal half of this lesion is well on the way to healing. The entire lesion seems to show continuous generation in the metaphysis, with bone destruction being converted to bone repair as the part containing the lesion becomes the shaft. As growth stops, the lesion may fill in and present as an osteoma.

AFIP Case No. 1158190: **B,** anteroposterior projection.

DIAGNOSIS AND GRADE.—Fibroxanthoma, tibia; growth rate IA.
LIFE INFORMATION.—Male, 12 years; well three years later.
LOCATION.—A sharply circumscribed lesion at the junction of the distal shaft and metaphysis, extending well into both areas.
SIZE.—7 × 3 × 2.5 cm.
MINERALIZATION OF TUMOR.—None.
DESTRUCTION.—Geographic; regular contour.
PROLIFERATION.—Thin rim of marginal sclerosis; just under 1 cm of expanded cortical shell laterally; faint septation.

DIFFERENTIAL DIAGNOSIS	PROBABILITY
Fibroxanthoma	.80
Chondromyxoid fibroma	.16
Cyst	.02

COMMENT: Note the broad zone of uninvolved bone between the edge of the lesion and the growth plate.

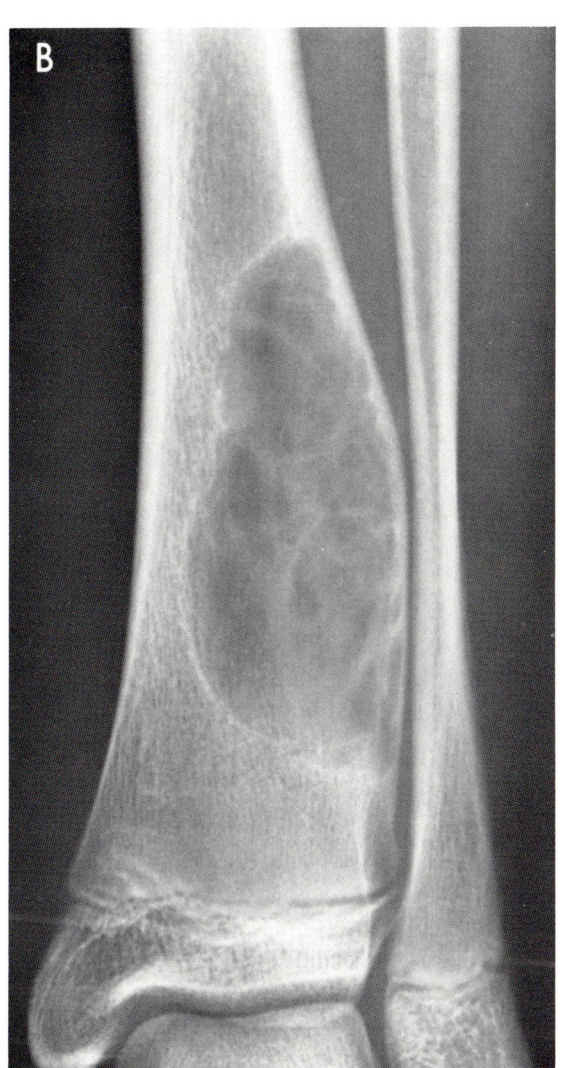
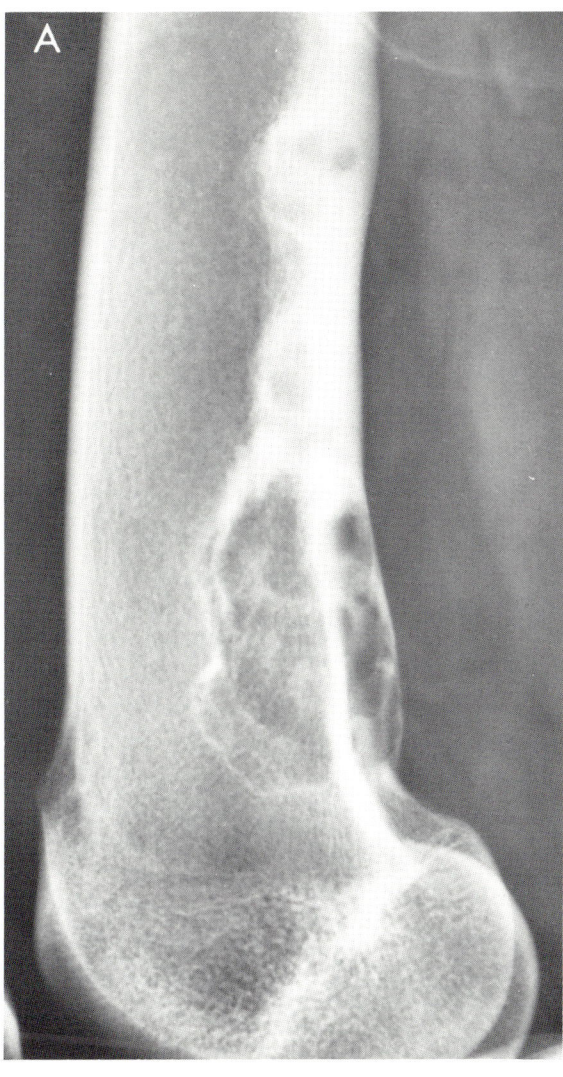

Figure 68 · Fibroxanthomas / 187

Figure 69.—Fibroxanthomas of the tibia and femur.

AFIP Case No. 1155055: **A,** anteroposterior projection.

DIAGNOSIS AND GRADE.—Fibroxanthoma, tibia; growth rate IA.
LIFE INFORMATION.—Female, 13 years; well two years later.
LOCATION.—A sharply circumscribed lesion centered slightly eccentrically in the distal metaphysis (in lateral projection, not shown), involving the epiphysis.
SIZE.—4 × 3 × 2 cm.
MINERALIZATION OF TUMOR.—None.
DESTRUCTION.—Geographic; lobulated contour.
PROLIFERATION.—Thin zone of marginal sclerosis surrounding the lesion; faint septate pattern.

DIFFERENTIAL DIAGNOSIS	PROBABILITY
Fibroxanthoma	.64
Chondromyxoid fibroma	.30
Cyst	.05
Osteoblastoma	< .01
Giant cell tumor	< .01
Fibrosarcoma	< .01

COMMENT: A large but fairly typical fibroxanthoma, with uninvolved area of bone between lesion and growth plate.

AFIP Case No. 1142240: **B,** lateral projection.

DIAGNOSIS AND GRADE.—Fibroxanthoma, midfemur growth rate IA.
LIFE INFORMATION.—Male, 9 years; survival unknown.
LOCATION.—A sharply circumscribed lesion in the distal shaft. (In an anterior view it was eccentrically centered.)
SIZE.—8 × 2.5 × 2.5 cm.
MINERALIZATION OF TUMOR.—None.
DESTRUCTION.—Geographic; slightly lobulated contour.
PROLIFERATION.—Narrow marginal zone of sclerosis; faint septation; slightly expanded cortical shell; enveloping thick layer of smooth laminated subperiosteal bone, showing backfill.

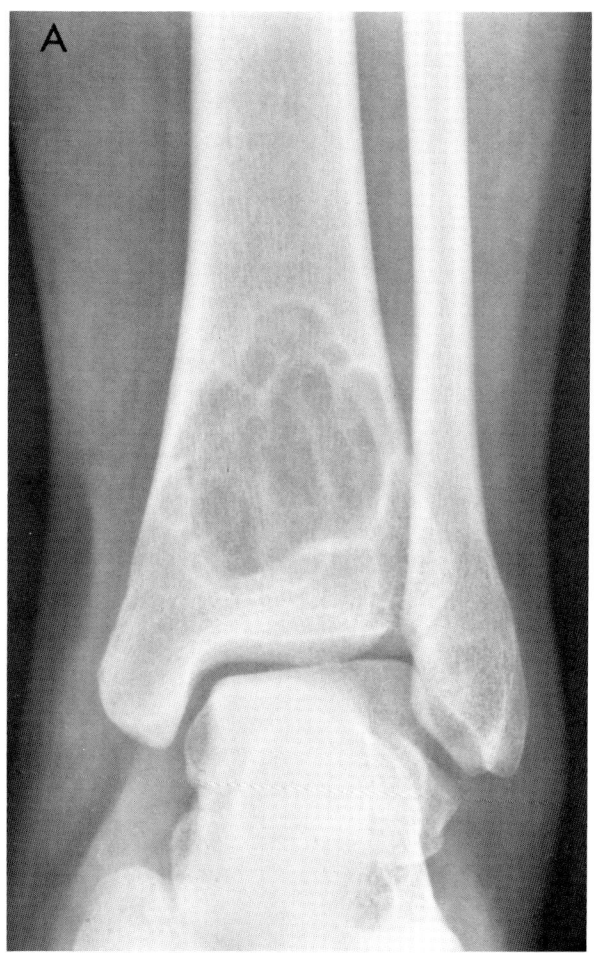
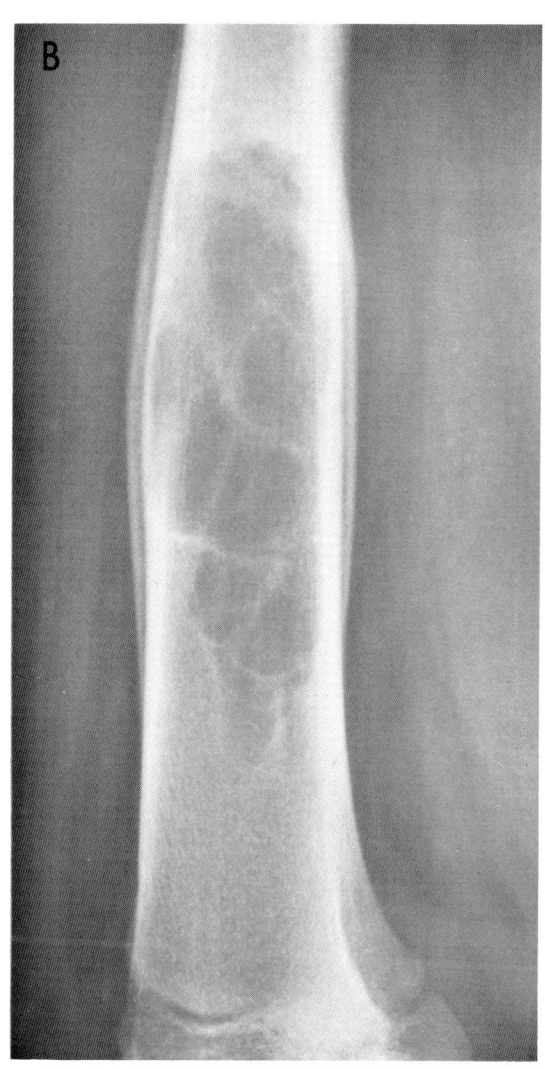

Differential Diagnosis	Probability
Fibroxanthoma	.68
Hemangio-, angiosarcoma	.10
Chondromyxoid fibroma	.07
Cyst	.07
Fibrosarcoma	.06
Chondrosarcoma	< .01
Ewing's sarcoma	< .01

COMMENT: The contributor's diagnosis was nonossifying fibroma. Fibroxanthoma, nonossifying fibroma and fibrous cortical defect appear to be radiologically and histologically the same.

Figure 69 · Fibroxanthomas

Figure 70.—Periosteal fibroma of the radius; fibroxanthoma of the metatarsal.

AFIP Case No. 1004238: **A,** posteroanterior projection.

> DIAGNOSIS AND GRADE.—Periosteal fibroma, radius; growth rate IC.
> LIFE INFORMATION. Male, 45 years; incidental finding after injury; well.
> LOCATION.—A circumscribed lesion in the medial cortex of the distal shaft and metaphysis.
> SIZE.—4 × 0.5 cm.
> MINERALIZATION OF TUMOR.—None.
> DESTRUCTION.—Shallow excavation of geographic pattern; regular contour.
> PROLIFERATION.—Subperiosteal new bone seems to form a partial shell over this fibrous lesion; coarse septal pattern (**arrow**).

DIFFERENTIAL DIAGNOSIS	PROBABILITY
Fibroxanthoma	.64
Fibrosarcoma	.21
Cartilaginous tumor	.10
Chondrosarcoma	.02

COMMENT: This lesion is presumably closely related to fibroxanthoma. The cortex beneath the lesion has been expanded medially or held in fixed position by a preexisting lesion while the rest of the bone has grown normally.

AFIP Case No. 1115976: **B,** anteroposterior projection.

> DIAGNOSIS AND GRADE.—Fibroxanthoma, metatarsal; growth rate IA.
> LIFE INFORMATION.—Male, 31 years; well four years later.
> LOCATION.—A small circumscribed lesion in the cortex of the proximal shaft of the middle metatarsal.
> SIZE.—2 cm × 5 mm.
> MINERALIZATION OF TUMOR.—None.
> DESTRUCTION.—Geographic; ragged contour.
> PROLIFERATION.—Thin, slightly expanded shell of periosteal new bone (**arrow**) enveloping the lesion.

DIFFERENTIAL DIAGNOSIS	PROBABILITY
Benign cartilaginous tumor	.99
Fibroxanthoma	< .01

COMMENT: An innocent-appearing lesion.

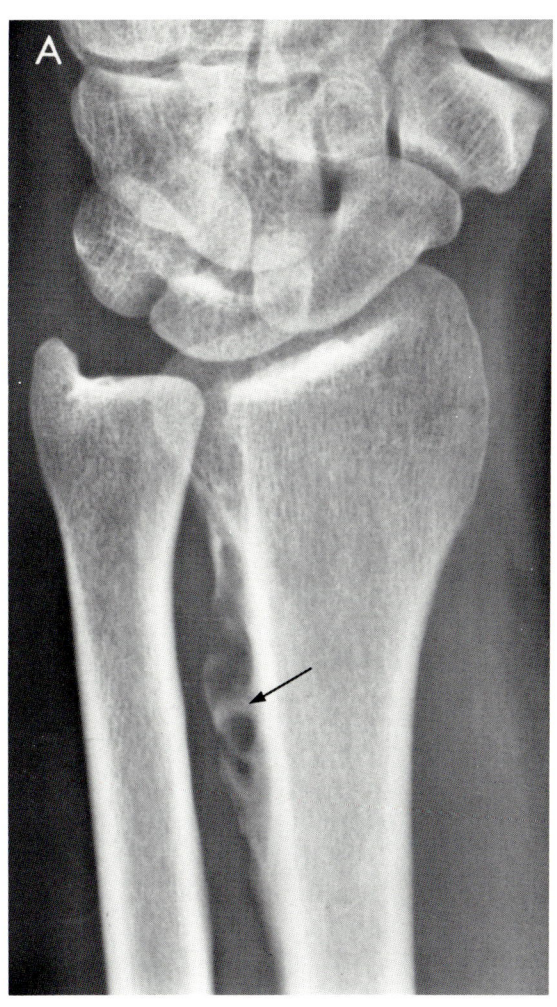
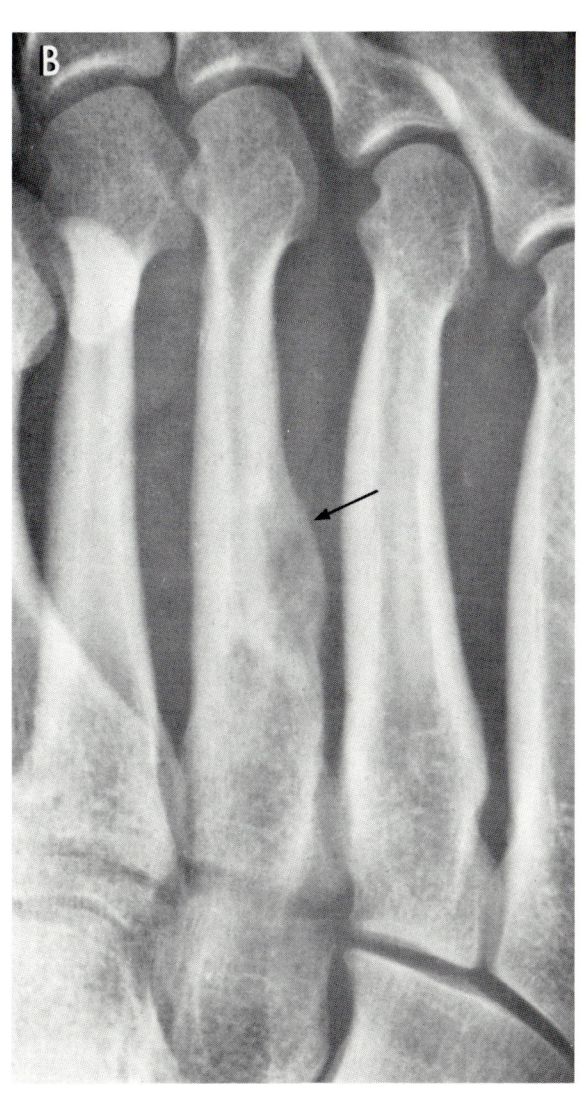

Figure 70 · Periosteal Fibroma; Fibroxanthoma / 191

Figure 71.—Fibroxanthoma of the femur.

AFIP Case No. 1156660: **A,** anteroposterior, and **B,** lateral views.

DIAGNOSIS AND GRADE.—Fibroxanthoma, femur; growth rate IA.

LIFE INFORMATION.—Male, 52 years; last known to be well; refused treatment after biopsy.

LOCATION.—A circumscribed cystic lesion involving the entire femoral head, neck and intertrochanteric region.

SIZE.—11 × 9 × 5 cm.

MINERALIZATION OF TUMOR.—None.

DESTRUCTION.—Geographic; lobulated contour; healed pathologic fracture.

PROLIFERATION.—Extensive septate proliferative response (soap-bubble appearance).

DIFFERENTIAL DIAGNOSIS	PROBABILITY
Giant cell tumor	.99
Fibrosarcoma	< .01
Chondromyxoid fibroma	< .01

COMMENT: The histologic material was typical of fibroxanthoma, but the size and location of the lesion are inconsistent with this diagnosis and typical of giant cell tumor. Actually, with giant cell tumor the tissues extending into the shaft are often fibrous and typical of fibroxanthoma; and note that the biopsy site here is indeed in the shaft portion of the lesion. In a patient of 52 with so much healing, giant cell tumor is a far better radiologic diagnosis than fibroxanthoma, which is not even considered in the computer differential diagnosis.

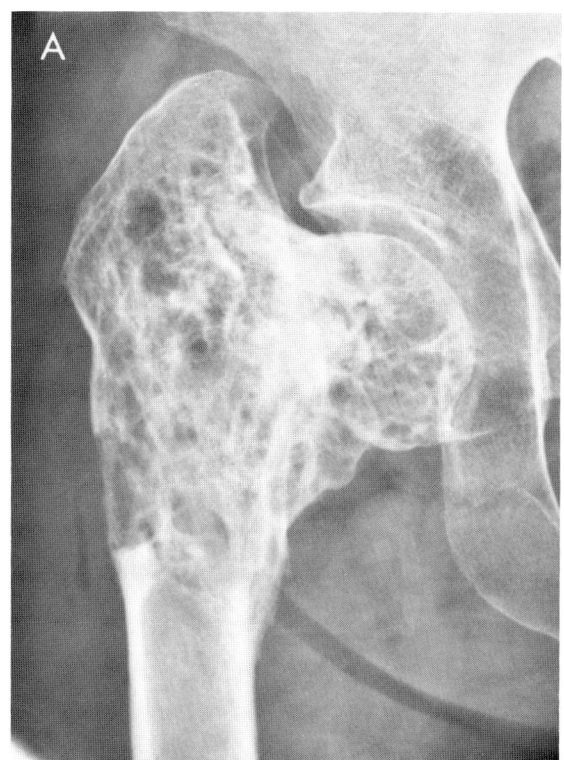
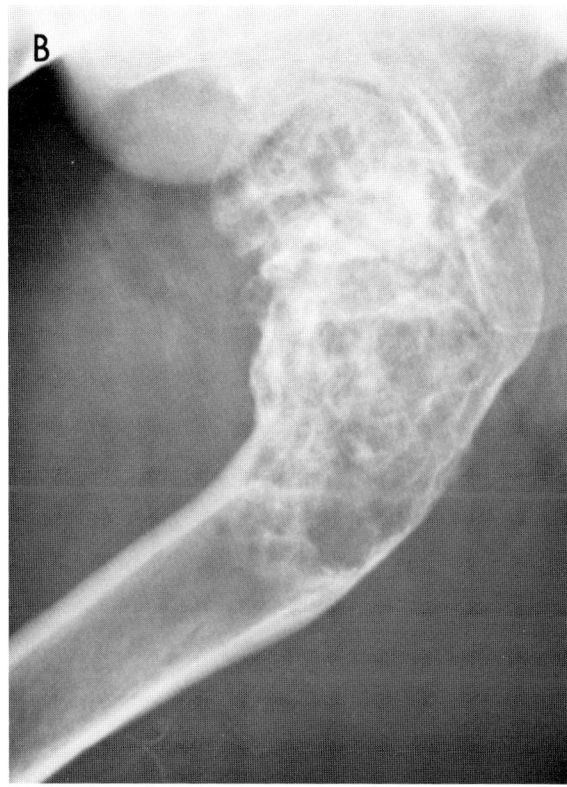

Figure 71 · Fibroxanthoma of Femur / 193

Figure 72.—Fibrous osteoma of the frontal sinus; ossifying fibroma of the antrum.

AFIP Case No. 1037533: **A,** posteroanterior projection.

DIAGNOSIS AND GRADE.—Fibrous osteoma, frontal sinus; growth rate IA-B-C.
LIFE INFORMATION.—Male, 24 years; survival unknown.
LOCATION.—An ill-defined lesion (**arrows**) in the frontal sinus.

SIZE.—4 × 4 cm.
MINERALIZATION OF TUMOR.—Focal, lumpy increased density.
DESTRUCTION.—None definite.
PROLIFERATION.—Medial superior orbital rim displaced laterally (**a**); portion of the sinus wall expanded into the orbit (**b**).

DIFFERENTIAL DIAGNOSIS	PROBABILITY
Ossifying fibroma	.99
Fibrosarcoma	< .01
Chondrosarcoma	< .01

COMMENT: Fibrous osteoma in the sinus may distort and balloon the structures it occupies.

AFIP Case No. 1048662: **B,** anteroposterior body section exposure.

DIAGNOSIS AND GRADE.—Ossifying fibroma, antrum; growth rate IA-B-C.
LIFE INFORMATION.—Male, 7 years; well three years later.
LOCATION.—A lesion filling the left antrum (**arrows**) and outlined by its walls.

SIZE.—4 × 3.5 cm.
MINERALIZATION OF TUMOR.—A hazy increase of density (ground glass) in the involved region, appearing to be at least partially due to cloudy tumor matrix mineralization.
DESTRUCTION.—None apparent.
PROLIFERATION.—The expanding tumor has displaced the floor of the orbit upward (**b**) and the lateral inferior and medial walls of the antrum outward. The antral wall (**arrows**) is thin and smooth, but seems intact around the perimeter.

DIFFERENTIAL DIAGNOSIS	PROBABILITY
Ossifying fibroma	.99
Fibrosarcoma	< .01
Chondrosarcoma	< .01

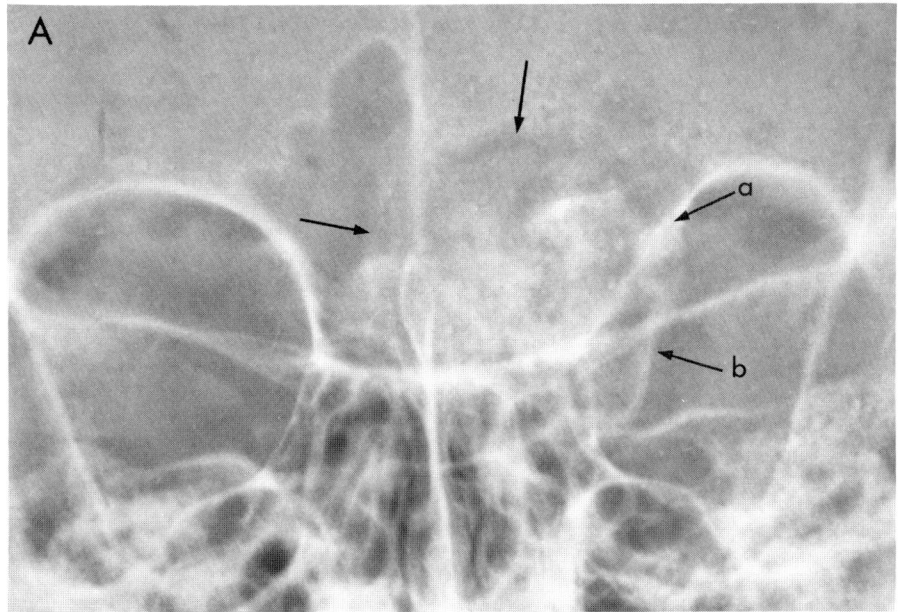

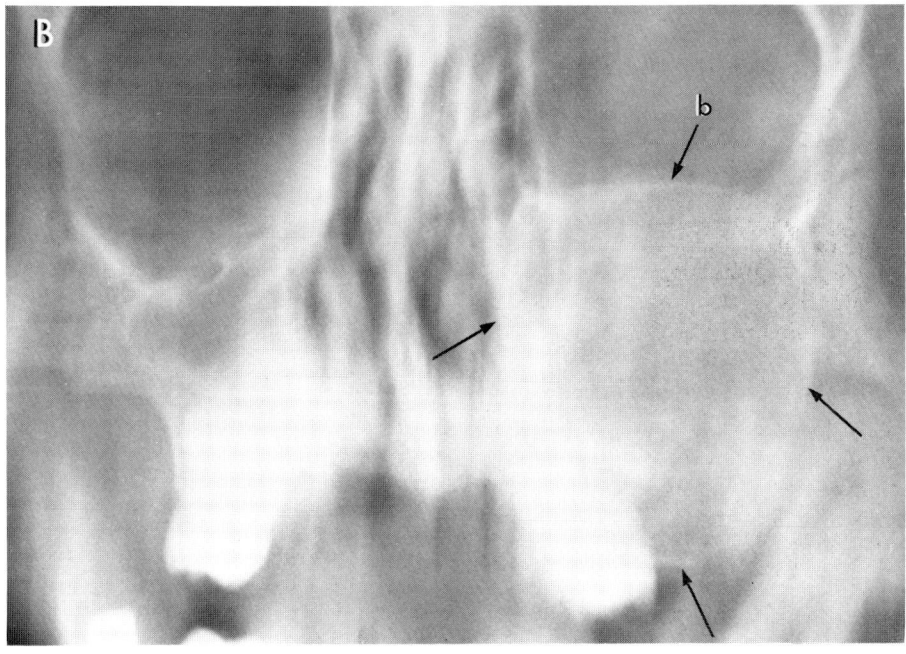

COMMENT: Growth rate is difficult to assess without bone destruction. Ossifying fibroma of the skull often distorts and balloons the structures it occupies. (See Fig. 48.)

Figure 72 · Osteoma and Fibroma of Nasal Sinuses

Figure 73.—Fibrous osteoma of the skull.

AFIP Case No. 1036261: Oblique tangential projection.

DIAGNOSIS AND GRADE.—Fibrous osteoma, skull; growth rate IA.
LIFE INFORMATION.—Male, 18 years; survival unknown.
LOCATION.—A circumscribed ballooning of the outer table over the parietal region.
SIZE.—6 × 2 cm.
MINERALIZATION OF TUMOR.—None.
DESTRUCTION.—Geographic; regular contour.
PROLIFERATION.—Inner table thickened; outer table expanded about 1 cm, quite thin (**arrows**) but completely enveloping the lesion.

DIFFERENTIAL DIAGNOSIS	PROBABILITY
Ossifying fibroma	.71
Fibrosarcoma	.24
Chondrosarcoma	.03

COMMENT: An atypical fibrous osteoma of the skull. It should be a fibrous lesion of bone. Fibrous dysplasia is not included by the computer in differential diagnosis.

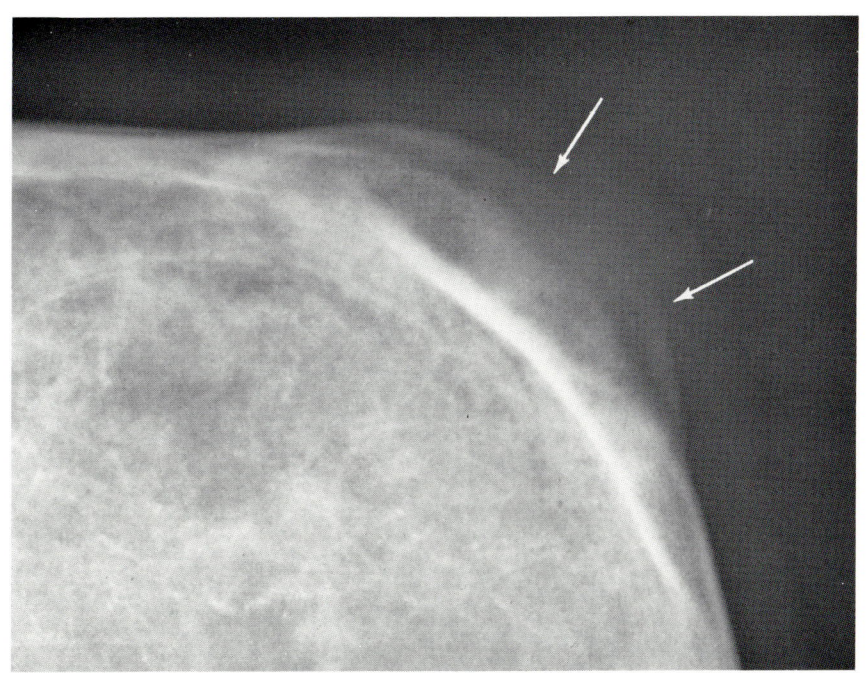

Figure 73 · Fibrous Osteoma of Skull / 197

Figure 74.—Cortical desmoids of the femur.

AFIP Case No. 1188917: **A,** lateral projection.

DIAGNOSIS AND GRADE.—Cortical desmoid, femur; growth rate IA.
LIFE INFORMATION.—Female, 16 years; last known to be well.
LOCATION.—A partially circumscribed lesion centered on the cortex of the lower third of the distal metaphysis posteriorly (**arrow**).

SIZE.—1.5 × 1 cm.
MINERALIZATION OF TUMOR.—None.
DESTRUCTION.—A shallow geographic excavation.
PROLIFERATION.—Slight sclerosis of the margin.

DIFFERENTIAL DIAGNOSIS	PROBABILITY
Cortical desmoid	100

COMMENT: This is a typical cortical desmoid.

AFIP Case No. 1105882: **B,** lateral projection.

DIAGNOSIS AND GRADE.—Cortical desmoid, femur; growth rate IA.
LIFE INFORMATION.—Male, 17 years; survival unknown.
LOCATION.—Small partially circumscribed lesion centered on the posterior cortex of the distal metaphysis (**arrow**).

SIZE.—2 × 1 cm.
MINERALIZATION OF TUMOR.—None.
DESTRUCTION.—Shallow excavation of geographic pattern; ragged contour.
PROLIFERATION.—Sclerosis of margin of destroyed area.

DIFFERENTIAL DIAGNOSIS	PROBABILITY
Cortical desmoid	.99
Soft tissue sarcoma	< .01
Fibrosarcoma	< .01

COMMENT: Another typical cortical desmoid.

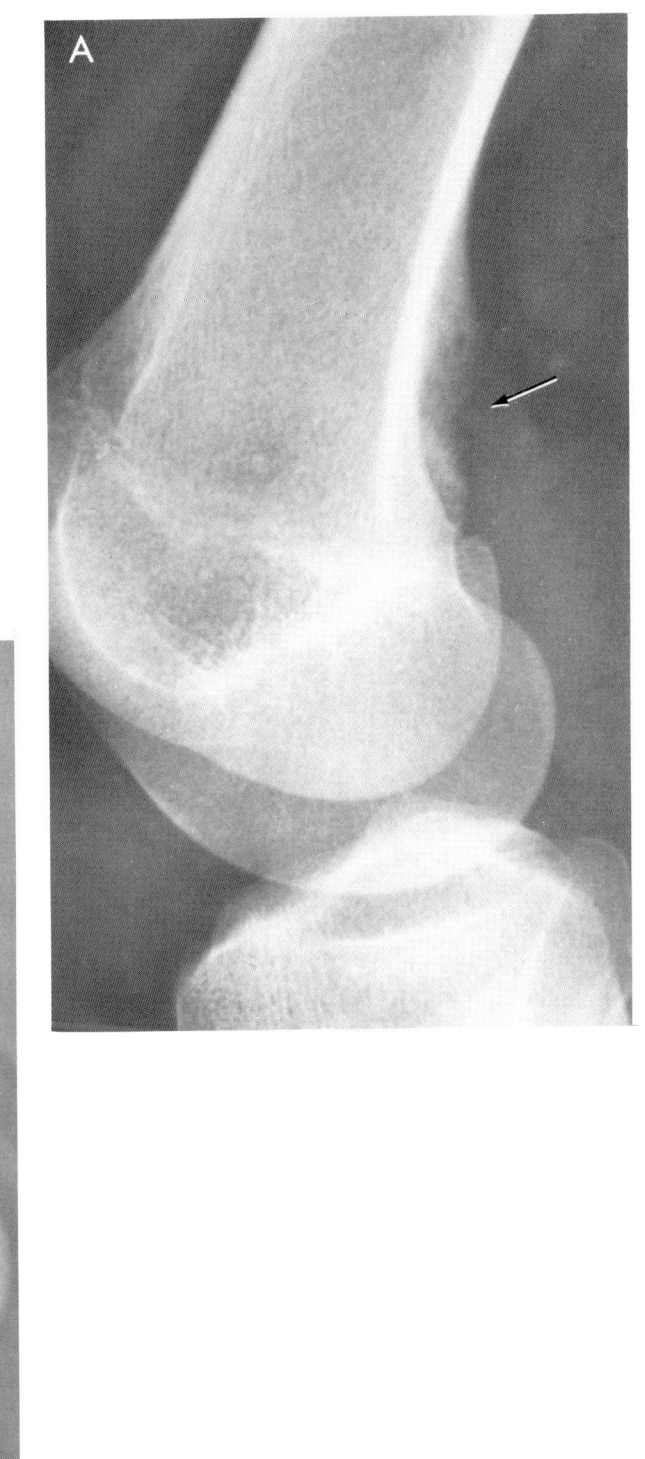
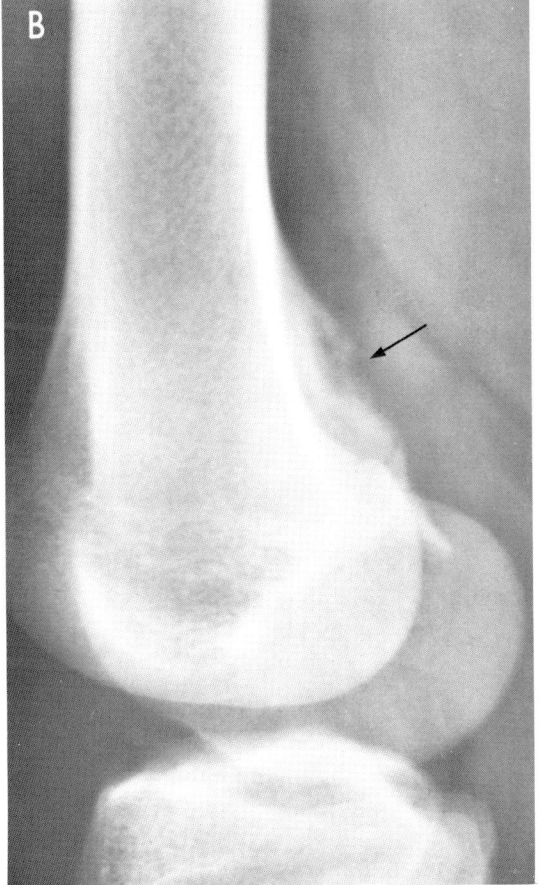

Figure 74 · Cortical Desmoids of Femur

Figure 75.—Cortical desmoids of the femur.

AFIP Case No. 1131478: **A,** anteroposterior projection.

DIAGNOSIS AND GRADE.—Cortical desmoid, femur; not graded.
LIFE INFORMATION.—Male, 12 years; well three years later.
LOCATION.—A poorly defined lesion centered on the medial cortex of the distal femoral metaphysis (**arrow**).
SIZE.—2 × 1 cm.
MINERALIZATION OF TUMOR.—New bone projecting from the surface of the cortex into the lesion has the appearance of periosteal new bone.
DESTRUCTION.—None.
PROLIFERATION.—None except that mentioned above.

DIFFERENTIAL DIAGNOSIS	PROBABILITY
Cortical desmoid	.99
Myositis ossificans	< .01
Soft tissue sarcoma	< .01

COMMENT: A variant of cortical desmoid, easy to diagnose because of location and size.

AFIP Case No. 1201001: **B,** anteroposterior body section exposure.

DIAGNOSIS AND GRADE.—Cortical desmoid, femur; not graded.
LIFE INFORMATION.—Female, 12 years; last known to be well.
LOCATION.—An ill-defined small lesion centered in the medial cortex of the distal femoral metaphysis (**arrow**).
SIZE.—2 × 1 cm.
MINERALIZATION OF TUMOR.—As in **A,** there is extension of periosteal bone into the soft tissue lesion.
DESTRUCTION.—None.
PROLIFERATION.—None, except as mentioned above.

DIFFERENTIAL DIAGNOSIS	PROBABILITY
Cortical desmoid	.98
Myositis ossificans	.01

COMMENT: A diagnosis easily recognized principally because of the location and very small size of the lesion.

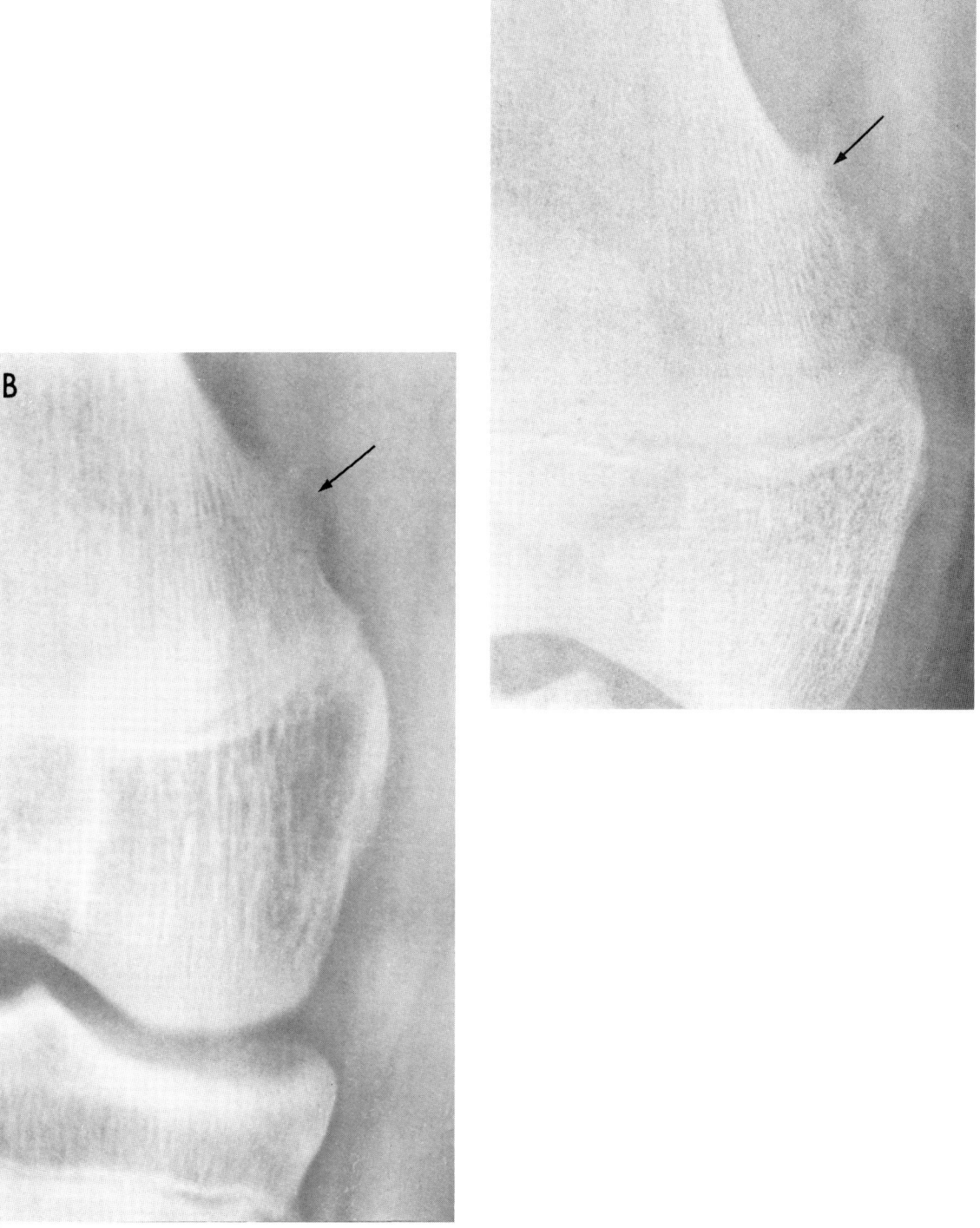

Figure 75 · Cortical Desmoids of Femur / 201

Figure 76.—Cortical desmoid of the femur.

AFIP Case No. 120002: Anteroposterior projection.

DIAGNOSIS AND GRADE.—Cortical desmoid, femur; growth rate IA.

LIFE INFORMATION.—Male, 9 years; last known to be well.

LOCATION.—A circumscribed small lesion arising in the medial cortex and subcortical bone of the distal femoral metaphysis (**arrow**).

SIZE.—2 × 1.5 cm.

MINERALIZATION OF TUMOR.—None.

DESTRUCTION.—Geographic; slight cortical erosion.

PROLIFERATION.—Sclerotic rim; irregular excrescence of cortical new bone, as seen in preceding cases.

DIFFERENTIAL DIAGNOSIS	PROBABILITY
Cortical desmoid	.97
Benign cartilaginous tumor	.02
Fibrosarcoma	< .01

COMMENT: Another variant of cortical desmoid, this one appearing very much like a fibroxanthoma or benign cortical defect.

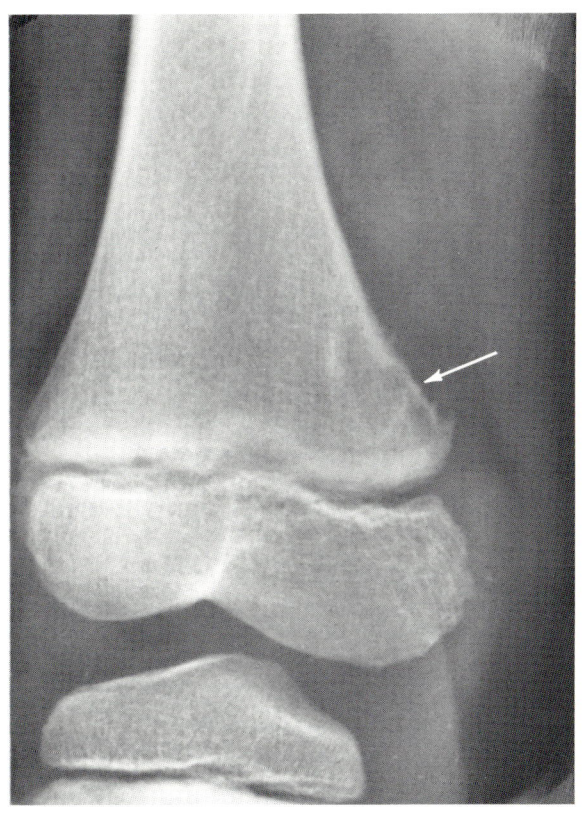

Figure 76 · Cortical Desmoid of Femur / 203

PART 4

Cartilaginous Tumors

Figure 77.—Chondrosarcoma of the ilium.

AFIP Case No. 1190741: **A,** anteroposterior view; **B,** roentgenogram of surgical specimen.

DIAGNOSIS AND GRADE.—Chondrosarcoma, ilium; not graded.

LIFE INFORMATION.—Female, 32 years; died three years after resection of a large abdominal mass arising from a small stalk on the right ilium.

LOCATION.—A very large extraosseous lesion occupying the hollow of the ilium and lower paraspinal area **(A, x)**.

SIZE.—12 × 15 cm.

MINERALIZATION OF TUMOR.—In **A,** mineralization is very difficult to see. Flocculent calcification (**a**) apparently overlies the superior iliac crest. **B** shows the typical flocculent calcification well.

DESTRUCTION.—Probable geographic area near the iliac crest laterally.

PROLIFERATION.—Sclerosis around the destroyed area in the iliac crest.

DIFFERENTIAL DIAGNOSIS	PROBABILITY
Chondrosarcoma	100

COMMENT: Destructive and proliferative changes in the ilium are difficult to evaluate. The suspected changes are in the area with the greatest amount of matrix mineralization. If present, they appear to be quite smooth and of erosive nature. It is interesting that such a large primary tumor can have so few changes in bone. The pelvis is the common site for chondrosarcoma without *any* changes in bone.

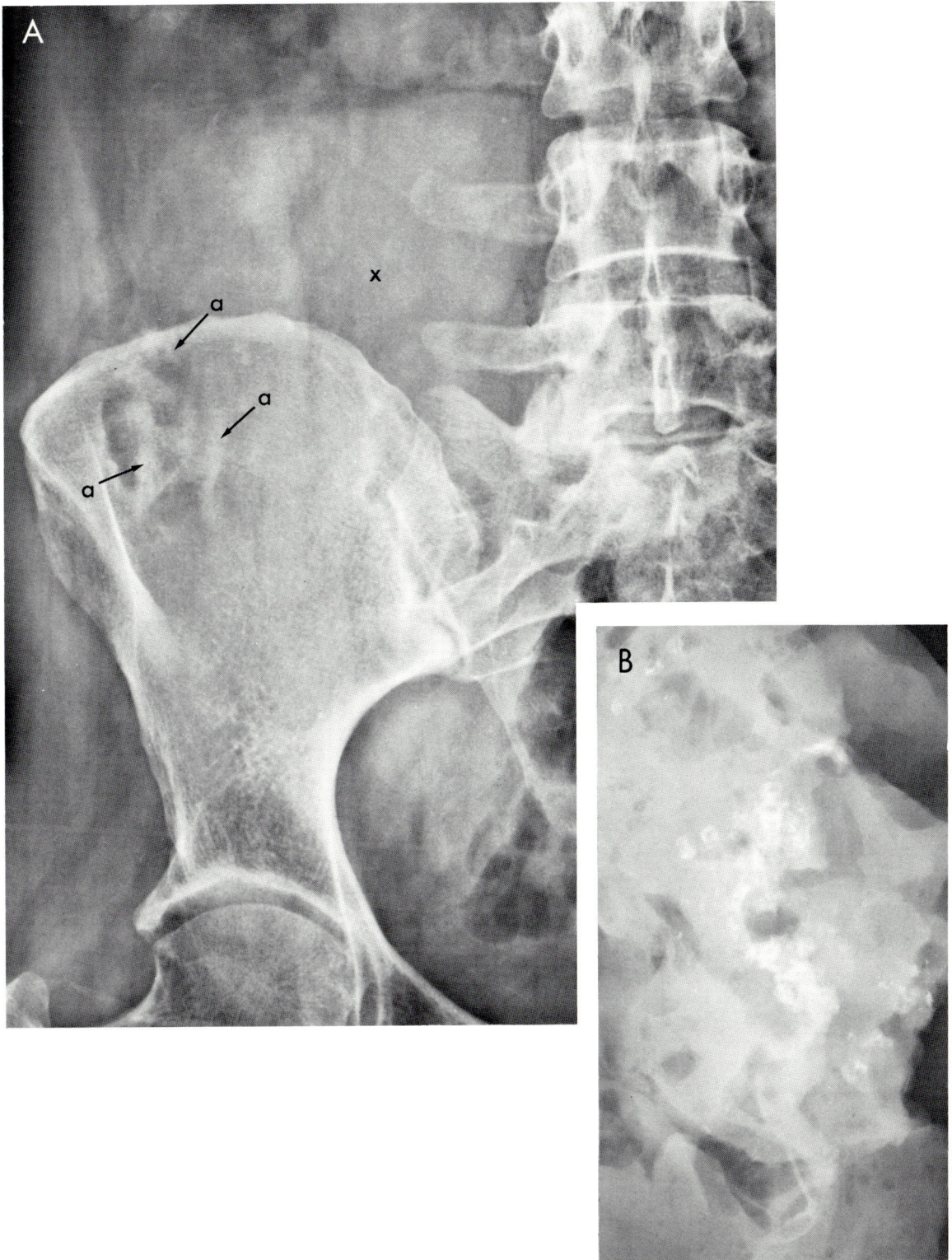

Figure 77 · Chondrosarcoma of Ilium

Figure 78.—Chondrosarcoma of the clavicle.

AFIP Case No. 9082676: Anteroposterior projection.

DIAGNOSIS AND GRADE.—Chondrosarcoma, clavicle; growth rate II.

LIFE INFORMATION.—Female, 27 years; well six years after diagnosis and resection.

LOCATION.—A large tumor of the distal end of the clavicle and the acromion.

SIZE.—10 × 10 cm.

MINERALIZATION OF TUMOR.—Floccules of calcified matrix (**x**) scattered throughout the center of the tumor.

DESTRUCTION.—Geographic, with moth-eaten edge in distal end of the clavicle (**a**); acromion and coracoid processes (**b**) partially destroyed; contour ragged.

PROLIFERATION.—Hyperostoses on the distal clavicle proximal to the tumor; several broad zones of dense sclerosis of bone surrounding the area of destruction; crescentic calcifications around the tumor, probably periosteal in origin.

DIFFERENTIAL DIAGNOSIS	PROBABILITY
Chondrosarcoma	100

COMMENT: As in Figure 82, the growth pattern presents a dynamic, exploding appearance. This tumor, present since age 7, is now so large that if the doubling time were only a year, the rate of increase would seem rapid.

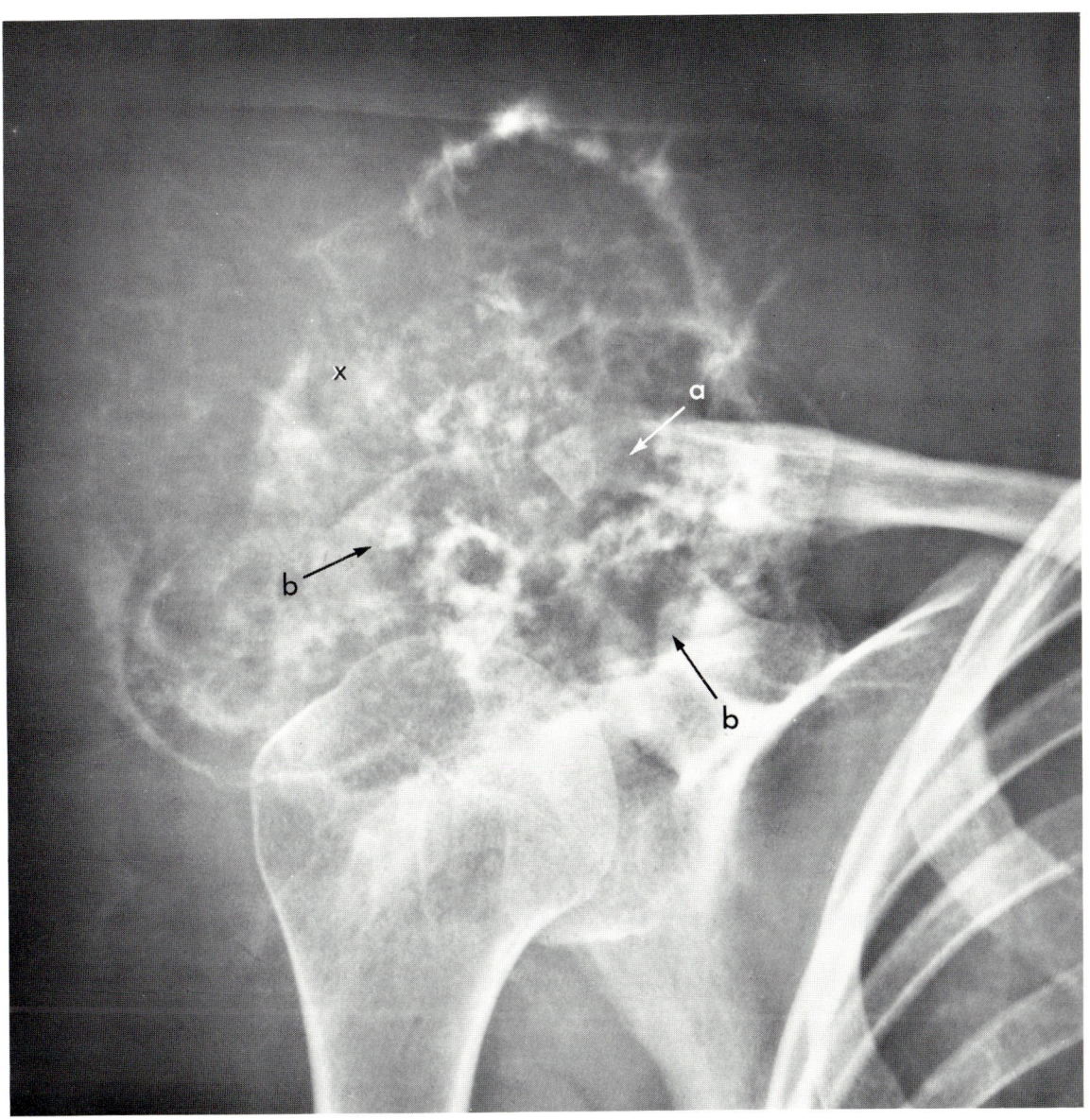

Figure 78 · Chondrosarcoma of Clavicle / 209

Figure 79.—Chondrosarcoma of the finger.

AFIP Case No. 1130060: **A,** posteroanterior, and **B,** lateral views.

DIAGNOSIS AND GRADE.—Chondrosarcoma, finger; growth rate IC.
LIFE INFORMATION.—Male, 59 years; died seven years later of metastases.
LOCATION.—A circumscribed lesion of the entire proximal phalanx; moderate extraosseous extension (**A, x**).

SIZE.—5 × 3 × 2 cm.
MINERALIZATION OF TUMOR.—One ring type floccule (**A, a**).
DESTRUCTION.—Geographic; reticulate moth-eaten contour; cortex penetrated dorsally (**B, b**).
PROLIFERATION.—Cortex of the proximal three-fourths of the first phalanx expanding around the tumor, with subperiosteal spiculation.

DIFFERENTIAL DIAGNOSIS	PROBABILITY
Chondrosarcoma	100

COMMENT: Four years after local treatment, midforearm amputation was required. A surprisingly strong probability for chondrosarcoma in a rare site.

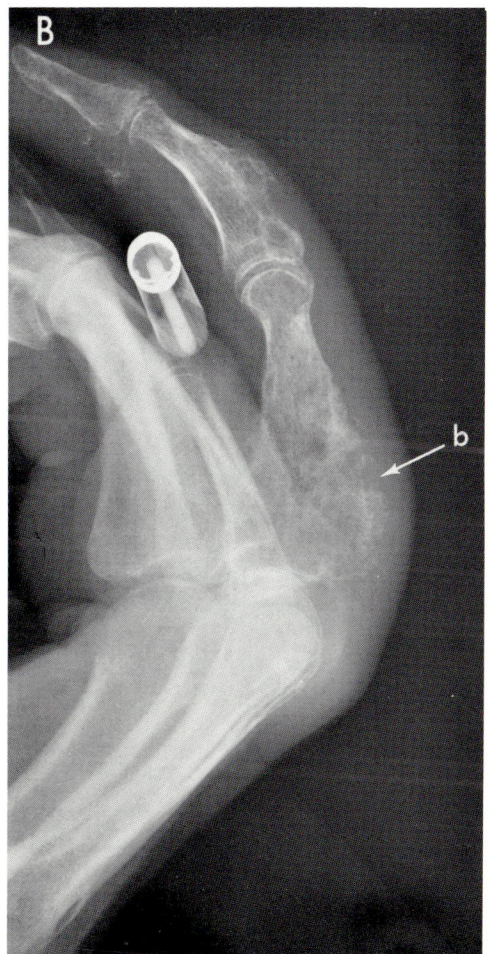
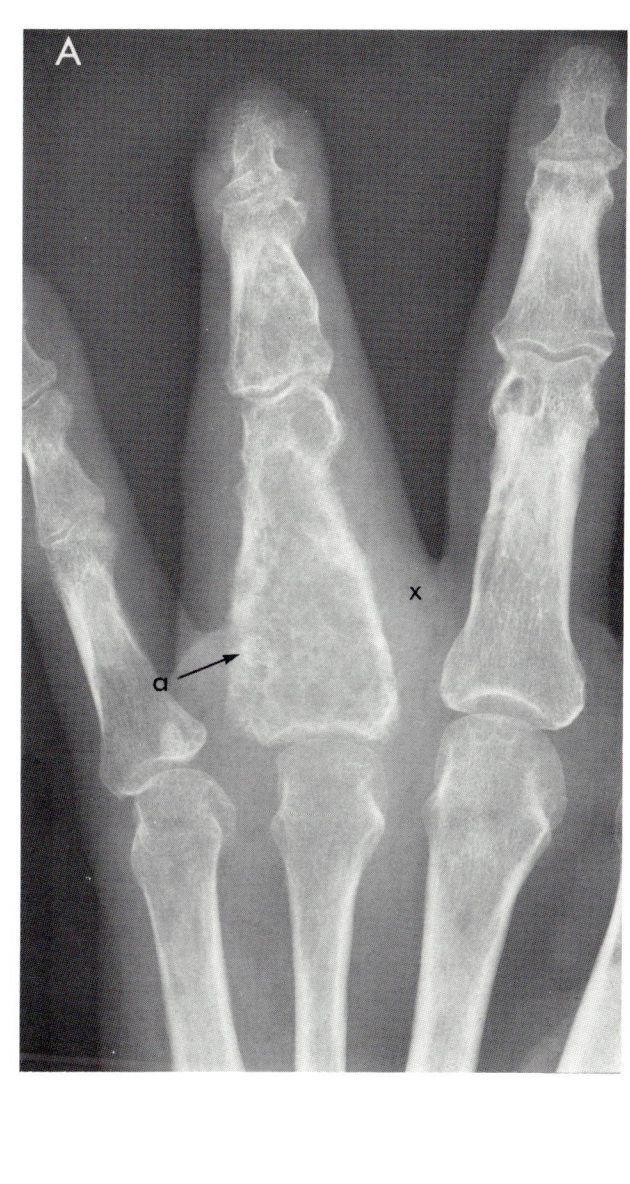

Figure 79 · Chondrosarcoma of Finger

Figure 80.—Chondrosarcoma arising in a calcified enchondroma in the femur.

AFIP Case No. 1109753: **A,** anteroposterior, and **B,** lateral views.

DIAGNOSIS AND GRADE.—Chondrosarcoma arising in calcified enchondroma, femur; growth rate IB.

LIFE INFORMATION. Female, 70 years; died of coronary disease five years after hip disarticulation.

LOCATION.—A circumscribed lesion centered in the proximal shaft of the femur extending into the intertrochanteric area; no extraosseous component.

SIZE.—10 × 4 × 4 cm.

MINERALIZATION OF TUMOR.—Dense floccules of calcified tumor matrix in the center of the lesion (**arrows**).

DESTRUCTION.—Geographic; lobulated contour; early cortical breakthrough laterally (**A, a**) and anteriorly.

PROLIFERATION.—Thick buttress at lower margin of the lesion (**A,b**); medial cortex slightly expanded over the lesion, appearing to encapsulate it (**A, c**).

DIFFERENTIAL DIAGNOSIS	PROBABILITY
Chondrosarcoma	.99
Fibrosarcoma	.01

COMMENT: An ordinary looking chondrosarcoma in a typical location.

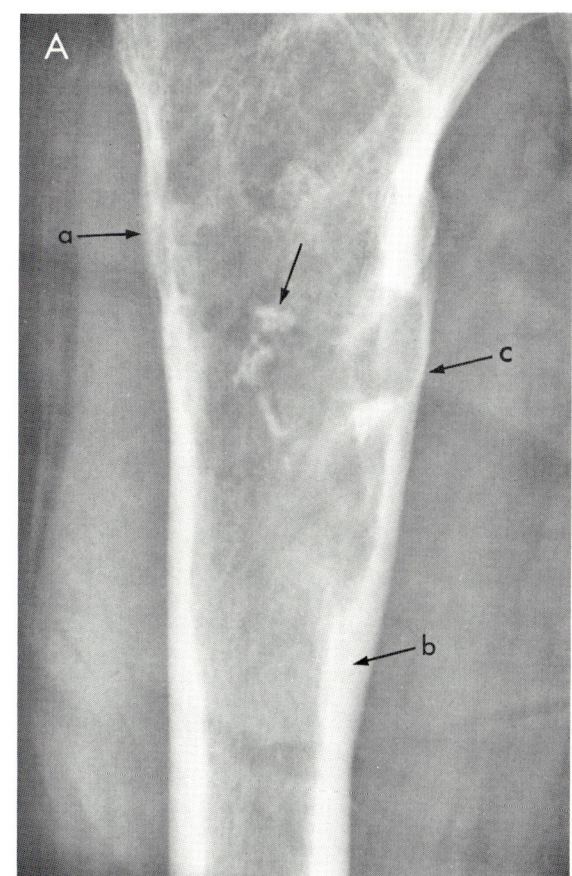
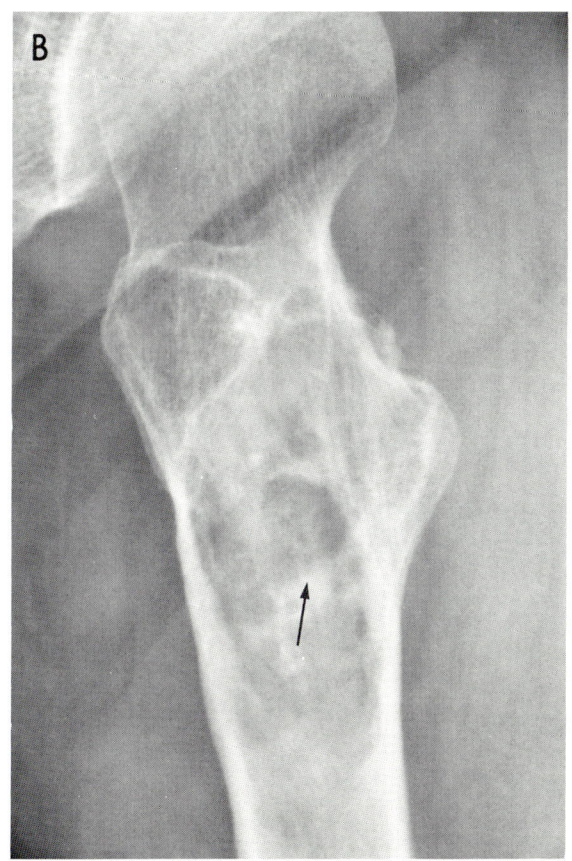

Figure 80 · Chondrosarcoma in Enchondroma of Femur / 213

Figure 81.—Chondrosarcoma of the pelvis.

AFIP Case No. 850094: Anteroposterior projection.

DIAGNOSIS AND GRADE.—Chondrosarcoma, pelvis; growth rate IC.

LIFE INFORMATION.—Male, 65 years; alive 11 years after onset.

LOCATION.—A circumscribed lesion in the acetabulum and pubis; a smaller circumscribed lesion in the ischium.

SIZE.—10 × 6 cm.

MINERALIZATION OF TUMOR.—Possibly a few floccules in the extreme upper end of the lesion and in the smaller ischial lesion.

DESTRUCTION.—Geographic; lobulated.

PROLIFERATION.—More than 1 cm of smooth expansion of the cortex medial to the acetabulum (**a**); dense sclerosis of medullary bone at upper margin of the tumor (**b**); faint septal pattern; amorphous periosteal response (**c**).

DIFFERENTIAL DIAGNOSIS	PROBABILITY
Chondrosarcoma	.99
Chondromyxoid fibroma	< .01
Fibrosarcoma	< .01

COMMENT: This large slowly growing lesion is freely invading the soft tissues in the obturator foramen and below the acetabulum. It is interesting to speculate whether the small satellite lesion in the ischium (**d**) arose de novo or as a metastasis from the primary—probably the former. The dense sclerosis in the upper end of the tumor is present where acetabular weight-bearing forces are brought to focus.

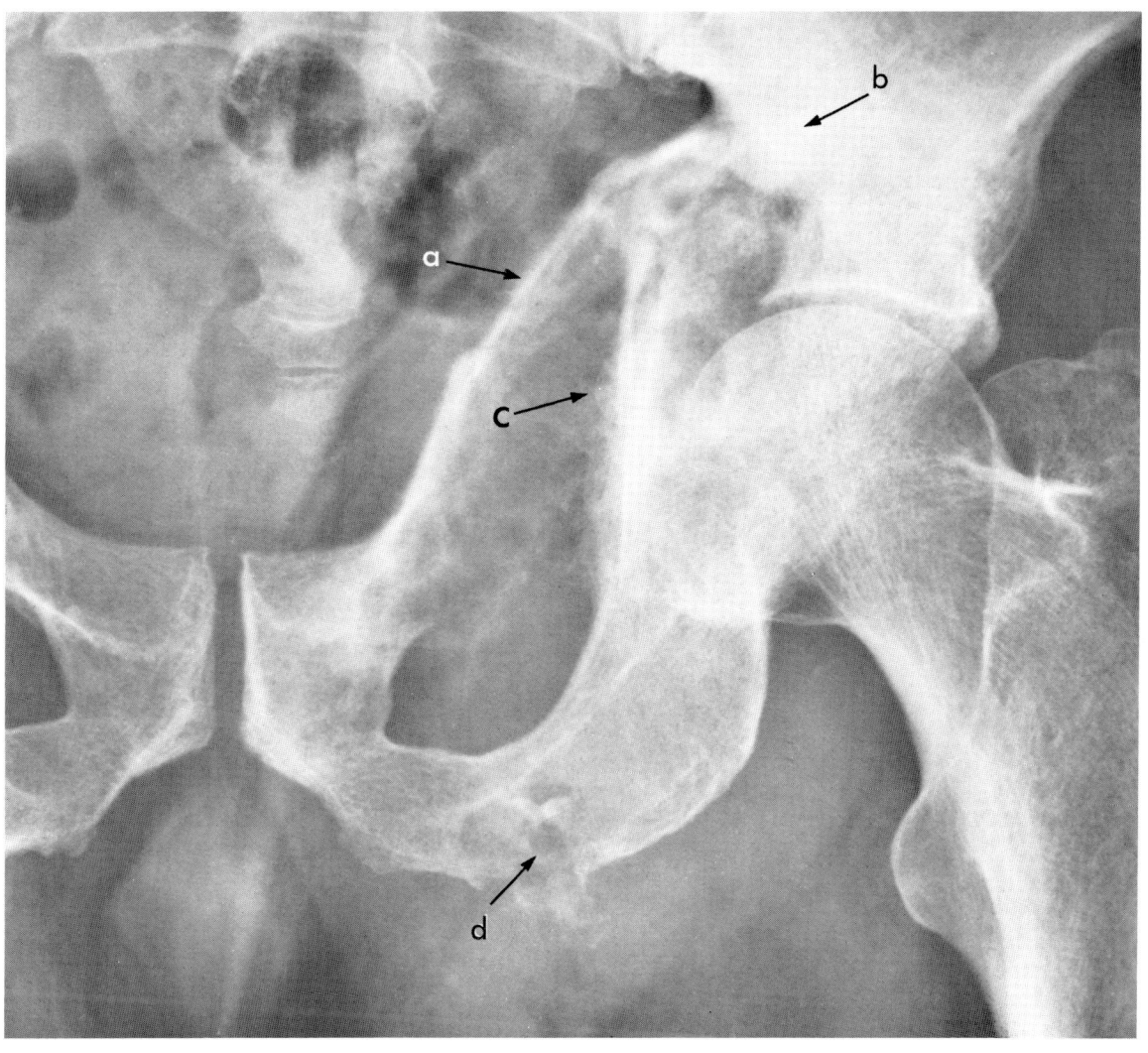

Figure 81 · Chondrosarcoma of Pelvis / 215

Figure 82.—Chondrosarcoma of the femur.

AFIP Case No. 1130957: Anteroposterior projection.

DIAGNOSIS AND GRADE.—Chondrosarcoma, femur; growth rate IC.

LIFE INFORMATION. Male, 54 years; died of metastases.

LOCATION.—A huge, partially circumscribed lesion involving the upper half of the femoral shaft; large extraosseous component.

SIZE.—30 × 15 cm.

MINERALIZATION OF TUMOR.—There are a few floccules of dense tumor bone (**a**) in the medullary portion. In the extraosseous component, numerous crescentic shadows of calcified, or possibly ossified, matrix (**arrows**) have an organized appearance, their convexities face outward from the tumor, and some are at the edge.

DESTRUCTION.—Geographic; slightly lobulated contour.

PROLIFERATION.—The cortex is symmetrically expanded more than 1 cm over the major length of the lesion. The cortical shell does not completely encapsulate the lesion and is thickened and supported by buttresses below (**b**). There are some sloping spicules of periosteal new bone medially (**c**).

DIFFERENTIAL DIAGNOSIS	PROBABILITY
Chondrosarcoma	.96
Fibrosarcoma	.03

COMMENT: The combination of expanded cortex, spicules and crescentic pattern of calcified matrix in the extraosseous component presents a dynamic image of an exploding tumor. At this stage of growth, more than a year after diagnosis, the tumor is undoubtedly enlarging rapidly.

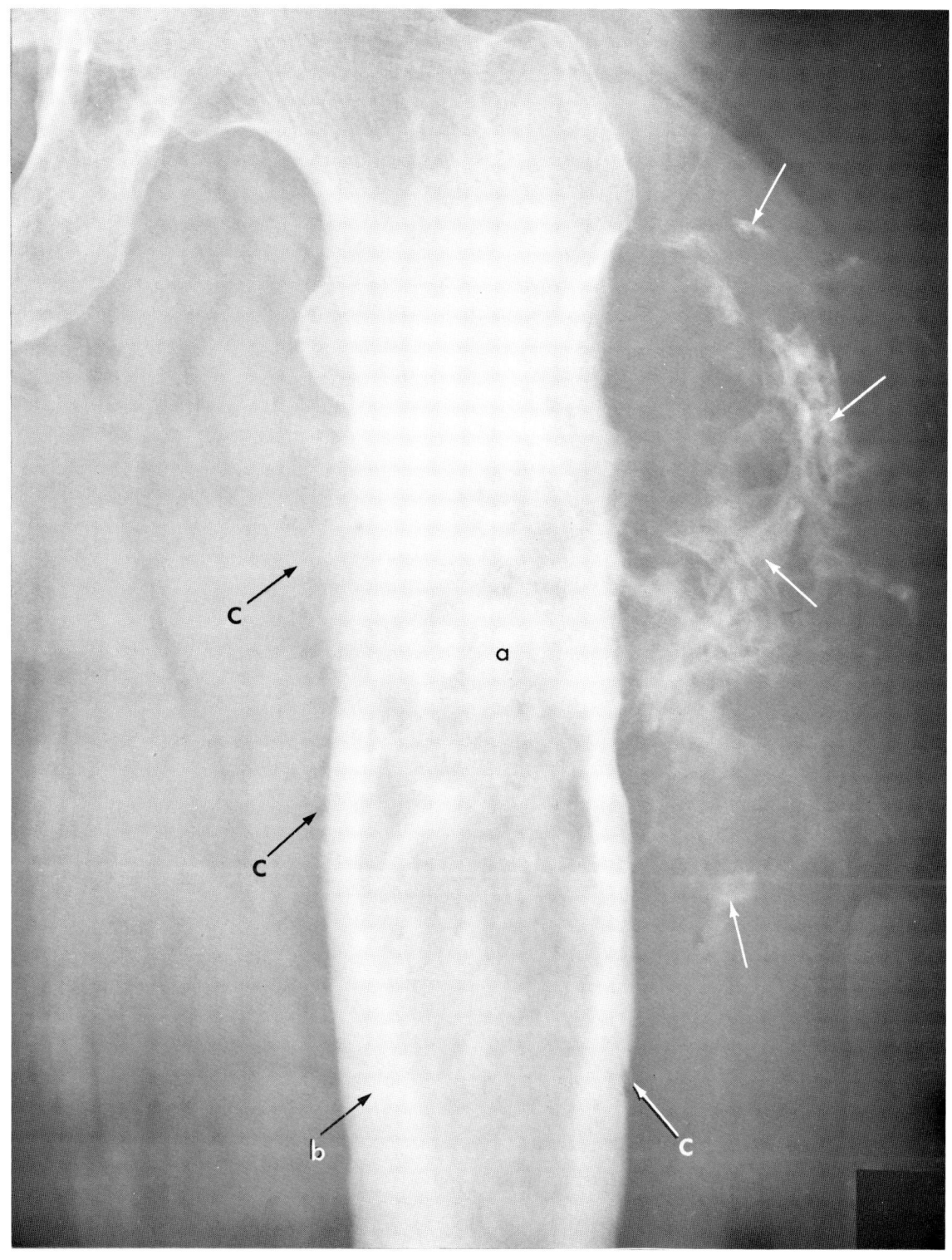

Figure 82 · Chondrosarcoma of Femur / 217

Figure 83.—Chondrosarcomas of the pubis and rib.

AFIP Case No. 1154401: **A,** anteroposterior projection.

DIAGNOSIS AND GRADE.—Chondrosarcoma, pubis; growth rate IB.

LIFE INFORMATION.—Male, 20 years; alive three years after onset.

LOCATION.—An extensive lesion in the pubis and ischium; no extraosseous component.

SIZE.—9 × 5 cm.

MINERALIZATION OF TUMOR.—Clouds, floccules and circles of calcified matrix scattered throughout the lesion.

DESTRUCTION.—Geographic; lobulated contour.

PROLIFERATION.—The cortex enveloping a major part of the lesion (**arrows**), expanded nearly 1 cm; marginal sclerosis near the acetabulum (**a**); an ill-defined septate pattern.

DIFFERENTIAL DIAGNOSIS	PROBABILITY
Chondrosarcoma	.96
Fibrosarcoma	.03

COMMENT: A typical slowly growing chondrosarcoma. Note the healed Legg-Perthes deformity on the left (**x**).

AFIP Case No. 1203575: **B,** anteroposterior projection.

DIAGNOSIS AND GRADE.—Chondrosarcoma, rib; not graded.

LIFE INFORMATION.—Male, 71 years; onset 13 years before.

LOCATION.—A large mass involving principally one rib (**x**) and soft tissues of the chest and flank.

SIZE.—Estimated 20 × 20 cm.

MINERALIZATION OF TUMOR.—Extensive flocculent calcification (**b**), circles (**c**) and some fairly solid areas of tumor matrix mineralization (**d**); crescentic patterns at the margin (**e**).

DESTRUCTION.—Obscured by tumor.

PROLIFERATION.—Obscured by tumor.

DIFFERENTIAL DIAGNOSIS	PROBABILITY
Chondrosarcoma	.96
Chondrosarcoma of mesenchymal or synovial origin	.03

COMMENT: Compare with Figure 86; one appears to be very slowly growing and the other rapidly, yet at the end, both are huge, necrotic and gas-containing.

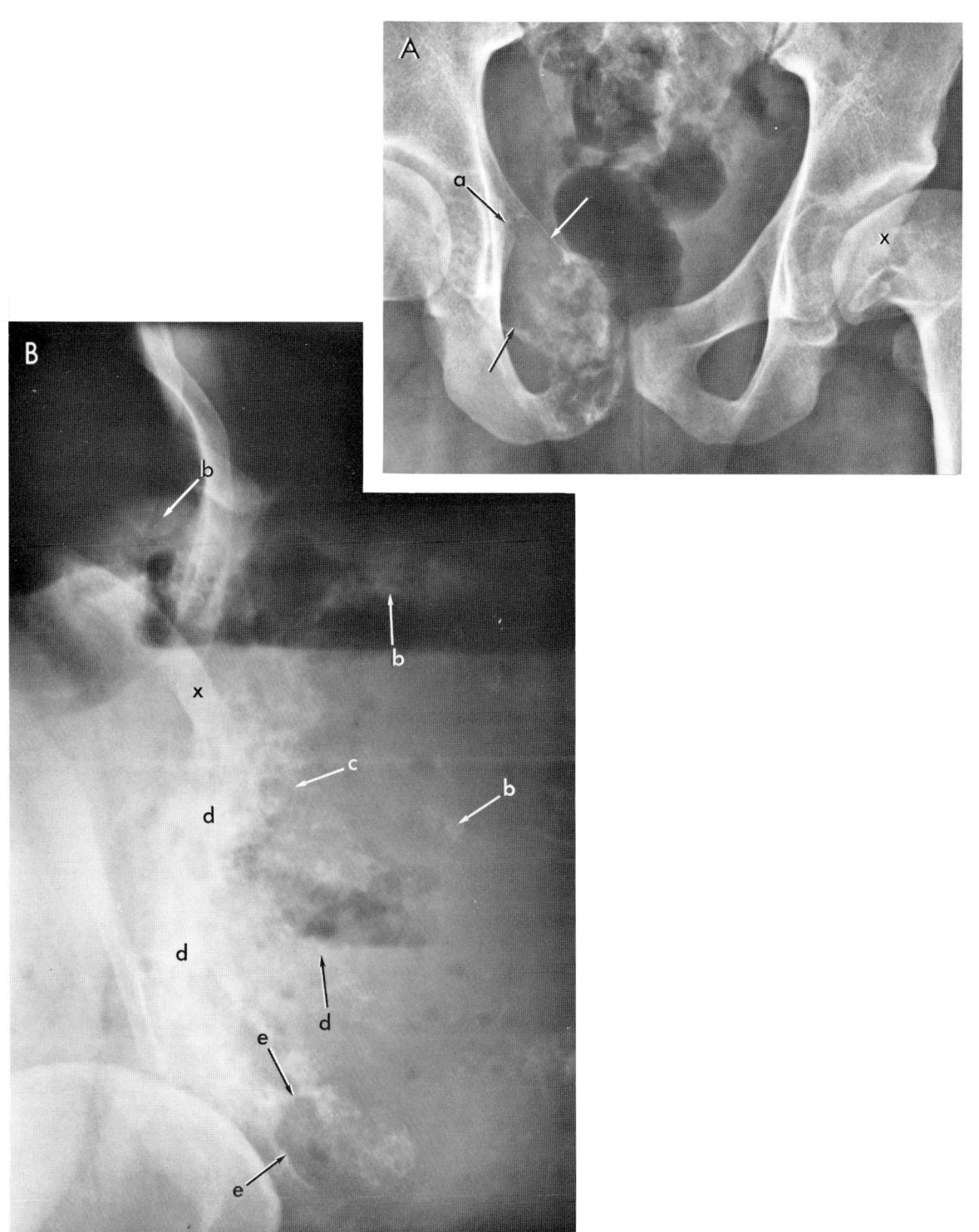

Figure 83 · Chondrosarcomas of Pubis and Rib / 219

Figure 84.—Chondrosarcoma arising in a calcified enchondroma in the humerus.

AFIP Case No. 1010529: Anteroposterior views—**A,** initial study; **B,** at 1 month; **C,** at 3½ months.

DIAGNOSIS AND GRADE.—Chondrosarcoma in calcified enchondroma, humerus; growth rate II.

LIFE INFORMATION.—Female, 71 years; lived 10 months after onset.

LOCATION.—Initially a circumscribed lesion in the proximal three-fourths of the shaft, metaphysis and epiphysis.

SIZE.—18 × 5 cm.

MINERALIZATION OF TUMOR.—Dense flocculent pattern of calcified matrix in center of the upper portion (**A, a**).

DESTRUCTION.—Generally geographic; moth-eaten areas.

PROLIFERATION.—Expanded shell with buttresses surrounds the focal lesion in midshaft; little other periosteal response.

One month later (**B**) a medial detached bone fragment (**b**) is being carried into axillary soft tissue by the tumor.

Three and one-half months later (**C**) tumor diameter is increased over 3 cm; continued rapid disintegration of upper half of humerus; some moth-eaten areas, but dissolution is unclear, the bone seeming to melt away; permeation hard to identify.

DIFFERENTIAL DIAGNOSIS	PROBABILITY
Chondrosarcoma	.95
Fibrosarcoma	.04
Osteosarcoma	< .01
Reticulum cell sarcoma	< .01

COMMENT: An exploding chondrosarcoma. A defect is first seen in the medial cortex of the metaphysis (**A, c**). In a month a fragment is detached and being *displaced* into soft tissues. Later, an entire cortical segment is displaced. Much of the destruction is geographic. It seems wise to predict behavior from the most aggressive portion of the lesion, and bone destruction in the humeral head seems of moth-eaten type.

An initial diagnosis was chondromyxoid fibroma, but the age group is wrong and we have yet to see one in a long bone which contains flocculent calcification. Another diagnosis was malignant giant cell tumor. There seem to be two separate new lesions arising at opposite ends of an old calcified enchondroma and growing at different rates.

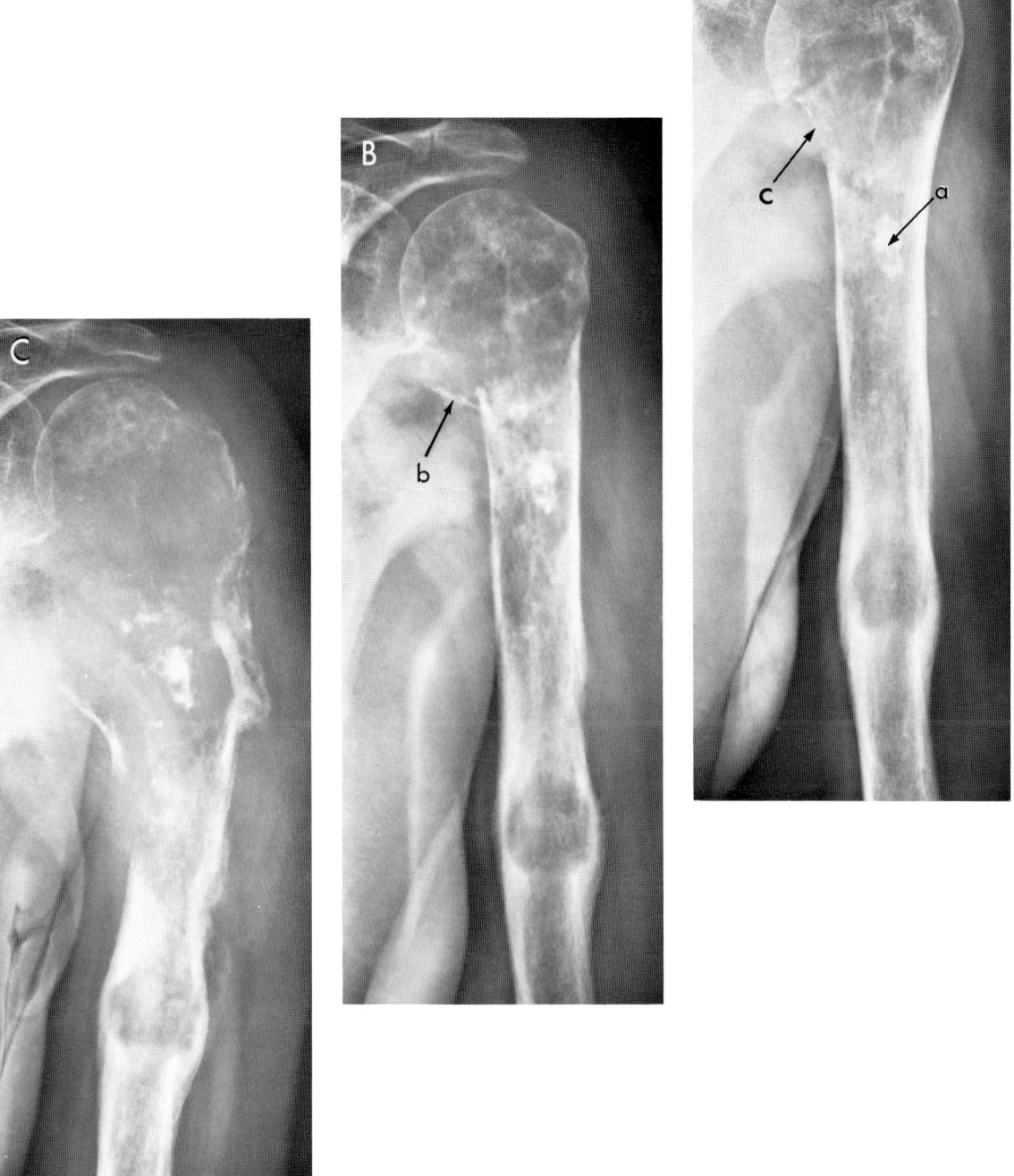

Figure 84 · Chondrosarcoma in Enchondroma of Humerus / 221

Figure 85.—Chondrosarcoma in a benign lesion of the femur.

AFIP Case No. 1181318: **A,** anteroposterior, and **B,** lateral views.

DIAGNOSIS AND GRADE.—Chondrosarcoma arising in antecedent benign lesion, femur; growth rate IC.

LIFE INFORMATION.—Female, 39 years; well two years after disarticulation.

LOCATION.—A circumscribed lesion centered eccentrically at the level of the fused growth plate of the lateral femoral condyle, extending anteriorly into the soft tissues. A second larger and more slowly growing lesion involves the entire distal end of the femur.

SIZE.—3 × 3 × 5 cm (including extraosseous extension).

MINERALIZATION OF TUMOR.—None identified in the tumor itself; in the older lesion are multiple floccules characteristic of calcification in cartilage (**arrows**).

DESTRUCTION.—Geographic; regular contour.

PROLIFERATION.—A dense zone of marginal sclerosis with amorphous periosteal response (**B, a**) when the tumor penetrates the cortex.

DIFFERENTIAL DIAGNOSIS	PROBABILITY
Fibrosarcoma	.55
Chondrosarcoma	.41
Cartilaginous tumor	.02
Chondromyxoid fibroma	< .01
Osteosarcoma	< .01

COMMENT: There was a long history of disease, with bowing of the leg noted at age 12. The lesion was first called giant cell tumor by the computer *because* only the destroyed area was described. The strong probability which resulted when flocculent calcification was added to information given to the computer was seriously eroded by the presence of amorphous periosteal response, much in favor of fibrosarcoma.

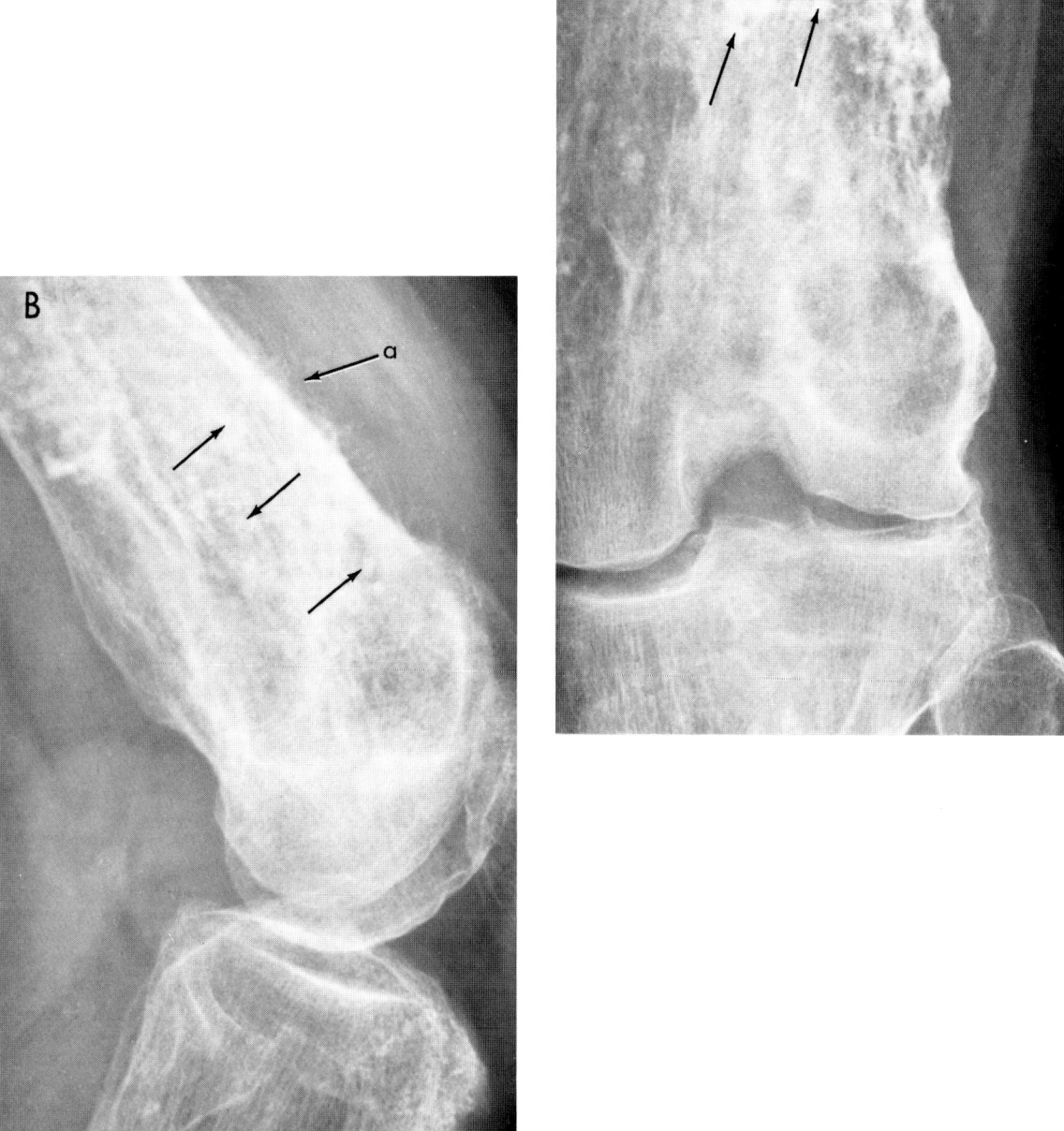

Figure 85 · Chondrosarcoma in Benign Lesion of Femur / 223

Figure 86.—Chondrosarcoma of the pelvis.

AFIP Case No. 1135837: Anteroposterior views—**A,** initial study; **B,** at seven weeks; **C,** at three months.

DIAGNOSIS AND GRADE.—Chondrosarcoma, pelvis; growth rate III.
LIFE INFORMATION.—Male, 20 years.
LOCATION.—The initial lesion is a relatively small diffuse tumor in the lateral aspect of the ilium; as time passes, there is rapid progression through the ilium and into the soft tissue (**B, arrow**).

SIZE.—Initially 8 × 4 cm; seven weeks later 12 × 10 cm; three months later 30 × 20 cm.

MINERALIZATION OF TUMOR.—From the beginning, there are collections of flocculent and cloudy calcified tumor matrix within the tumor.

DESTRUCTION.—Permeative pattern.

PROLIFERATION.—Perhaps some mottled reparative response in spongy bone, but more probably calcified tumor matrix.

DIFFERENTIAL DIAGNOSIS	PROBABILITY
Osteosarcoma	.78
Chondrosarcoma	.20
Ewing's sarcoma	< .01
Fibrosarcoma	< .01
Reticulum cell sarcoma	< .01

COMMENT: This tumor grows extraordinarily rapidly for a chondrosarcoma and, in **C,** contains extensive necrosis and gas (**x**). The patient's youth and the aggressive growth are much in favor of osteosarcoma.

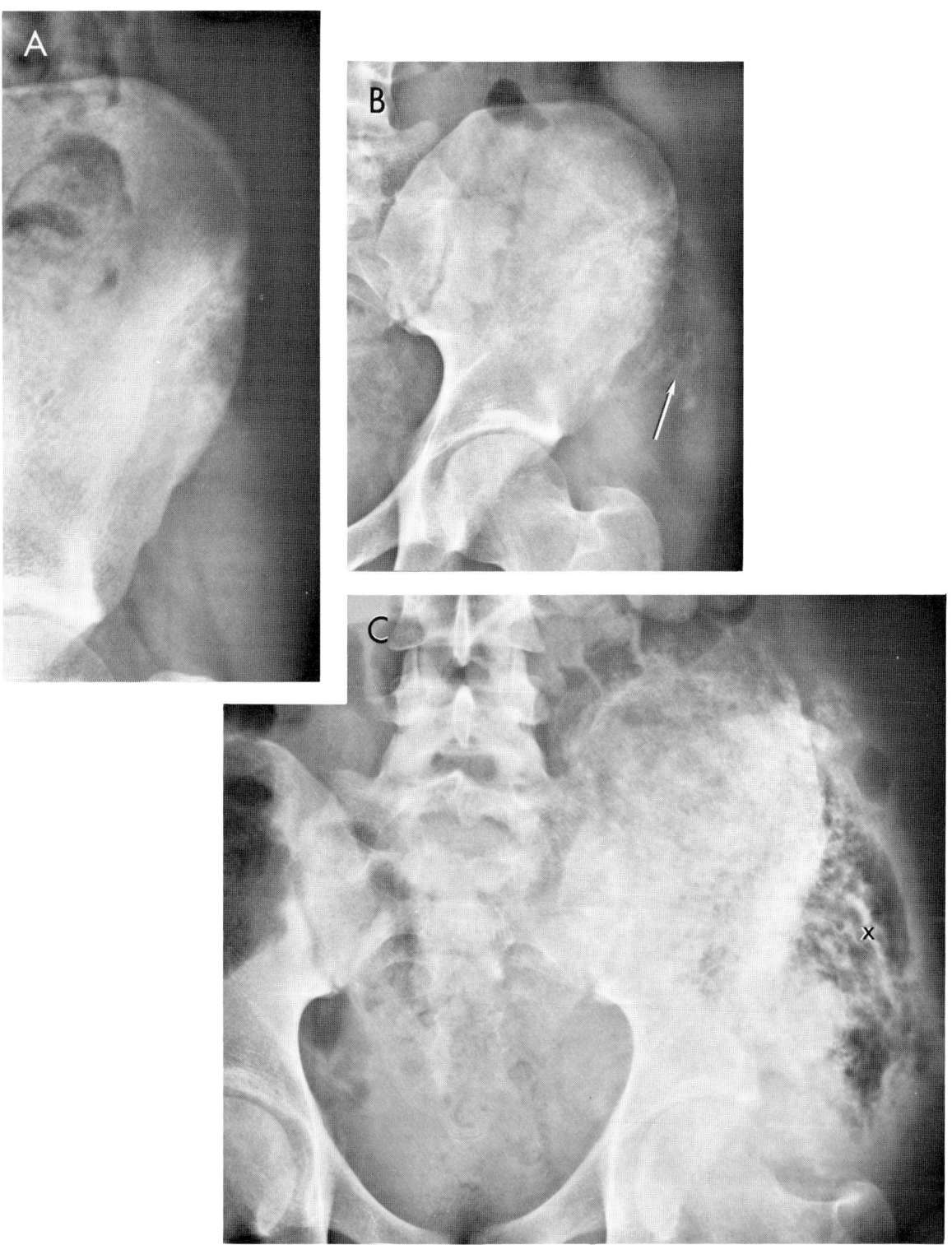

Figure 86 · Chondrosarcoma of Pelvis / 225

Figure 87.—Chondrosarcoma of the astragalus.

AFIP Case No. 1182899: **A,** anteroposterior view initially; **B,** anteroposterior, and **C,** lateral projections four years later.

DIAGNOSIS AND GRADE.—Chondrosarcoma, astragalus; not graded.

LIFE INFORMATION.—Male, 30 years; well seven years after onset.

LOCATION.—A diffuse lesion arising on the medial surface, ultimately with large extraosseous component.

SIZE.—Initially a vaguely outlined shell just below the medial malleolus, about 2 × 1 cm.

MINERALIZATION OF TUMOR.—None initially.

DESTRUCTION.—A small geographic excavation on the medial surface with smooth regular base (**A, a**).

PROLIFERATION.—Narrow zone of bone sclerosis around the destroyed area, with very thin shell of periosteal bone.

Four years later (**B** and **C**), size has increased to 4 × 3 × 2 cm, the lesion now involving both bone and soft tissues (**arrows**), with heavily calcified matrix (**x**).

DIFFERENTIAL DIAGNOSIS	PROBABILITY
Benign cartilaginous tumor	.97
Chondrosarcoma	.02

COMMENT: Initial diagnosis was bone cyst, with chondrosarcoma not diagnosed until four years after onset of symptoms. The computer has difficulty deciding between a benign and a malignant cartilaginous tumor.

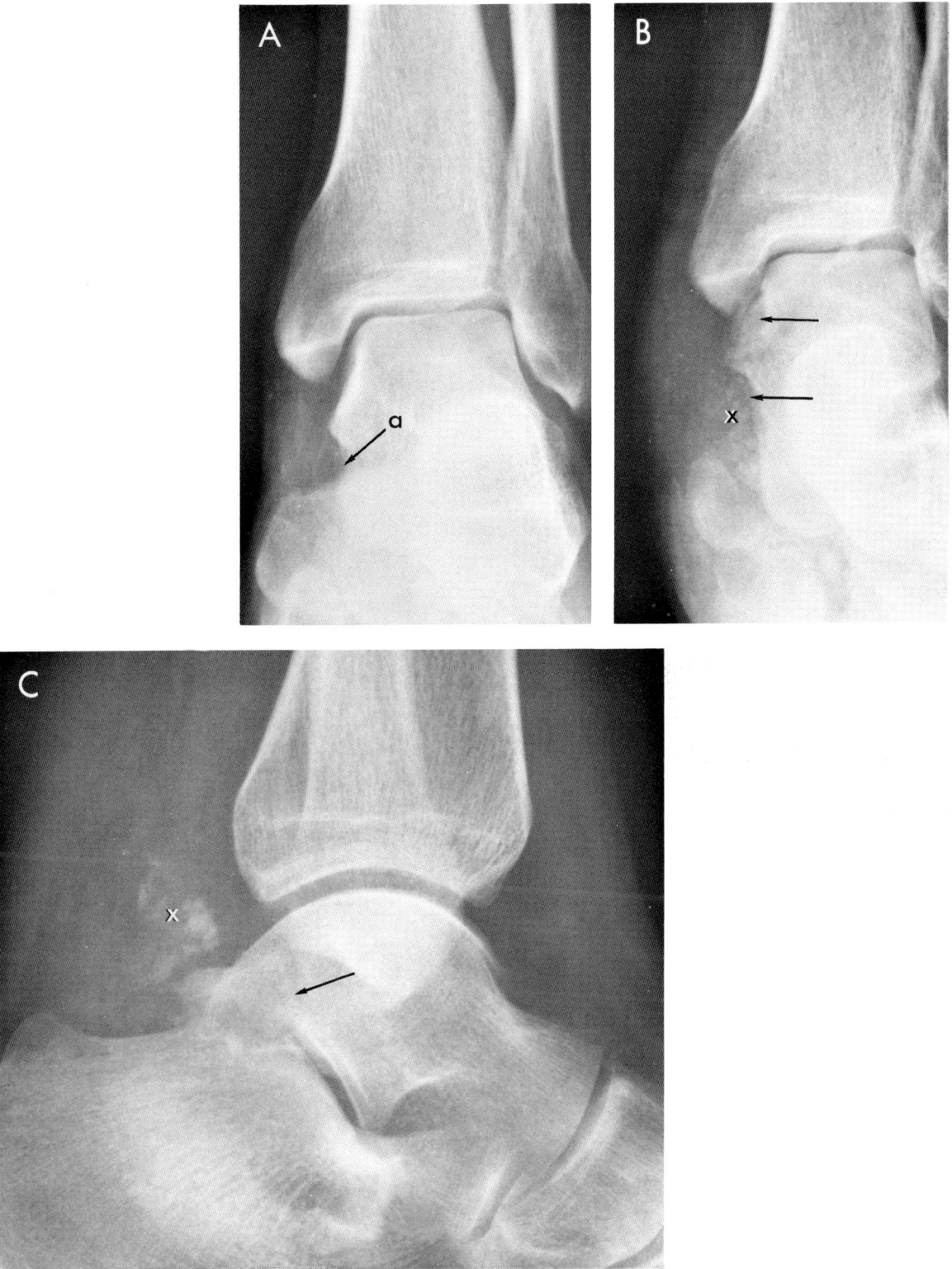

Figure 87 · Chondrosarcoma of Astragalus / 227

Figure 88.—Chondrosarcomas of the rib and tibia.

AFIP Case No. 1194779: **A,** anteroposterior projection.

DIAGNOSIS AND GRADE.—Chondrosarcoma, rib; growth rate III.

LIFE INFORMATION.—Male, 19 years; lesion first noted on intravenous pyelogram; survived about 18 months.

LOCATION.—A large ill-defined lesion involving the twelfth rib.

SIZE.—11 × 5 cm.

MINERALIZATION OF TUMOR.—Lumps, clouds and floccules of calcified tumor matrix throughout (**arrows**); no crescentic matrix shadows.

DESTRUCTION.—Permeative, largely obscured by calcified tumor matrix.

PROLIFERATION.—Questionable mottled proliferative change.

DIFFERENTIAL DIAGNOSIS	PROBABILITY
Osteosarcoma	.98
Chondrosarcoma	.01

COMMENT: Radiologic differentiation of osteosarcoma and chondrosarcoma is difficult here, although the characteristics in either instance are those of a highly malignant tumor. Because mottling was questionable, it was omitted in the computer analysis, following the policy that *questionable findings not be included.*

AFIP Case No. 1142139: **B,** lateral, and **C,** anteroposterior views.

DIAGNOSIS AND GRADE.—Chondrosarcoma, tibia; growth rate IC.

LIFE INFORMATION.—Female, 15 years; survival unknown.

LOCATION.—A diffuse eccentric lesion in the proximal third of the proximal metaphysis; large extraosseous component.

SIZE.—Estimated 4 × 4 × 4 cm.

MINERALIZATION OF TUMOR.—None definite.

DESTRUCTION.—Single lamina of periosteal new bone with Codman's triangle (**a**); above, a crescentic shadow (**B, b**) at edge of tumor is assumed, in absence of tumor matrix mineralization elsewhere, to be periosteal; intramedullary proliferation not clear.

DIFFERENTIAL DIAGNOSIS	PROBABILITY
Osteosarcoma	.99
Chondrosarcoma	< .01

COMMENT: For evaluation of growth rate the type of bone destruction is largely unknown. The best case can be made for geographic bone destruction, but the active periosteal response and large extraosseous component imply a more aggressive lesion.

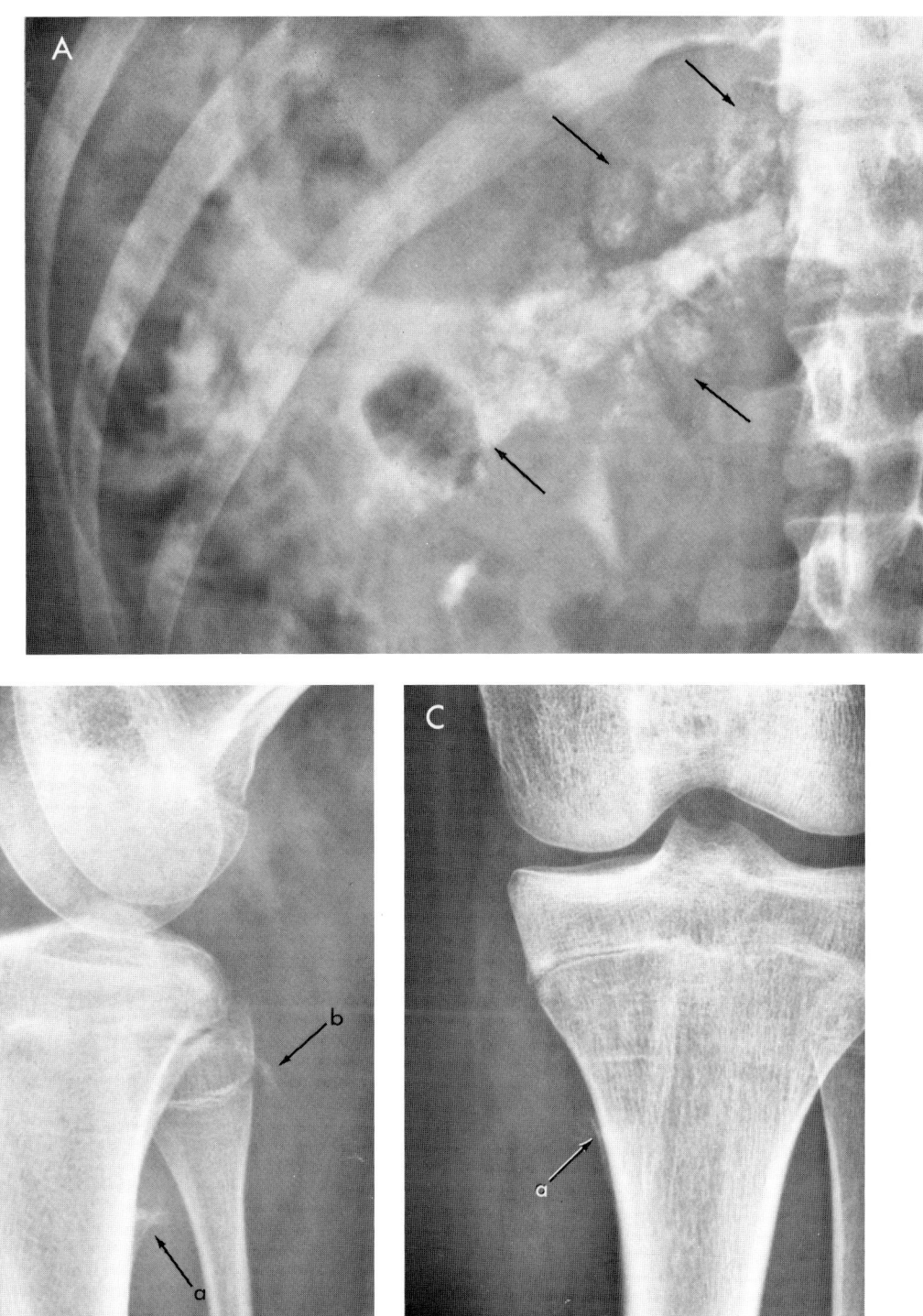

Figure 88 · Chondrosarcomas of Rib & Tibia / 229

Figure 89.—Chondrosarcoma of the femur.

AFIP Case No. 1170056: Anteroposterior views—**A,** initial study; **B,** five weeks later; **C,** one year later.

DIAGNOSIS AND GRADE.—Chondrosarcoma, femur; growth rate IC.

LIFE INFORMATION.—Male, 20 years; died 20 months after treatment.

LOCATION.—Initially, an ill-defined lesion in the medial condyle, centered in the distal third of the metaphysis.

SIZE.—Initially, estimated 4 × 4 cm.

MINERALIZATION OF TUMOR.—With growth, progressively larger amounts of flocculent and cloudy tumor bone.

DESTRUCTION.—Initially, destruction apparently early geographic, largely reduction of spongy bone, and difficult to visualize (**A, arrows**).

PROLIFERATION.—Slight irregular periosteal response at first.

Five weeks later (**B**), after biopsy, the lesion is much better circumscribed, with definite extraosseous component (**b**) and clearly geographic pattern with ragged contour. A dense broad zone of reactive sclerosis (**a**) has developed around the destroyed area (**x**) and a single lamina of periosteal new bone has appeared (**c**).

One year later (**C**) the tumor is now 15 × 12 cm. Large amounts of flocculent and cloudy tumor bone (**d**). The basic pattern is still geographic, but with moth-eaten components laterally (**x**). The single lamina has consolidated, and much of the marginal reactive response has disappeared.

	DIFFERENTIAL DIAGNOSIS	PROBABILITY
Exam. 1	Osteosarcoma	1.00
Exam. 2	Osteosarcoma	.95
	Chondrosarcoma	.02
	Fibrosarcoma	.01

COMMENT: The clue to early diagnosis here is the rather large area of cancellous bone reduction. The computer is at least consistent in its analysis of this lesion.

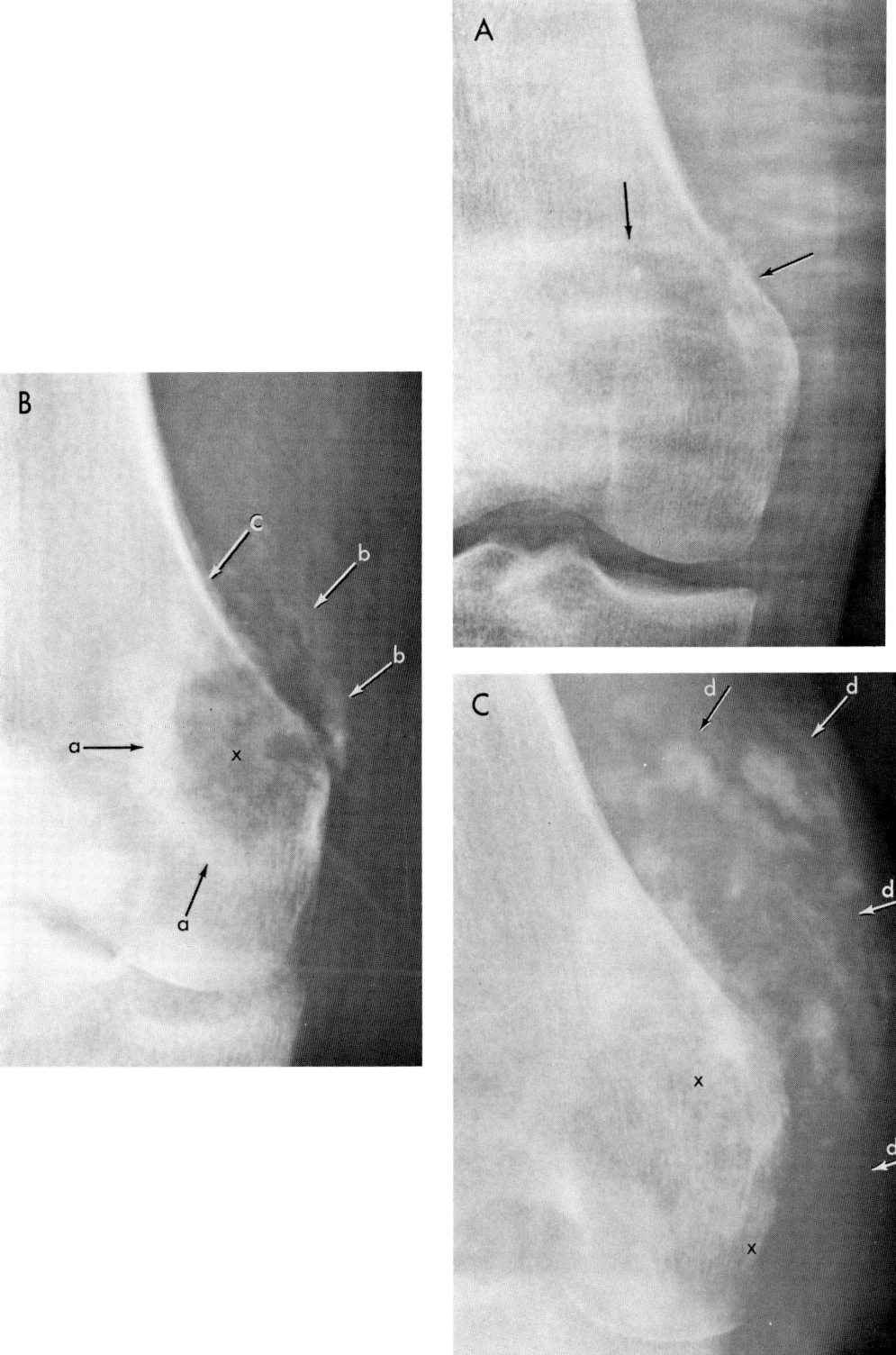

Figure 89 · Chondrosarcoma of Femur / 231

Figure 90.—Chondrosarcoma of the pelvis.

AFIP Case No. 1100836: Anteroposterior projection.

DIAGNOSIS AND GRADE.—Chondrosarcoma, pelvis; growth rate III.
LIFE INFORMATION.—Male, 53 years; survived about two months.
LOCATION.—A diffuse lesion involving the acetabulum and lower ilium, with large soft tissue component in the pelvis (**arrows**).
SIZE.—10 × 8 cm.
MINERALIZATION OF TUMOR.—None.
DESTRUCTION.—Permeative; reduction of cancellous bone (**a**).
PROLIFERATION.—A few mottled foci in the acetabular roof (**b**).

DIFFERENTIAL DIAGNOSIS	PROBABILITY
Reticulum cell sarcoma	.94
Fibrosarcoma	.02
Chondrosarcoma	.01
Osteosarcoma	.01

COMMENT: A typical example of permeative destruction in that most osseous landmarks are retained despite diffuse involvement. Such destruction is far more typical of reticulum cell sarcoma than of chondrosarcoma. This, plus absence of matrix mineralization, created the strong probability for reticulum cell sarcoma.

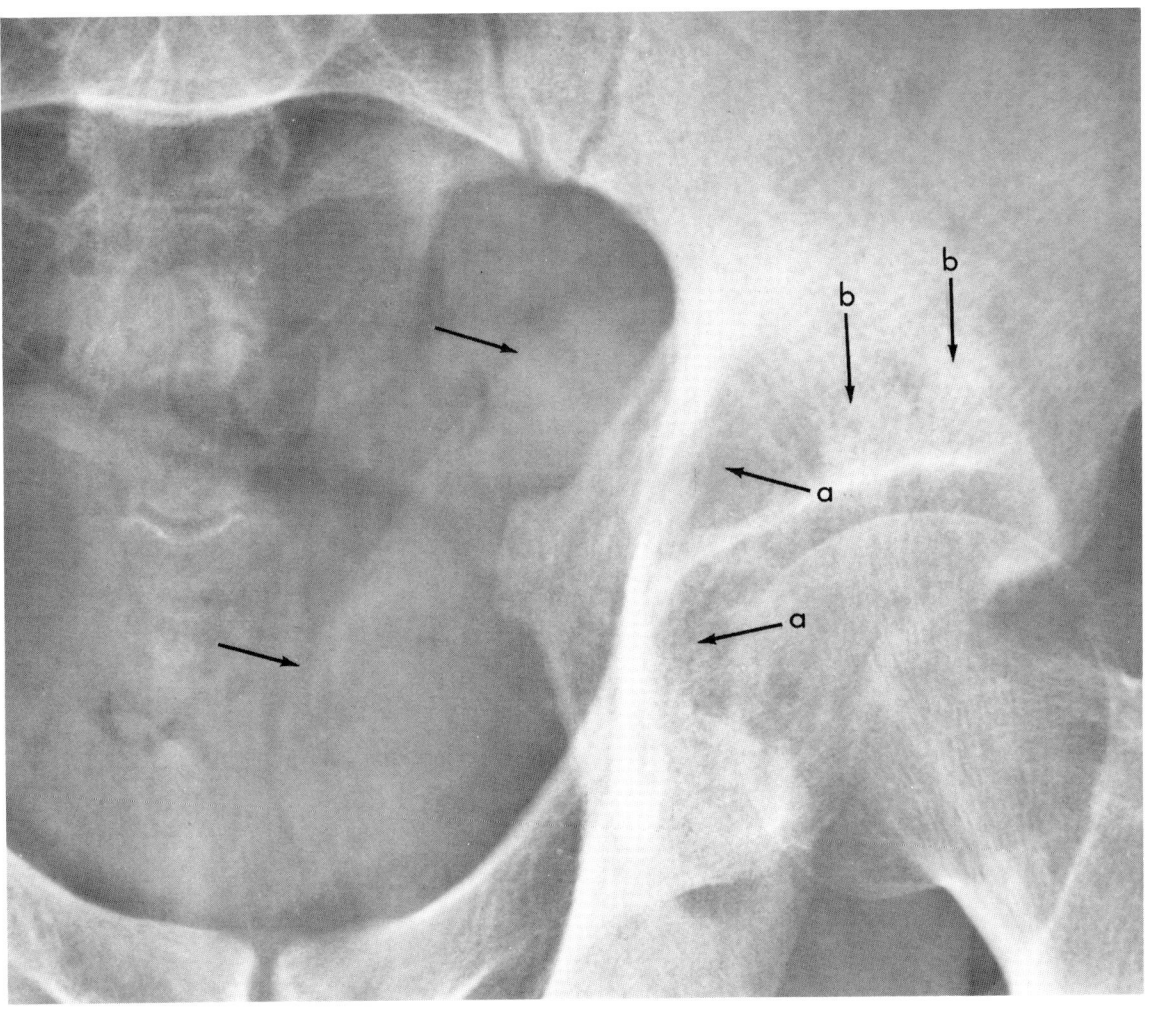

Figure 90 · Chondrosarcoma of Pelvis / 233

Figure 91.—Chondrosarcoma of the pelvis.

AFIP Case No. 1138139: Anteroposterior projection.

DIAGNOSIS AND GRADE.—Chondrosarcoma, pelvis; growth rate III.

LIFE INFORMATION.—Male, 52 years; survived three months after hemipelvectomy.

LOCATION.—A diffuse lesion of the pubis (**a**) with large extraosseous component (**arrows**) demonstrated by displacement of the opacified bladder (**x**).

SIZE.—12 × 10 cm.

MINERALIZATION OF TUMOR.—None.

DESTRUCTION.—Permeative pattern with penetration of the cortex; pathologic fracture (**b**).

PROLIFERATION.—A single thick, slightly irregular lamina of periosteal new bone on the superior surface of the pubis (**c**).

DIFFERENTIAL DIAGNOSIS	PROBABILITY
Reticulum cell sarcoma	.94
Fibrosarcoma	.02
Chondrosarcoma	.01
Osteosarcoma	.01

COMMENT: There is nothing to identify this lesion conclusively as chondrosarcoma. As in Figure 90, the absence of matrix mineralization and presence of the permeative pattern of destruction strongly favor the probability for reticulum cell sarcoma in this age group. Even so, I believe I would have placed chondrosarcoma first because of the large pelvic mass, which I have not seen in reticulum cell sarcoma in this location.

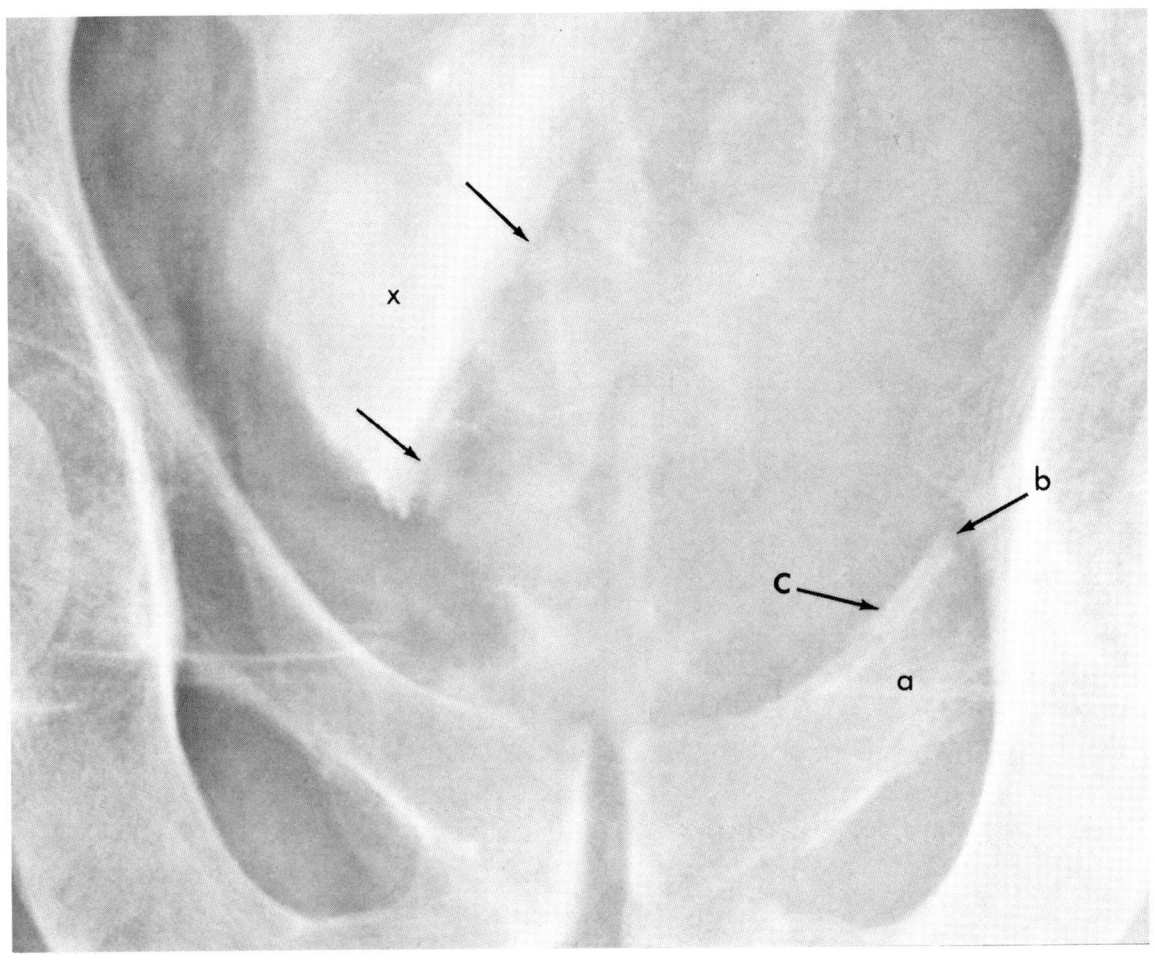

Figure 91 · Chondrosarcoma of Pelvis / 235

Figure 92.—Chondroblastomas of the humerus and tibia.

AFIP Case No. 1074141: **A,** anteroposterior projection.

DIAGNOSIS AND GRADE.—Chondroblastoma, humerus; growth rate IB.

LIFE INFORMATION.—Male, 16 years; well 42 months later.

LOCATION.—A circumscribed lesion centered in the proximal epiphysis, extending through the growth plate to adjacent edge of the metaphysis; no extraosseous component.

SIZE.—5 × 3.5 cm.

MINERALIZATION OF TUMOR.—Suggestion of flocculent calcification.

DESTRUCTION.—Geographic; regular contour.

PROLIFERATION.—Thin zone of marginal sclerosis (**a**); cortex, expanded more than 1 cm laterally, enveloping the tumor; periosteal new bone thick and irregular over expanded portion of the tumor (**b**); dense hyperostosis on lateral cortex of the metaphysis (**c**).

DIFFERENTIAL DIAGNOSIS	PROBABILITY
Chondroblastoma	100

COMMENT: The radiographic pattern is typical, especially with hyperostosis of the adjacent shaft.

AFIP Case No. 1162659: **B,** anteroposterior view.

DIAGNOSIS AND GRADE.—Chondroblastoma, tibia; growth rate IC.

LIFE INFORMATION.—Male, 13 years.

LOCATION.—A small circumscribed lesion centered eccentrically in the proximal epiphysis (**arrow**).

SIZE.—1.5 × 1 cm.

MINERALIZATION OF TUMOR.—Several dense floccules of tumor mineralization in the center of the lesion.

DESTRUCTION.—Geographic; regular contour; tumor penetrating the cortex laterally (**d**).

PROLIFERATION.—Distinct marginal sclerosis; no periosteal response in the involved bone.

DIFFERENTIAL DIAGNOSIS	PROBABILITY
Chondroblastoma	100

COMMENT: Evidence of tumor matrix mineralization is quite definite.

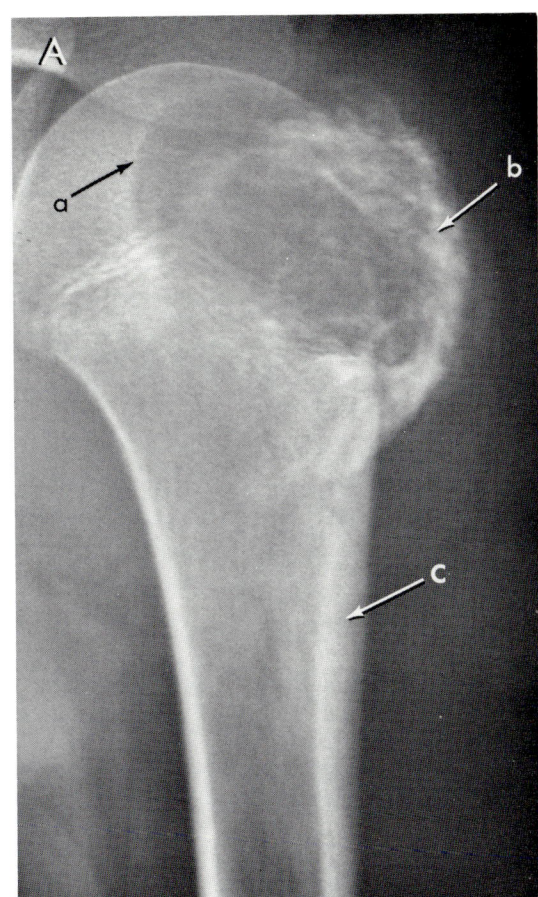
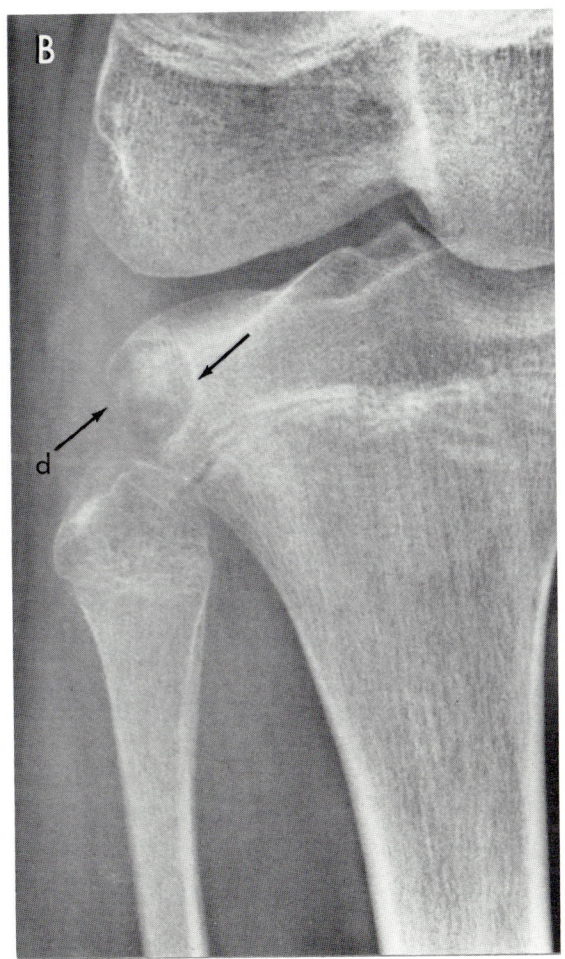

Figure 92 · Chondroblastomas of Humerus & Tibia

Figure 93.—Chondroblastomas of the tibia and humerus.

AFIP Case No. 909973: **A,** anteroposterior projection.

DIAGNOSIS AND GRADE.—Cystic chondroblastoma, tibia; growth rate IA.
LIFE INFORMATION.—Male, 23 years.
LOCATION.—A small circumscribed lesion centered eccentrically at the fused growth plate in the proximal tibia, extending into epiphysis and metaphysis; no extraosseous component.
SIZE.—3 × 2.5 cm.
MINERALIZATION OF TUMOR.—None definite; several foci of increased density along the upper edge may represent flocculent calcification but are indistinguishable from the proliferative response.
DESTRUCTION.—Geographic; regular contour.
PROLIFERATION.—Dense sclerotic rim; no periosteal response.

DIFFERENTIAL DIAGNOSIS	PROBABILITY
Chondroblastoma	100

COMMENT: The heaviness of the marginal sclerosis gives a healed appearance.

AFIP Case No. 1154610: **B,** anteroposterior projection.

DIAGNOSIS AND GRADE.—Chondroblastoma, humerus; growth rate IB.
LIFE INFORMATION.—Male, estimated 20 years.
LOCATION.—A small circumscribed lesion in the proximal epiphysis (**arrow**).
SIZE.—1.5 × 1 cm.
MINERALIZATION OF TUMOR.—None.
DESTRUCTION.—Geographic; regular contour.
PROLIFERATION.—No apparent sclerosis of bone at the margin; hyperostotic wedge of subperiosteal new bone along lateral metaphysis, remote from primary lesion (**a**).

DIFFERENTIAL DIAGNOSIS	PROBABILITY
Chondroblastoma	100

COMMENT: With the hyperostosis, a typical chondroblastoma in the most common location.

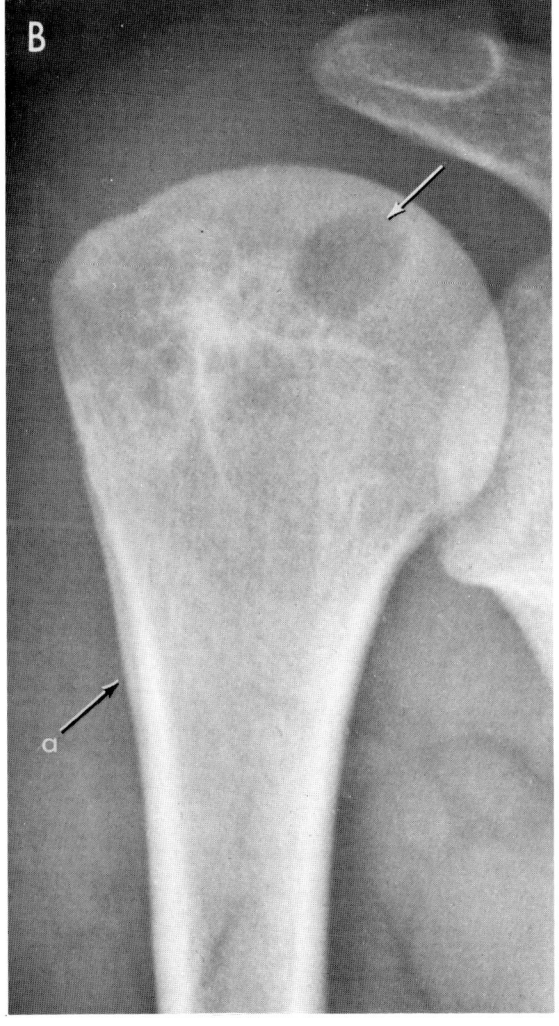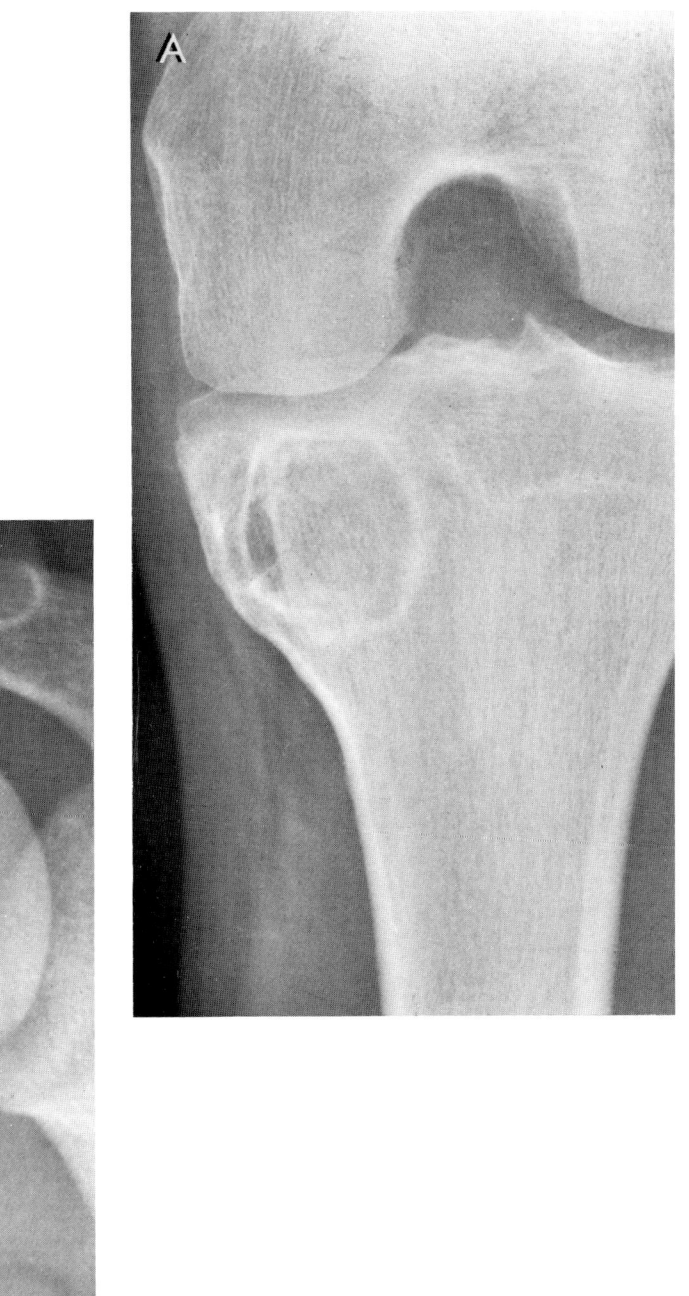

Figure 93 · Chondroblastomas of Tibia & Humerus

Figure 94.—Chondroblastoma of the femur.

AFIP Case No. 1053068: **A,** anteroposterior, and **B,** lateral views.

DIAGNOSIS AND GRADE.—Chondroblastoma, femur; growth rate IA.
LIFE INFORMATION.—Female, estimated 14 years; well five years after onset.
LOCATION.—A circumscribed lesion centered in the distal epiphysis.

SIZE.—2 × 2 × 2 cm.
MINERALIZATION OF TUMOR.—In **B,** suggestive evidence of matrix mineralization in the form of floccules.
DESTRUCTION.—Geographic; regular contour.
PROLIFERATION.—Narrow but dense sclerotic rim (**arrows**) around the lesion, plus dense hyperostosis of new bone on the medial surface of the metaphysis (**A, a**).

DIFFERENTIAL DIAGNOSIS	PROBABILITY
Chondroblastoma	.99

COMMENT: Matrix mineralization is present often enough to be a useful sign in diagnosis of chondroblastoma. The wedge of periosteal new bone located, as here, remote from the lesion is also common.

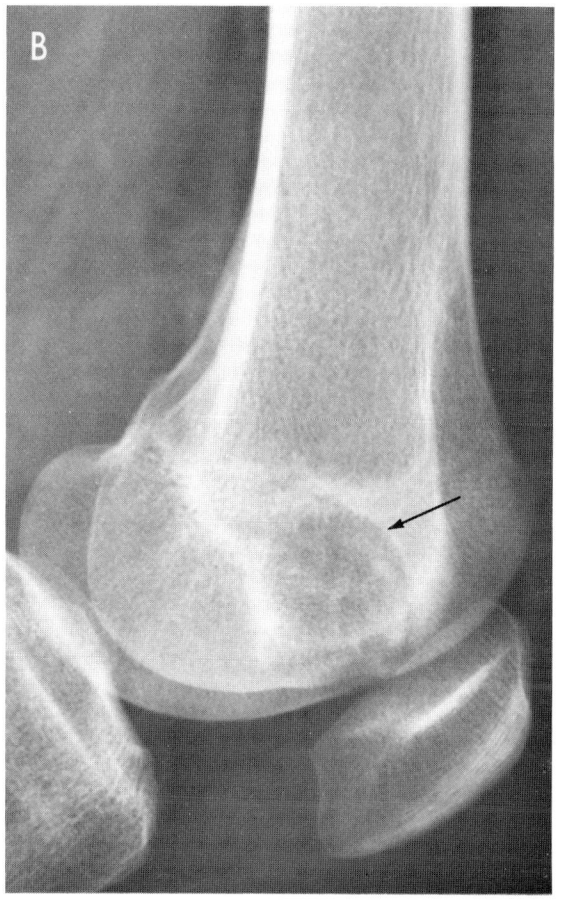
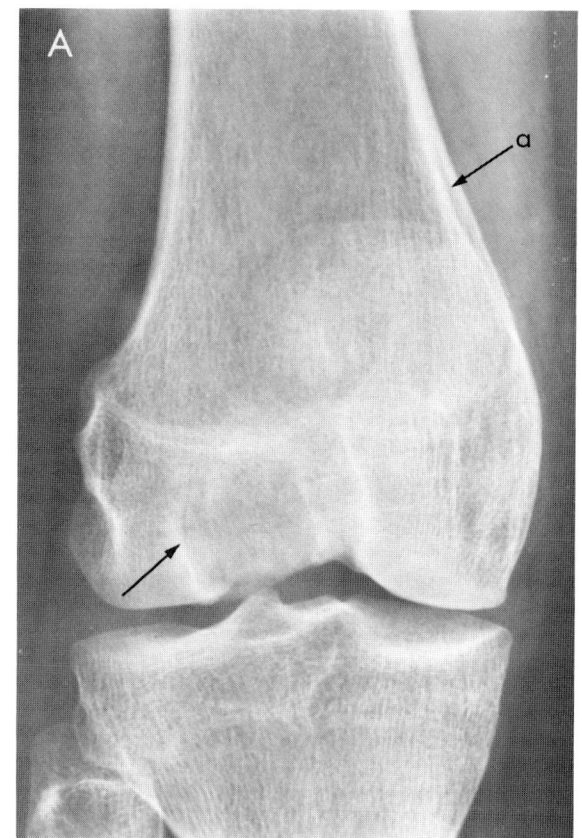

Figure 94 · Chondroblastoma of Femur / 241

Figure 95.—Chondroblastomas of the femur.

AFIP Case No. 1142245: **A,** anteroposterior exposure.

DIAGNOSIS AND GRADE.—Chondroblastoma, femur; growth rate IA.
LIFE INFORMATION.—Male, 15 years; survival unknown.
LOCATION.—A circumscribed lesion centered in the proximal epiphysis of the femoral head, apparently extending into the metaphysis.

SIZE.—2.5 × 2.5 × 2.5 cm.
MINERALIZATION OF TUMOR.—None definite; single fleck of increased density near the lower edge of the tumor (**a**).
DESTRUCTION.—Geographic; regular contour.
PROLIFERATION.—A thin dense sclerotic zone (**arrow**) around the margin of the tumor.

DIFFERENTIAL DIAGNOSIS	PROBABILITY
Chondroblastoma	.99
Cartilaginous tumor	< .01

COMMENT: A typical chondroblastoma of the femoral capital epiphysis. It is visible largely because of the sclerotic rim.

AFIP Case No. 1099859: **B,** anteroposterior projection.

DIAGNOSIS AND GRADE.—Chondroblastoma, greater trochanter; growth rate IA.
LIFE INFORMATION.—Male, estimated 20 years.
LOCATION.—A circumscribed lesion in the greater trochanter; no visible extraosseous component.

SIZE.—2.5 × 2 cm.
MINERALIZATION OF TUMOR.—Possible floccule.
DESTRUCTION.—Geographic; slightly lobulated contour.
PROLIFERATION.—Definite narrow sclerosis around entire lesion (**arrow**); heavier sclerosis medially; hyperostosis in shaft below the lesion (**b**).

DIFFERENTIAL DIAGNOSIS	PROBABILITY
Chondroblastoma	.99
Benign cartilaginous tumor	< .01

COMMENT: The defect in the lateral cortex is secondary to biopsy. The greater trochanter is a favorite site for chondroblastoma.

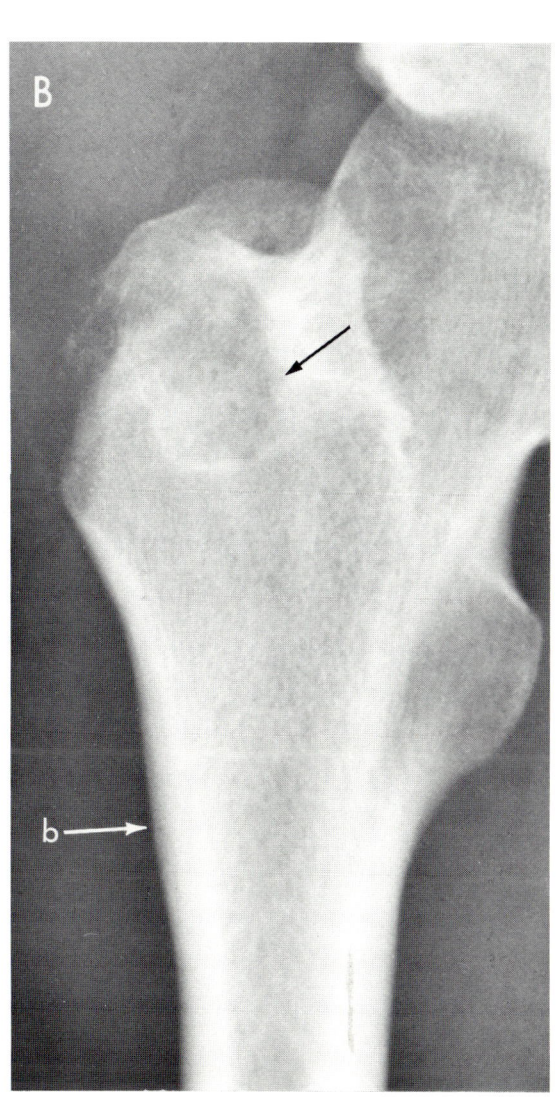
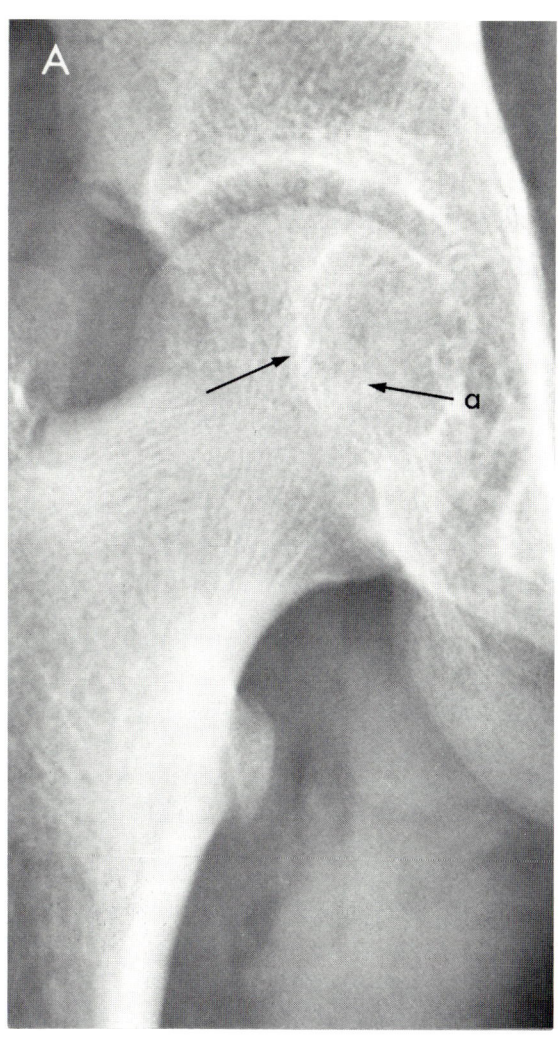

Figure 95 · Chondroblastomas of Femur / 243

Figure 96.—Chondroblastoma of the tibia.

AFIP Case No. 1180671: **A,** lateral initial view; **B,** lateral, and **C,** anteroposterior views 10 months later.

DIAGNOSIS AND GRADE.—Chondroblastoma, tibia; growth rate IC.

LIFE INFORMATION.—Male, 11 years; alive and well.

LOCATION.—Initially a circumscribed lesion centered eccentrically at the level of the growth plate, involving the epiphysis below and metaphysis above.

SIZE.—Initially 2 × 2 cm.

MINERALIZATION OF TUMOR.—None.

DESTRUCTION.—Geographic; regular contour. Initially the cortex is totally penetrated (**A, arrow**).

PROLIFERATION.—Narrow zone of marginal sclerosis (**A, a**).

Ten months later (**B** and **C**) the tumor, now 5 × 4 × 3 cm, is much more circumscribed; the cortex, slightly expanded, encapsulates the tumor completely.

DIFFERENTIAL DIAGNOSIS	PROBABILITY
Chondroblastoma	.99
Chondrosarcoma	< .01

COMMENT: The early lesion seems more aggressive, with complete loss of cortex anteriorly; it is quite typical of chondroblastoma. Later it is completely enveloped by cortex (**B** and **C, arrows**) but extends a bit farther into the metaphysis than usual for chondroblastoma (**B, b**). Histologically this was a rare duplex tumor, the part in the metaphysis having cellular characteristics and behavior of giant cell tumor, while the tumor in the epiphysis was characteristic of chondroblastoma in both cell type and behavior.

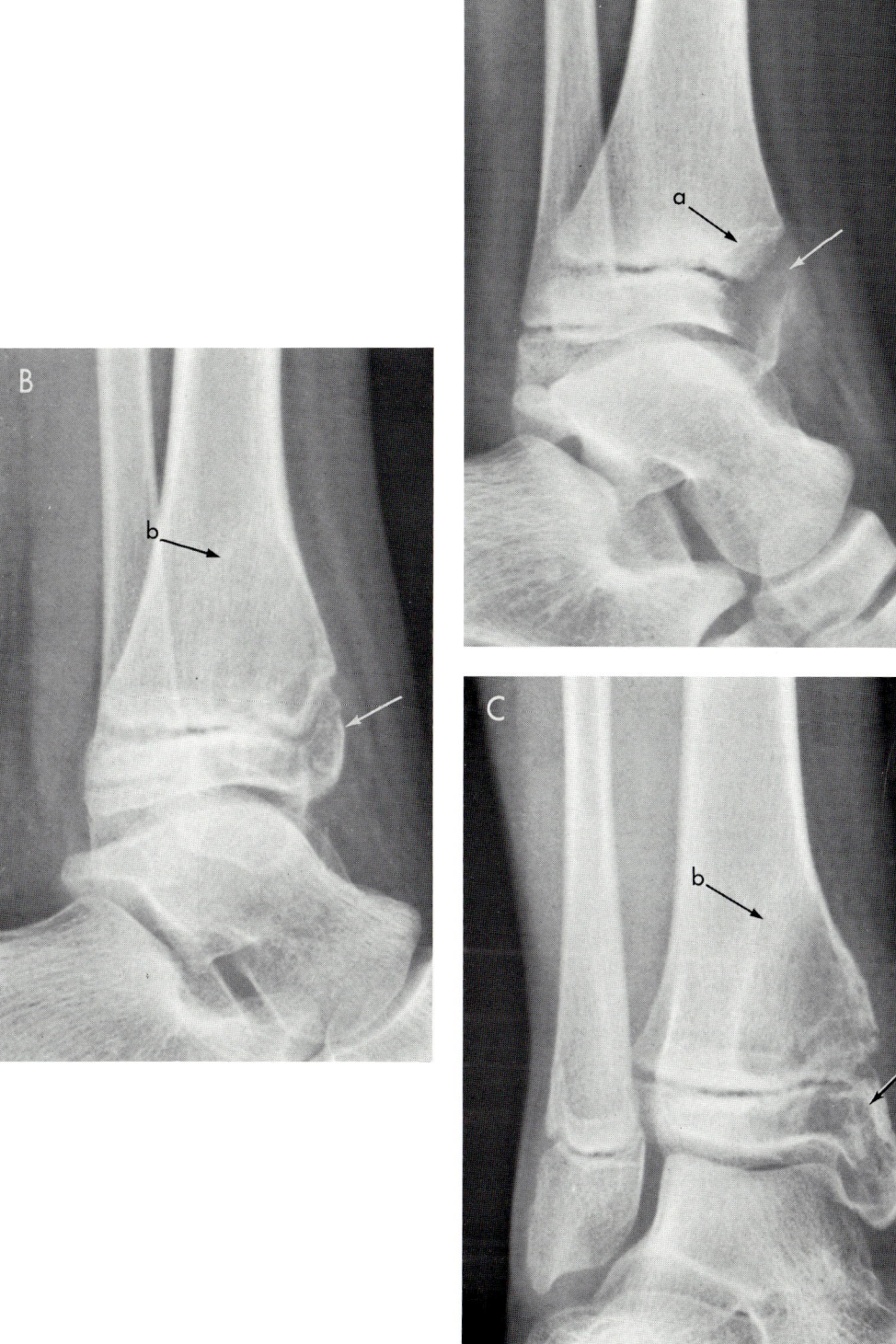

Figure 96 · Chondroblastoma of Tibia / 245

Figure 97.—Chondroblastoma of the femur; periosteal chondroma of the toe.

AFIP Case No. 909010: **A,** anteroposterior projection.

DIAGNOSIS AND GRADE.—Chondroblastoma, femur; growth rate IA.
LIFE INFORMATION.—Male, 18 years.
LOCATION.—A circumscribed lesion centered in the epiphysis of the medial femoral condyle.
SIZE.—1.5 × 1 cm.
MINERALIZATION OF TUMOR.—Questionable fleck of tumor matrix mineralization in center of the lesion (**arrow**).
DESTRUCTION.—Geographic; regular contour.
PROLIFERATION.—Faint sclerosis of bone at the edge of the tumor, particularly between tumor and cortex.

DIFFERENTIAL DIAGNOSIS	PROBABILITY
Chondroblastoma	.99
Chondrosarcoma	< .01
Benign cartilaginous tumor	< .01

COMMENT: Another common location for chondroblastoma.

AFIP Case No. 1173043: **B,** anteroposterior projection.

DIAGNOSIS AND GRADE.—Periosteal chondroma, toe; growth rate IC.
LIFE INFORMATION.—Male, 47 years.
LOCATION.—A largely extraosseous lesion centered parosteally in the medial cortex of the distal phalanx of the second toe.
SIZE.—2 × 1.5 cm.
MINERALIZATION OF TUMOR.—Floccules and clouds of tumor matrix throughout the lesion (**x**).
DESTRUCTION.—Geographic erosion of cortex from without; regular contour.
PROLIFERATION.—Dense sclerosis of the edge of bone underlying the lesion.

DIFFERENTIAL DIAGNOSIS	PROBABILITY
Benign cartilaginous tumor	100

COMMENT: This much mineralization in a periosteal chondroma is quite unusual.

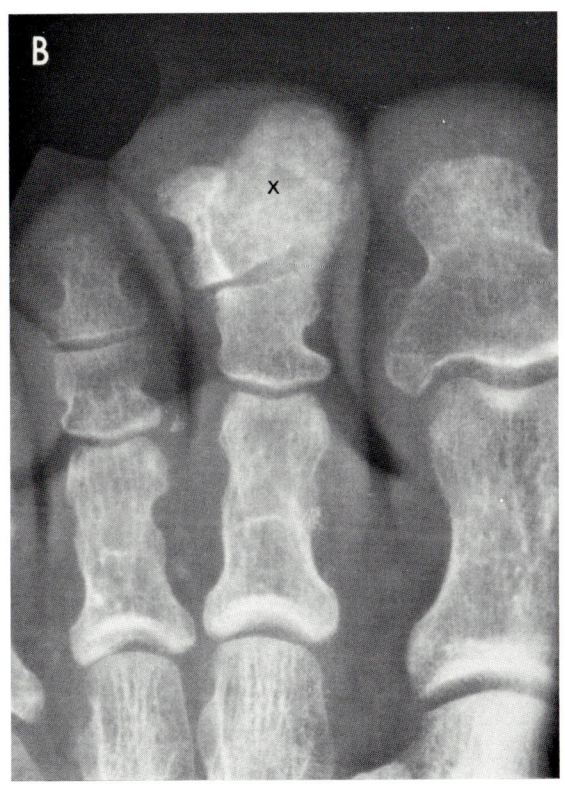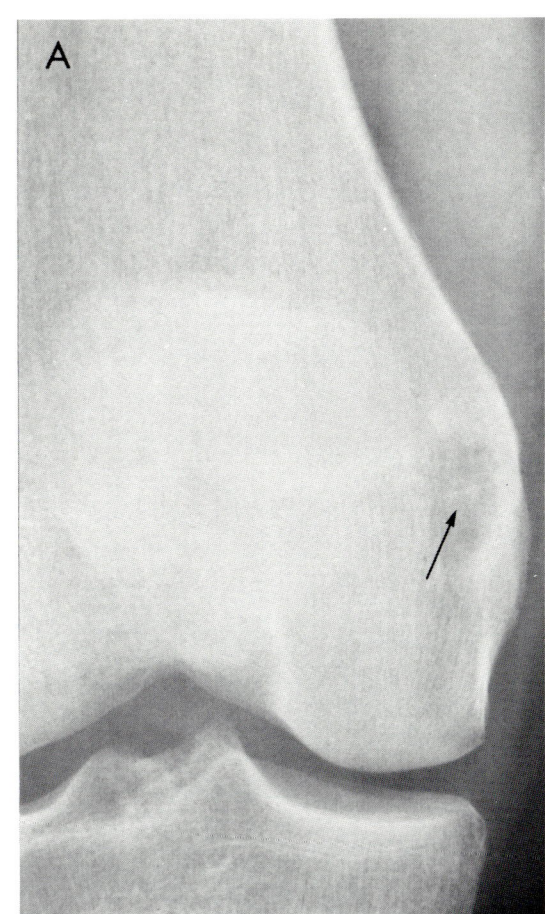

Figure 97 · Chondroblastoma; Periosteal Chondroma / 247

Figure 98.—Periosteal chondroma of the toe; synovial chondroma of the finger.

AFIP Case No. 1187793: **A,** anteroposterior projection.

DIAGNOSIS AND GRADE.—Periosteal chondroma, toe; growth rate IC.
LIFE INFORMATION.—Female, 43 years.
LOCATION.—A small circumscribed lesion centered on the cortex of the medial aspect of the distal phalanx of the great toe.
SIZE.—1 × 0.5 cm.
MINERALIZATION OF TUMOR.—None.
DESTRUCTION.—Shallow geographic saucerized erosion of the cortex (**arrow**) from without.
PROLIFERATION.—Faint zone of sclerosis underlying the lesion; a small fragment of bone near the edge of the extraosseous component, probably of periosteal origin.

DIFFERENTIAL DIAGNOSIS	PROBABILITY
Benign cartilaginous tumor	.99
Chondrosarcoma	< .01

COMMENT: A typical periosteal chondroma. The suggestion of periosteal shell is against the diagnosis of epithelial inclusion cyst or glomus tumor.

AFIP Case No. 1015416: **B,** anteroposterior view.

DIAGNOSIS AND GRADE.—Synovial chondroma, finger; growth rate IC.
LIFE INFORMATION.—Male, 32 years.
LOCATION.—A circumscribed lesion centered on the anteromedial cortex of the middle phalanx of the third finger.
SIZE.—1.2 cm × 5 mm.
MINERALIZATION OF TUMOR.—None.
DESTRUCTION.—Geographic, eroded from without; regular contour.
PROLIFERATION.—Faint zone of bone sclerosis around the edge of the lesion (**arrow**); small buttress at the lower margin with faint septation (**a**).

DIFFERENTIAL DIAGNOSIS	PROBABILITY
Benign cartilaginous tumor	.99
Villonodular	< .01
Fibroma	< .01

COMMENT: The rather extensive bone erosion bespeaks a chondroma of periosteal rather than synovial origin.

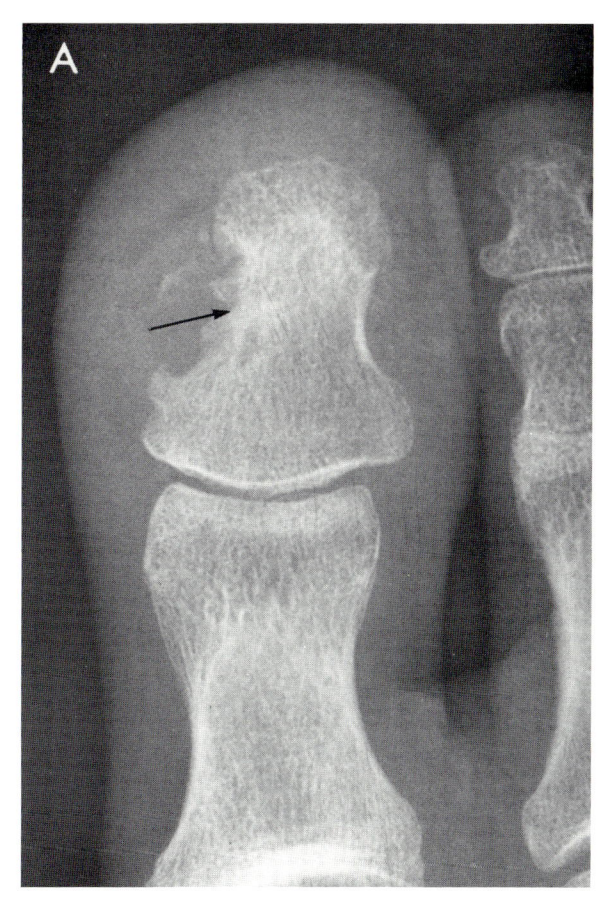
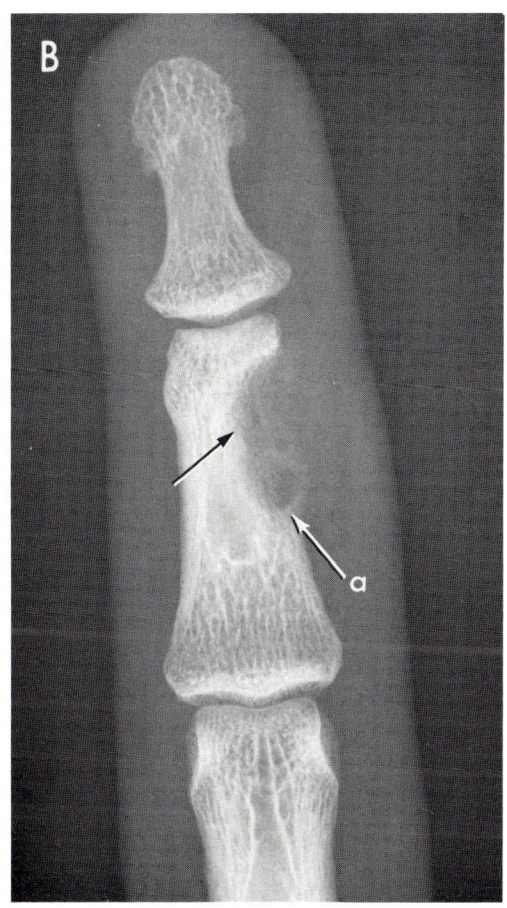

Figure 98 · Periosteal and Synovial Chondroma / 249

Figure 99.—Chondromas of the tibia and humerus.

AFIP Case No. 1135669: **A,** anteroposterior projection.

DIAGNOSIS AND GRADE.—Chondroma, tibia; growth rate 1A.
LIFE INFORMATION.—Female, 19 years; well 11 years later.
LOCATION.—A sharply circumscribed lesion eccentrically centered beneath the medial cortex of the distal metaphysis; no extraosseous component.
SIZE.—2.5 × 1.5 × 1.5 cm.
MINERALIZATION OF TUMOR.—Numerous small, sharply delineated floccules in the substance of the lesion.
DESTRUCTION.—Geographic; lobular contour.
PROLIFERATION.—Dense, broad marginal sclerosis; cortex expanded above the lesion, encapsulating it completely.

DIFFERENTIAL DIAGNOSIS	PROBABILITY
Benign cartilaginous tumor	.99
Chondrosarcoma	< .01

COMMENT: This is a favorite location for chondromyxoid fibroma.

AFIP Case No. 1219380: **B,** anteroposterior projection.

DIAGNOSIS AND GRADE.—Cortical chondroma, humerus; growth rate IA.
LIFE INFORMATION.—Male, 15 years.
LOCATION.—Focal circumscribed lesions in the medial cortex of the proximal shaft and metaphysis; no extraosseous component.
SIZE.—9 × 1.7 cm.
MINERALIZATION OF TUMOR.—A few dense floccules in the tumor substance.
DESTRUCTION.—Several discrete geographic areas, tending to be confluent; lobulated contours; pathologic fracture through the lesion.
PROLIFERATION.—Dense, irregular sclerosis of bone around margins of the cystic areas; a thin shell of slightly expanded bone over the periosteal surface appears to encapsulate the tumor.

DIFFERENTIAL DIAGNOSIS	PROBABILITY
Benign cartilaginous tumor	.96
Chondrosarcoma	.02
Fibrosarcoma	< .01

COMMENT: Since this lesion appears to replace the cortex completely, with a periosteal shell of new bone separating it from soft tissues laterally, the classification of cortical rather than periosteal chondroma has been used.

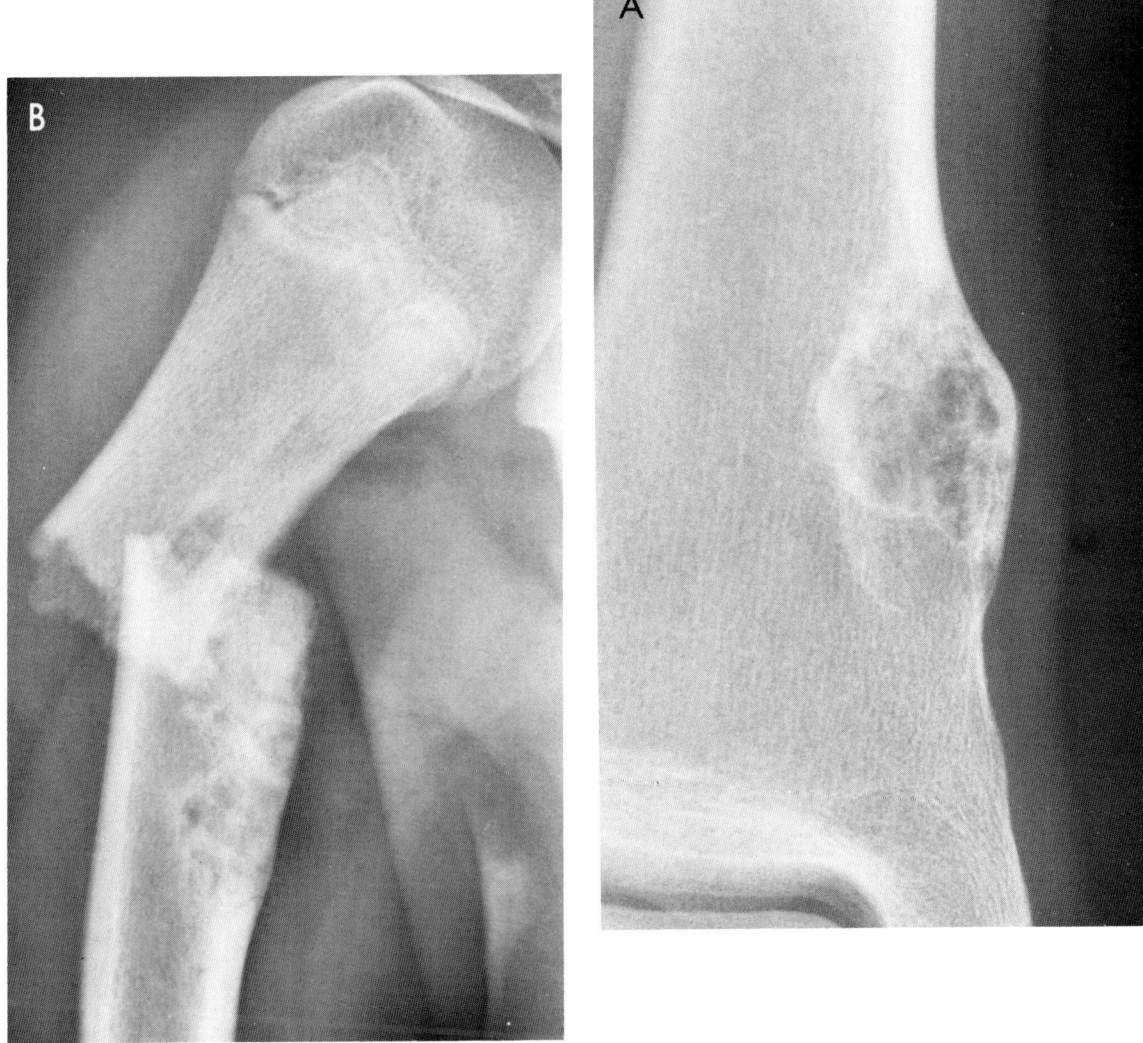

Figure 99 · Chondromas of Tibia and Humerus / 251

Figure 100.—Periosteal chondroma of the clavicle.

AFIP Case No. 1044761: Anteroposterior projection.

DIAGNOSIS AND GRADE.—Periosteal chondroma, clavicle; not graded.

LIFE INFORMATION.—Male, 37 years; well on last contact.

LOCATION.—A well-defined lesion arising on the superior surface of the distal metaphysis of the clavicle.

SIZE.—4 × 4 cm.

MINERALIZATION OF TUMOR.—Numerous flecks and rings of densely calcified tumor matrix; no crescentic mineralization at the margin of the soft tissue lesion.

DESTRUCTION.—None.

PROLIFERATION.—None.

DIFFERENTIAL DIAGNOSIS	PROBABILITY
Chondrosarcoma	.88
Benign cartilaginous tumor	.11

COMMENT: This moderately sized chondroma has a static appearance. The computer is unable to distinguish between a benign and a malignant cartilaginous tumor when there is little or no bone involvement; nor am I. Compare with Figure 78, *a*.

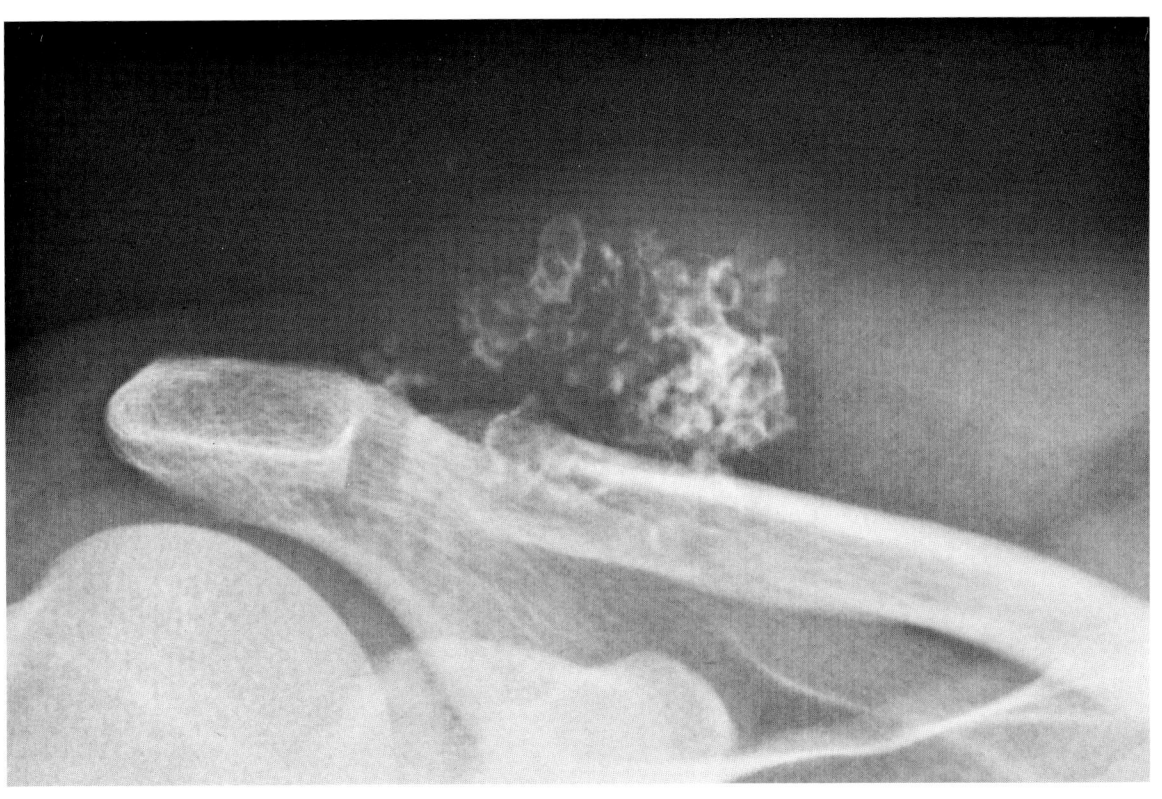

Figure 100 · Periosteal Chondroma of Clavicle / 253

Figure 101.—Enchondroma of the dorsal spine; benign chondroma of the thumb.

AFIP Case No. 1154288: **A,** anteroposterior, and **B,** lateral views.

DIAGNOSIS AND GRADE.—Enchondroma, dorsal spine; growth rate IA.
LIFE INFORMATION.—Male, 22 years.
LOCATION.—A circumscribed lesion involving the body of D8.
SIZE.—4 × 2 × 3 cm.
MINERALIZATION OF TUMOR.—Several dense floccules of calcified matrix in the substance of the tumor.
DESTRUCTION.—Probably geographic, although the pattern has been disturbed by the compression fracture.
PROLIFERATION.—Some sclerosis of upper and lower vertebral plates.

DIFFERENTIAL DIAGNOSIS	PROBABILITY
Osteoblastoma	.96
Chordoma	.02
Fibrosarcoma	< .01
Chondrosarcoma	< .01

COMMENT: This enchondroma contains flocculent calcification, which is very helpful in diagnosis of this unusual lesion. I do not agree with the computer differential diagnosis.

AFIP Case No. 904008: **C,** lateral projection.

DIAGNOSIS AND GRADE.—Chondroma (benign), thumb; growth rate IA.
LIFE INFORMATION.—Male, 67 years; died of intercurrent disease.
LOCATION.—A circumscribed periosteal tumor attached to the distal cortex of the proximal phalanx.
SIZE.—3 × 1.5 cm.
MINERALIZATION OF TUMOR.—The main substance of the tumor appears to consist of trabeculated bone, with a cap of calcified cartilage. The intrinsic bone of the tumor is fused to underlying bone without intervening cortex. Long cleavage plane.
DESTRUCTION.—None.
PROLIFERATION.—None.

DIFFERENTIAL DIAGNOSIS	PROBABILITY
Osteochondroma	.99
Myositis ossificans	< .01

COMMENT: Most of the tumor appears to be mature bone. If chondrosarcomatous elements are present, they must be in the cartilage cap.

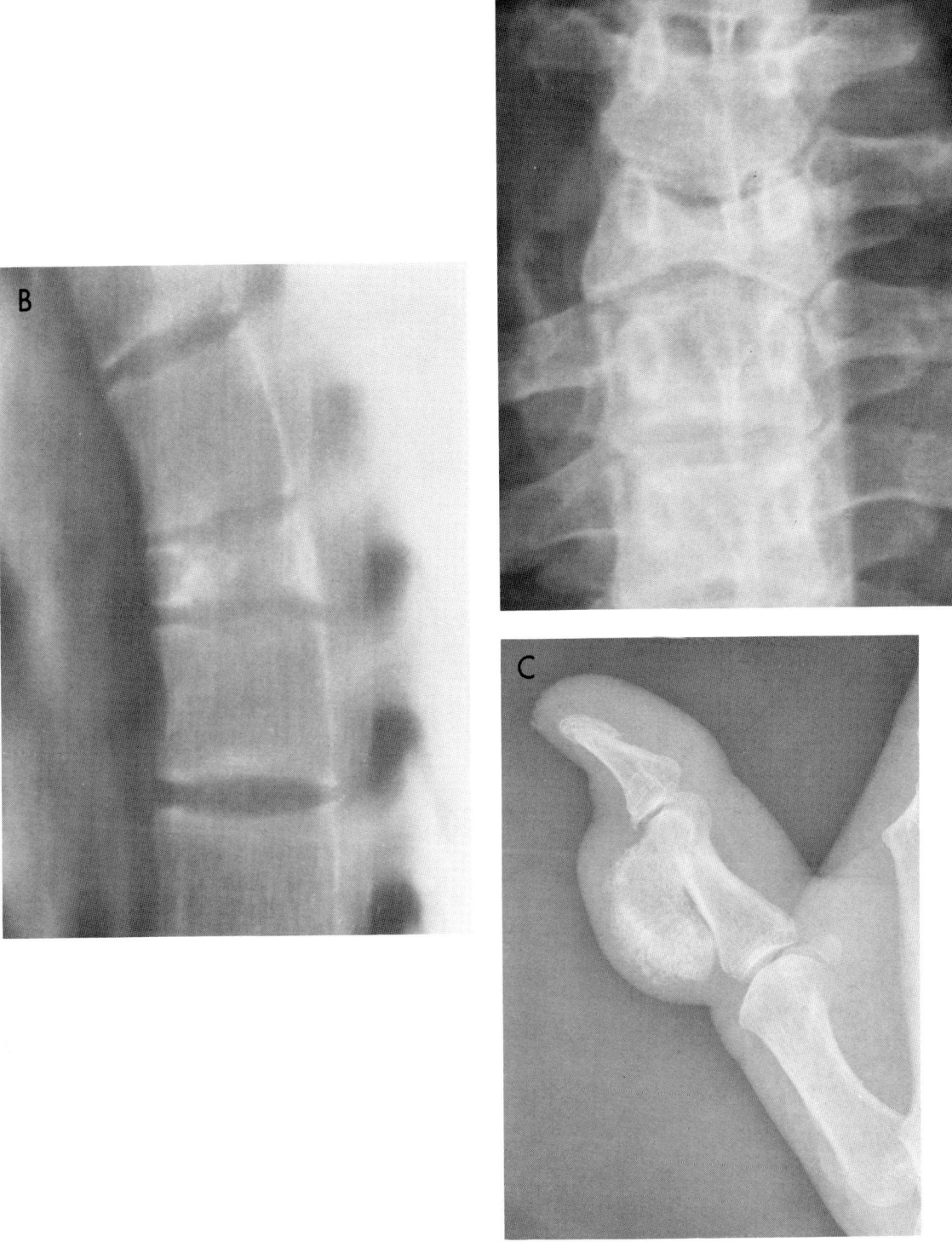

Figure 101 · Enchondroma; Chondroma / 255

PART 5

Osseous Tumors

Figure 102.—Osteosarcomas of the tibia.

AFIP Case No. 1115991: **A,** anteroposterior projection.

DIAGNOSIS AND GRADE.—Osteosarcoma, tibia; growth rate III.
LIFE INFORMATION.—Male, 19 years; alive 3½ years later.
LOCATION.—A lesion centered eccentrically in the proximal metaphysis, involving the epiphysis and adjacent soft tissues.

SIZE.—6 × 5 cm.
MINERALIZATION OF TUMOR.—Lumps and clouds of tumor bone throughout.
DESTRUCTION.—Permeative; total penetration of cortex.
PROLIFERATION.—Ill-defined spicular pattern (**x**) extending into soft tissue mass.

DIFFERENTIAL DIAGNOSIS	PROBABILITY
Osteosarcoma	100

COMMENT: A typical and diagnosable osteosarcoma. Note that the tumor bone is more solid in and near the epiphysis than in the center.

AFIP Case No. 1071103: **B,** anteroposterior projection.

DIAGNOSIS AND GRADE.—Osteosarcoma, tibia; growth rate III.
LIFE INFORMATION.—Male, estimated 10 years; died within year of diagnosis.
LOCATION.—Diffuse lesion centered eccentrically in the proximal metaphysis, extending into the shaft but not the epiphysis.

SIZE.—9 × 6 cm.
MINERALIZATION OF TUMOR.—One solid area of tumor bone in proximal end of tumor, with lumps and clouds in the remainder; extraosseous extension contains clouds, but is nearly radiolucent.
DESTRUCTION.—Permeative pattern.
PROLIFERATION.—Lateral metaphysial cortex covered by dense hyperostosis of laminated bone (**a**); medially, Codman's triangle (**b**), some nondescript spiculation.

DIFFERENTIAL DIAGNOSIS	PROBABILITY
Osteosarcoma	100

COMMENT: A highly typical, easily diagnosed, very malignant osteosarcoma. Whether or not the dense hyperostosis laterally resulted from earlier slow growth is a question.

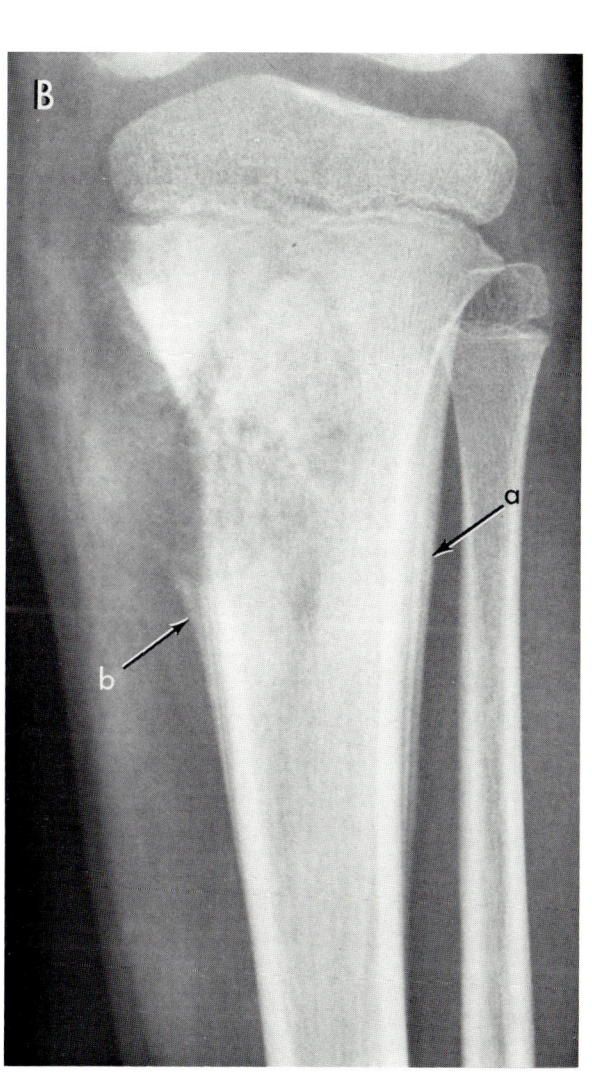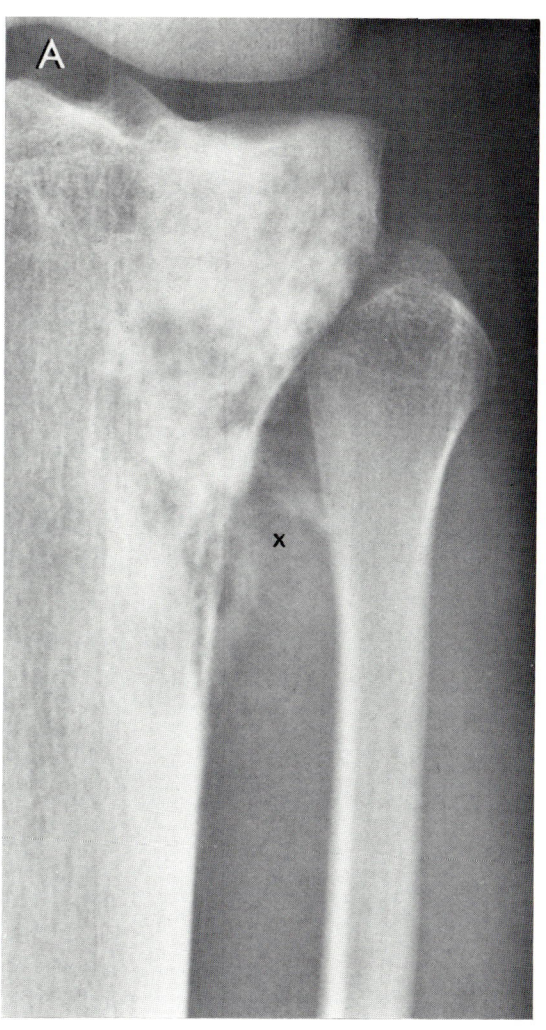

Figure 102 · Osteosarcomas of Tibia

Figure 103.—Osteosarcoma of the tibia.

AFIP Case No. 1072069: Anteroposterior projection.

DIAGNOSIS AND GRADE.—Osteosarcoma, tibia; growth rate III.

LIFE INFORMATION.—Female, 14 years; lived two years after onset.

LOCATION.—An ill-defined lesion centered centrally in the proximal metaphysis of the tibia, extending into the epiphysis and down into the shaft.

SIZE.—8 × 5 × 4 cm.

MINERALIZATION OF TUMOR.—Lumps and clouds of tumor bone in an intramedullary location.

DESTRUCTION.—Permeative pattern, if present (**arrow**), is largely obscured by the matrix mineralization.

PROLIFERATION.—None.

DIFFERENTIAL DIAGNOSIS	PROBABILITY
Osteosarcoma	100

COMMENT: This osteosarcoma is typical in that the tumor bone tends to obscure destructive and other kinds of change.

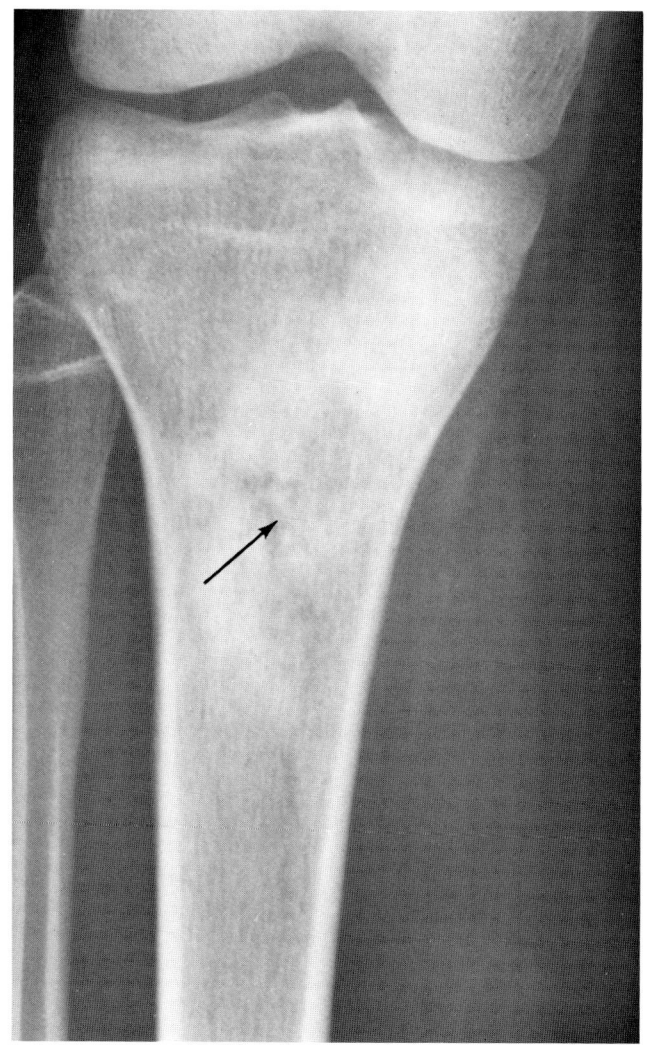

Figure 103 · Osteosarcoma of Tibia

Figure 104.—Osteosarcoma of one femur with metastatis in opposite femur.

AFIP Case No. 1102907: Anteroposterior views of left and right femora.

Left Leg Lesion

>   DIAGNOSIS AND GRADE.—Osteosarcoma, left femur; growth rate III.
>   LIFE INFORMATION.—Male, 4½ years; lived five months after diagnosis.
>   LOCATION.—A poorly circumscribed lesion centered in and involving the distal metaphysis and shaft.
>
>   SIZE.—6 × 4 cm.
>   MINERALIZATION OF TUMOR.—Lumps and clouds of tumor bone throughout.
>   DESTRUCTION.—Ill-defined vague loss of cortical bone, of a type often associated with permeative bone destruction, though the pattern is not identifiable here (compare density with cortex in right femur).
>   PROLIFERATION.—Codman's triangle (**a**).

Right Leg Lesion

>   DIAGNOSIS AND GRADE.—Osteosarcoma (metastatic), right femur; growth rate probably III.
>   LOCATION.—Extensive involvement of distal metaphysis to growth plate.
>
>   SIZE.—3 × 4 cm.
>   MINERALIZATION OF TUMOR.—Lumps of tumor bone in the metaphysis adjacent to the growth plate; clouds more proximally.
>   DESTRUCTION.—Vague reduction of cancellous bone (**arrows**) plus focal areas of ill-defined destruction.
>   PROLIFERATION.—Dense masses against the growth plate, possibly a proliferative response.

DIFFERENTIAL DIAGNOSIS	PROBABILITY
Osteosarcoma	100

>   COMMENT: Onset of illness was two weeks prior to this examination, when the patient fell and bumped his knee. This could be diagnosed as multicentric osteosarcoma but almost certainly is an example of tumor metastasizing to another bone. There were additional lesions in the proximal humeri.

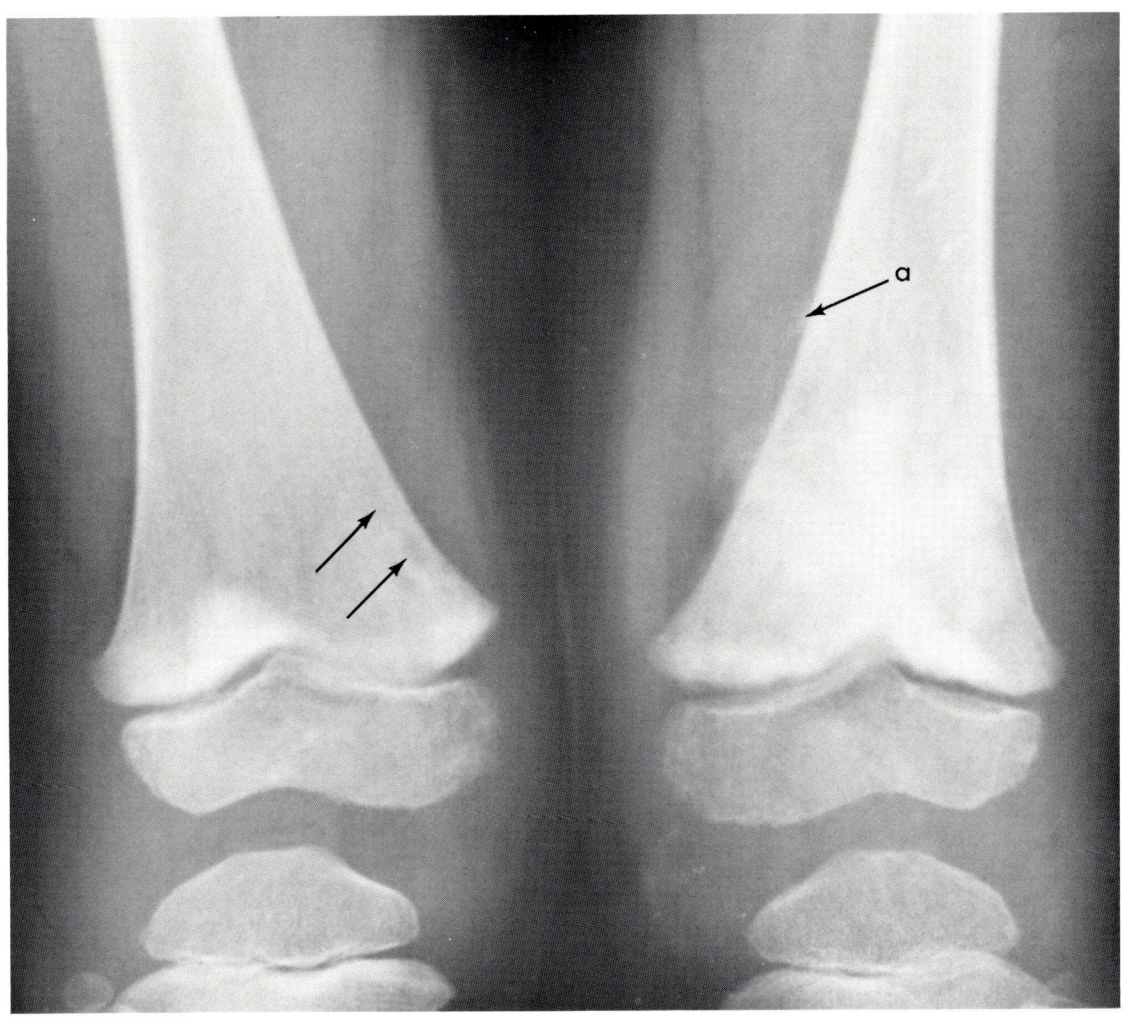

Figure 104 · Osteosarcoma & Metastasis / 263

Figure 105.—Osteosarcoma of the femur.

AFIP Case No. 1185558: Anteroposterior projection.

DIAGNOSIS AND GRADE.—Osteosarcoma, femur; growth rate IC.

LIFE INFORMATION.—Female, 8 years; lived 16 months after onset, 10 months following diagnosis.

LOCATION.—A small circumscribed lesion centered eccentrically in the distal metaphysis; reaches the growth plate but does not invade the epiphysis.

SIZE.—3 × 2 × 2 cm.

MINERALIZATION OF TUMOR.—Probably none (see Comment and Proliferation).

DESTRUCTION.—Geographic center, moth-eaten lower margin; contour generally regular; penetration of cortex laterally (**arrow**).

PROLIFERATION.—Broad zone of sclerosis around the medial edge of the tumor (**a**); several small foci of increased density, possibly reactive rather than tumor bone.

DIFFERENTIAL DIAGNOSIS	PROBABILITY
Osteosarcoma	100

COMMENT: Diagnosis in this case may depend on whether the foci of increased density are called tumor bone or reactive response. The choice is between osteosarcoma and Ewing's sarcoma.

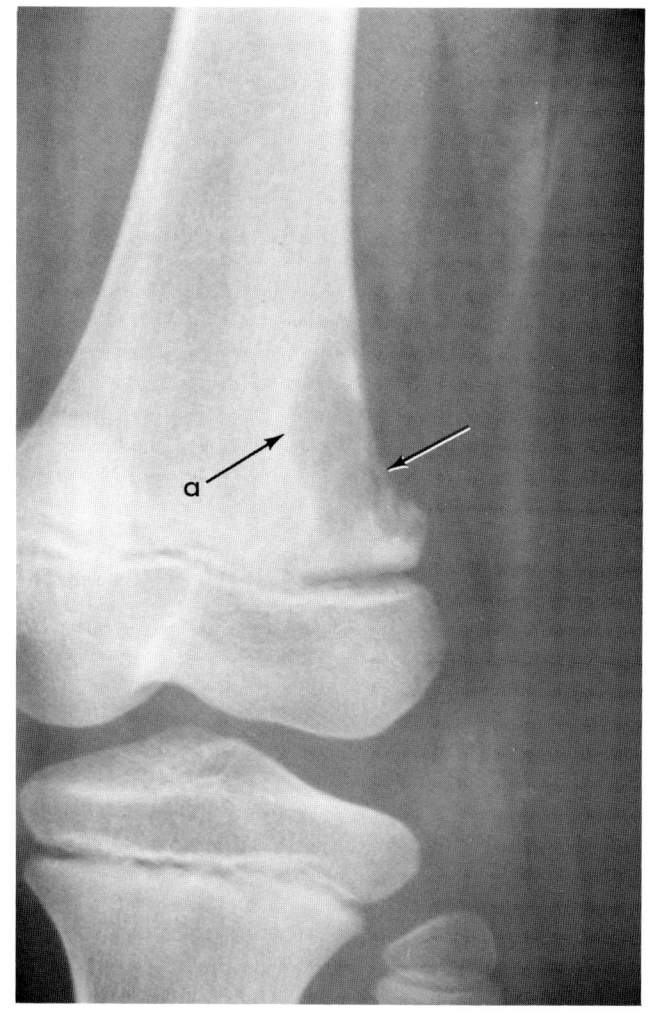

Figure 105 · Osteosarcoma of Femur / 265

Figure 106.—Osteosarcoma of the femur.

AFIP Case No. 1051392: Anteroposterior projection.

DIAGNOSIS AND GRADE.—Osteosarcoma, femur; growth rate III.

LIFE INFORMATION.—Male, 19 years; survived two years after onset.

LOCATION.—A large, fairly circumscribed lesion based on the medial cortex of the midfemoral shaft.

SIZE.—20 × 7 × 9 cm.

MINERALIZATION OF TUMOR.—Lumps, clouds and consolidated rays of tumor bone in the upper half of the extraosseous mass; in the lower half, lumps, floccules and short segments of linear ossified matrix at the edge of the mass.

DESTRUCTION.—Permeative; total penetration of cortex (**arrows**).

PROLIFERATION.—Extensive sunburst spiculation; hyperostosis of the cortex beneath the tumor; amorphous periosteal response.

DIFFERENTIAL DIAGNOSIS	PROBABILITY
Osteosarcoma	.99

COMMENT: A pattern highly specific for osteosarcoma. Bone sections of such tumors show the medullary canal filled with tumor, even though its presence is not clearly indicated in the radiograph. The lower half of the soft tissue part of the tumor looks more like chondrosarcoma than osteosarcoma and may be growing at a different rate. Spicule formation in tumors begins as normal bone, but spaces between spicules may backfill or consolidate with tumor bone.

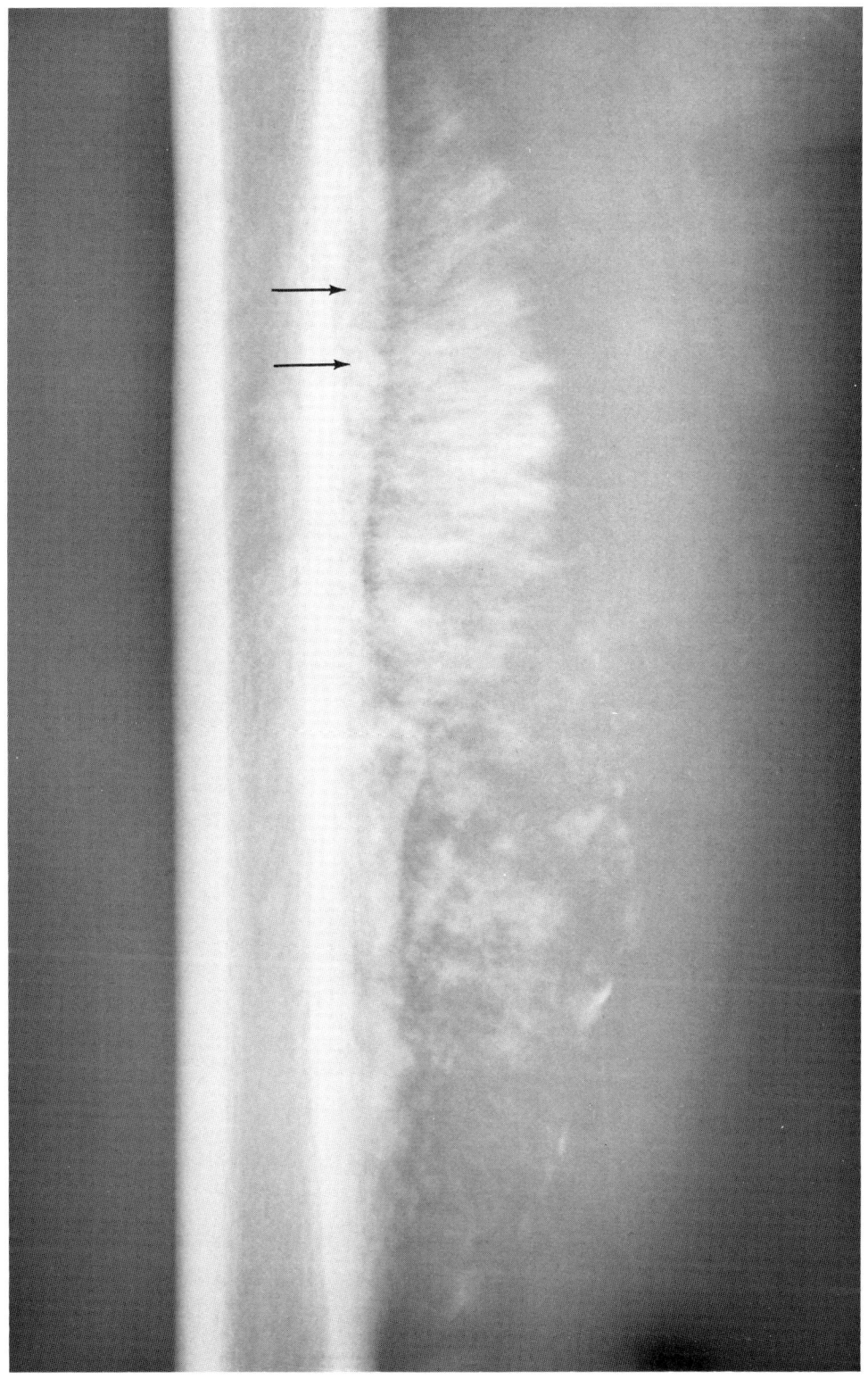

Figure 106 · Osteosarcoma of Femur / 267

Figure 107.—Osteosarcoma of the humerus.

AFIP Case No. 1102182: Anteroposterior projection.

DIAGNOSIS AND GRADE.—Osteosarcoma, humerus; growth rate III.

LIFE INFORMATION.—Male, 39 years; lived five months after onset.

LOCATION.—A large well-defined lesion centered on the medial cortex of the proximal metaphysis, extending up into the epiphysis, down into the shaft; large extraosseous component.

SIZE.—11 × 10 cm.

MINERALIZATION OF TUMOR.—Dense lumps and clouds of tumor bone inside and outside the cortex; small cleavage plane.

DESTRUCTION.—Probably permeative, largely obscured by the tumor matrix (**arrow**).

PROLIFERATION.—None.

DIFFERENTIAL DIAGNOSIS	PROBABILITY
Osteosarcoma	.99
Fibrosarcoma	< .01
Chondrosarcoma	< .01

COMMENT: In the evaluation of bone destruction in this case it is clear that the cortex ultimately disappears into the heart of the tumor bone. Absence of a sharp line of demarcation and apparent gradual fading of density suggest permeative bone destruction. The tumor may have arisen inside the bone, despite centering on the cortex.

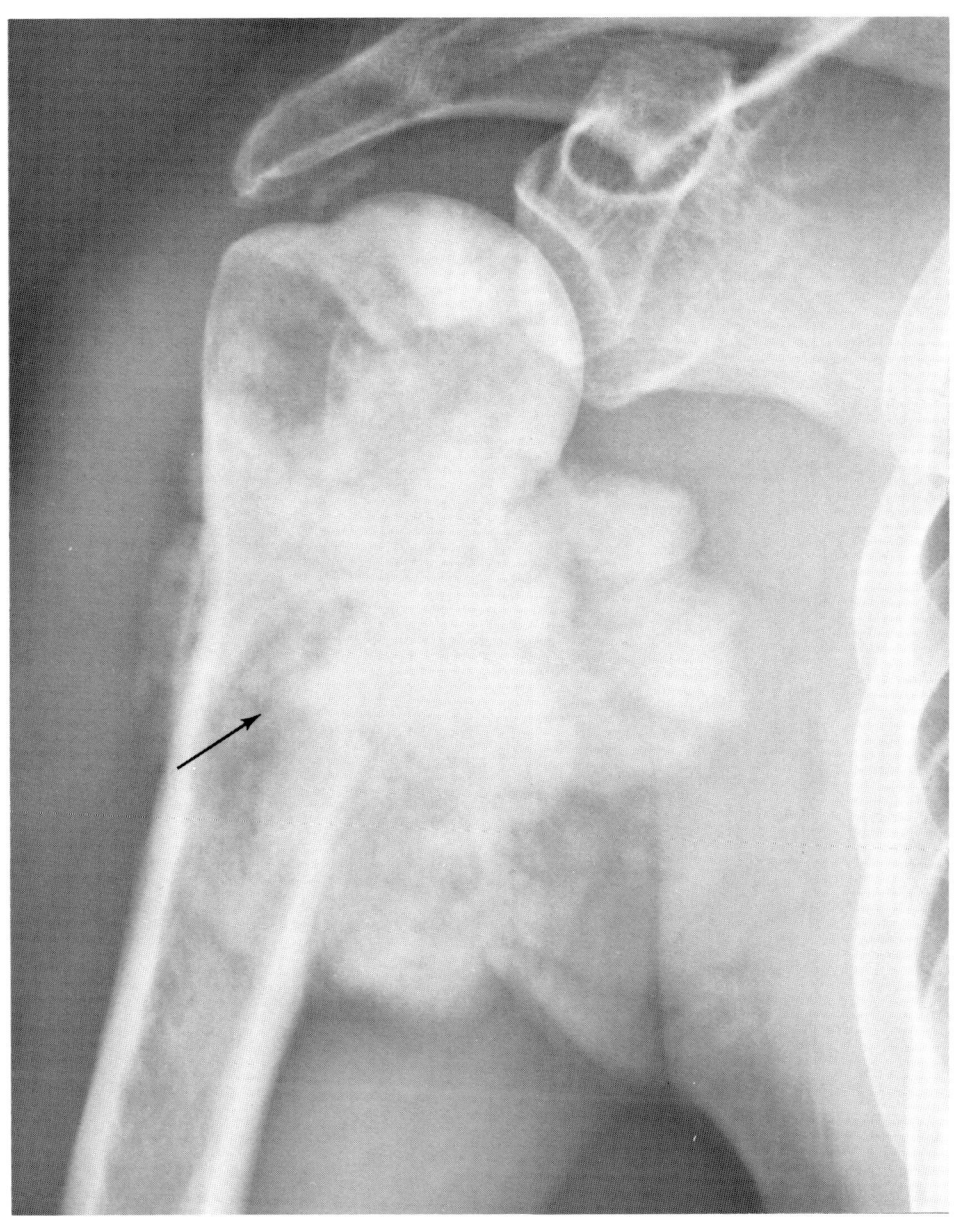

Figure 107 · Osteosarcoma of Humerus

Figure 108.—Osteosarcoma of the femur.

AFIP Case No. 1115305: **A,** anteroposterior, and **B,** lateral views.

DIAGNOSIS AND GRADE.—Osteosarcoma, femur; growth rate II.

LIFE INFORMATION.—Female, 28 years; died of metastases within four years.

LOCATION.—An ill-defined lesion centered eccentrically in the distal femoral metaphysis.

SIZE.—6 × 4 cm.

MINERALIZATION OF TUMOR.—None definitely present.

DESTRUCTION.—Moth-eaten pattern; total penetration of the cortex.

PROLIFERATION.—Moderate reactive sclerosis around the edge of the tumor; mottled increased density throughout, apparently an accentuation of trabecular density due to deposition of appositional new bone (**a**) rather than lumps of tumor bone.

DIFFERENTIAL DIAGNOSIS	PROBABILITY
Osteosarcoma	.99
Fibrosarcoma	< .01

COMMENT: Histologic diagnosis included malignant fibroxanthoma and liposarcoma. Radiographically it has the characteristics of a moderately aggressive tumor.

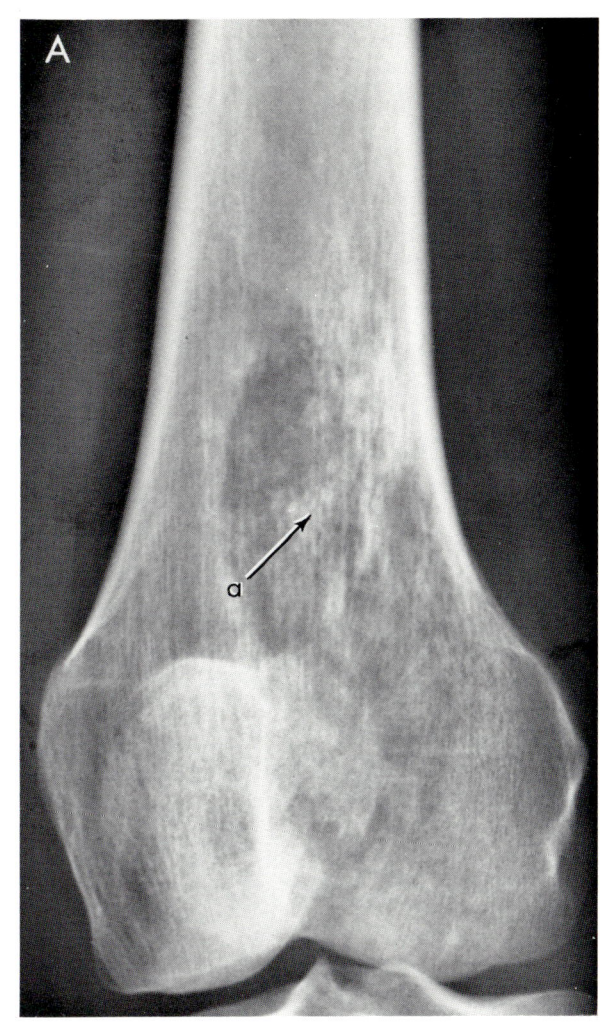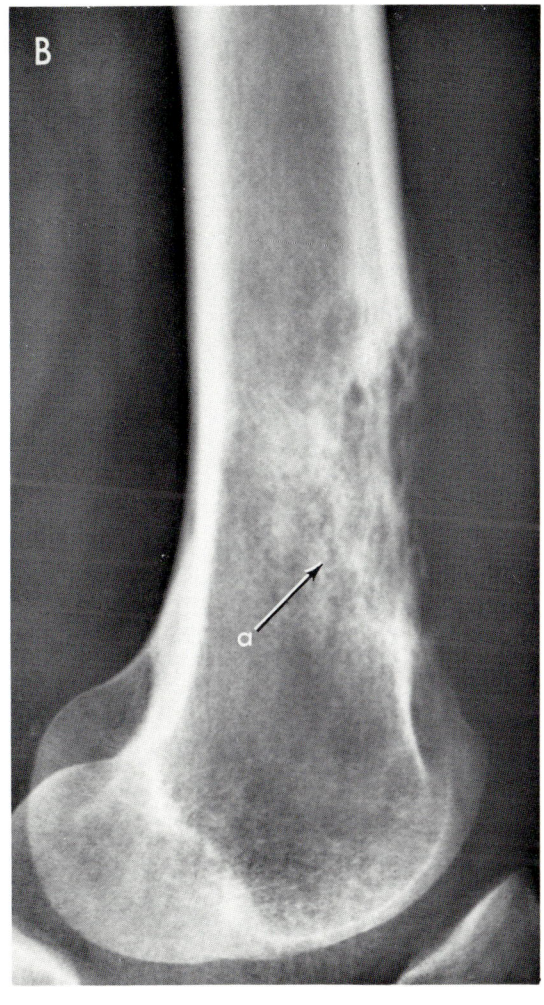

Figure 108 · Osteosarcoma of Femur / 271

Figure 109.—Osteosarcoma of the tibia.

AFIP Case No. 1081977: Anteroposterior views—**A,** initially; **B,** five months later, after radiation therapy.

DIAGNOSIS AND GRADE.—Osteosarcoma, tibia; growth rate IC.

LIFE INFORMATION.—Female, 15 years; alive 12 years after onset, following radiation therapy, amputation and resection of pulmonary metastasis.

LOCATION.—Fairly circumscribed lesion centered eccentrically in the peripheral third of the proximal metaphysis, extending into the epiphysis; no apparent extraosseous extension.

SIZE.—4 × 3 cm.

MINERALIZATION OF TUMOR.—Initially, clouds of intramedullary tumor bone (**a**).

DESTRUCTION.—Geographic; indistinct contour; incomplete penetration of cortex (**b**); vague reduction of cancellous bone (**B, c**).

PROLIFERATION.—Amorphous periosteal response over center of lesion.

Five months later (**B**) the cloudy bone has consolidated into lumpy and solid tumor bone under the influence of radiation therapy.

DIFFERENTIAL DIAGNOSIS	PROBABILITY
Osteosarcoma	.92
Fibrosarcoma	.07

COMMENT: One of the smaller, slower growing varieties of osteosarcoma which has some radiologic characteristics of fibrosarcoma. It is interesting that the tumor bone becomes more dense after radiation therapy.

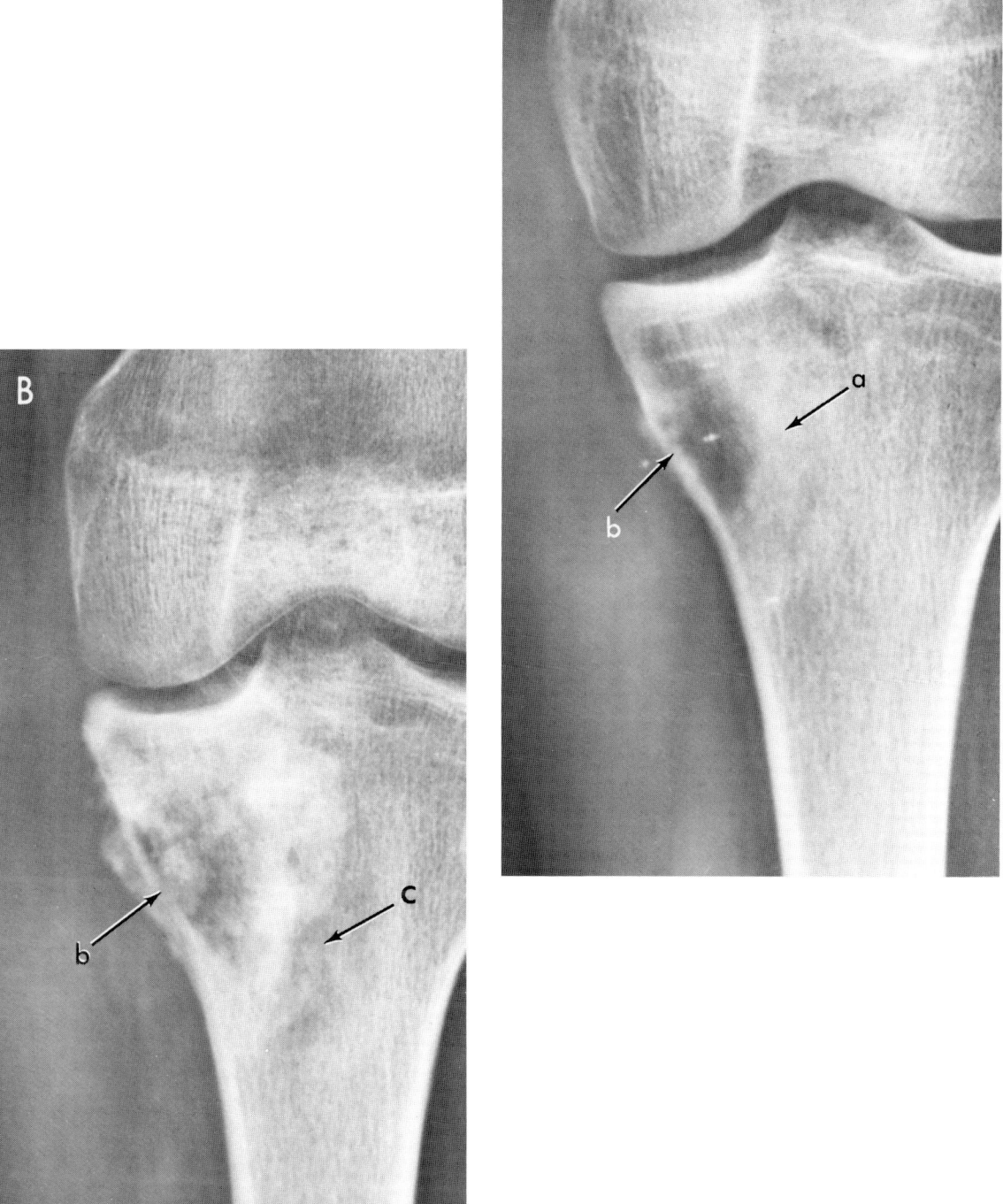

Figure 109 · Osteosarcoma of Tibia / 273

Figure 110.—Osteosarcoma of the humerus.

AFIP Case No. 1058661: Anteroposterior projection.

DIAGNOSIS AND GRADE.—Osteosarcoma, humerus; growth rate III.

LIFE INFORMATION.—Female, 19 years; survival unknown.

LOCATION.—A diffuse lesion centered in the proximal shaft of the humerus, extending well into the metaphysis and soft tissues.

SIZE.—10 × 4 cm.

MINERALIZATION OF TUMOR.—None.

DESTRUCTION.—Permeative throughout.

PROLIFERATION.—Several laminae of periosteal new bone (**arrow**), with Codman's triangle and possibly a few spicules.

DIFFERENTIAL DIAGNOSIS	PROBABILITY
Osteosarcoma	.38
Ewing's sarcoma	.36
Reticulum cell sarcoma	.25
Fibrosarcoma	< .01
Chondrosarcoma	< .01

COMMENT: A highly malignant tumor of bone without specific identifying characteristics.

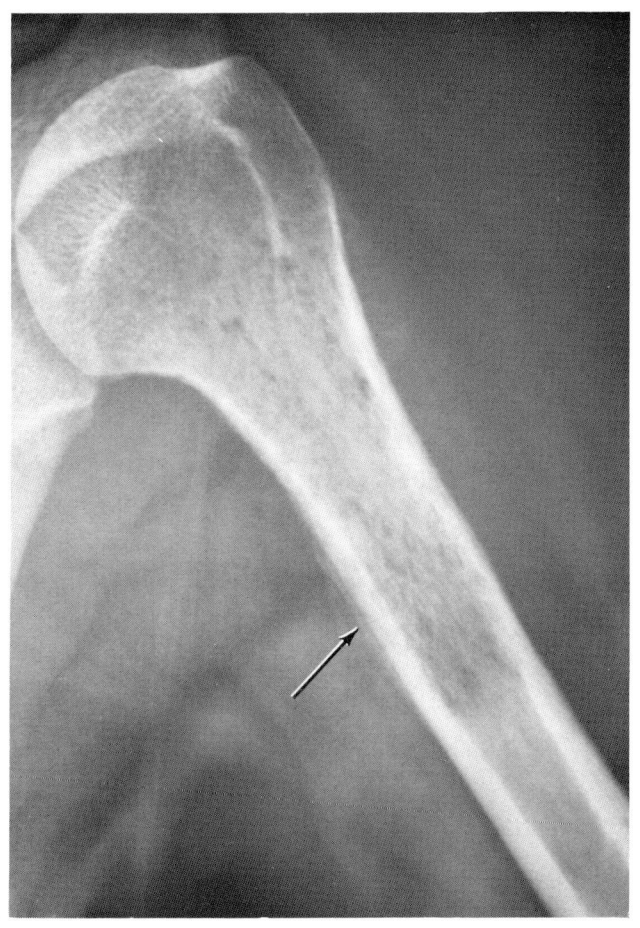

Figure 110 · Osteosarcoma of Humerus / 275

Figure 111.—Osteosarcoma of the femur.

AFIP Case No. 1165589: **A,** anteroposterior, and **B,** lateral views.

DIAGNOSIS AND GRADE.—Osteosarcoma, femur; growth rate IC.

LIFE INFORMATION.—Female, 8 years; symptoms for three weeks before diagnosis; lived five months after onset.

LOCATION.—A circumscribed appearing lesion located slightly eccentrically in the lower femoral shaft; extraosseous extension.

SIZE.—6 × 3 × 2 cm.

MINERALIZATION OF TUMOR.—One fairly large lump of matrix mineralization near the superior edge of the tumor (**a**); the remainder radiolucent.

DESTRUCTION.—Geographic; edges of the destroyed area fairly sharply defined; a suggestion of permeated pattern around the periphery but not definite; the cortex totally penetrated medially (**A, b**).

PROLIFERATION.—Three quadrants of the cortex enveloped in dense hyperostosis; the fourth side penetrated by tumor and flanked by two huge buttresses.

DIFFERENTIAL DIAGNOSIS	PROBABILITY
Fibrosarcoma	.61
Osteosarcoma	.32
Chondrosarcoma	.06

COMMENT: The size of the tumor and extent of the periosteal reaction indicate that the tumor had been present for a considerable time before this examination. There are at least five distinct laminae of periosteal new bone (**B, c**) which make up one of the hyperostoses. These suggest a fairly long duration despite the short clinical history. There is no question that the basic pattern of bone destruction is geographic, the evidence for permeation not being convincing. Despite the lumpy tumor mineralization the manifestations of slow growth downgrade the diagnosis of osteosarcoma.

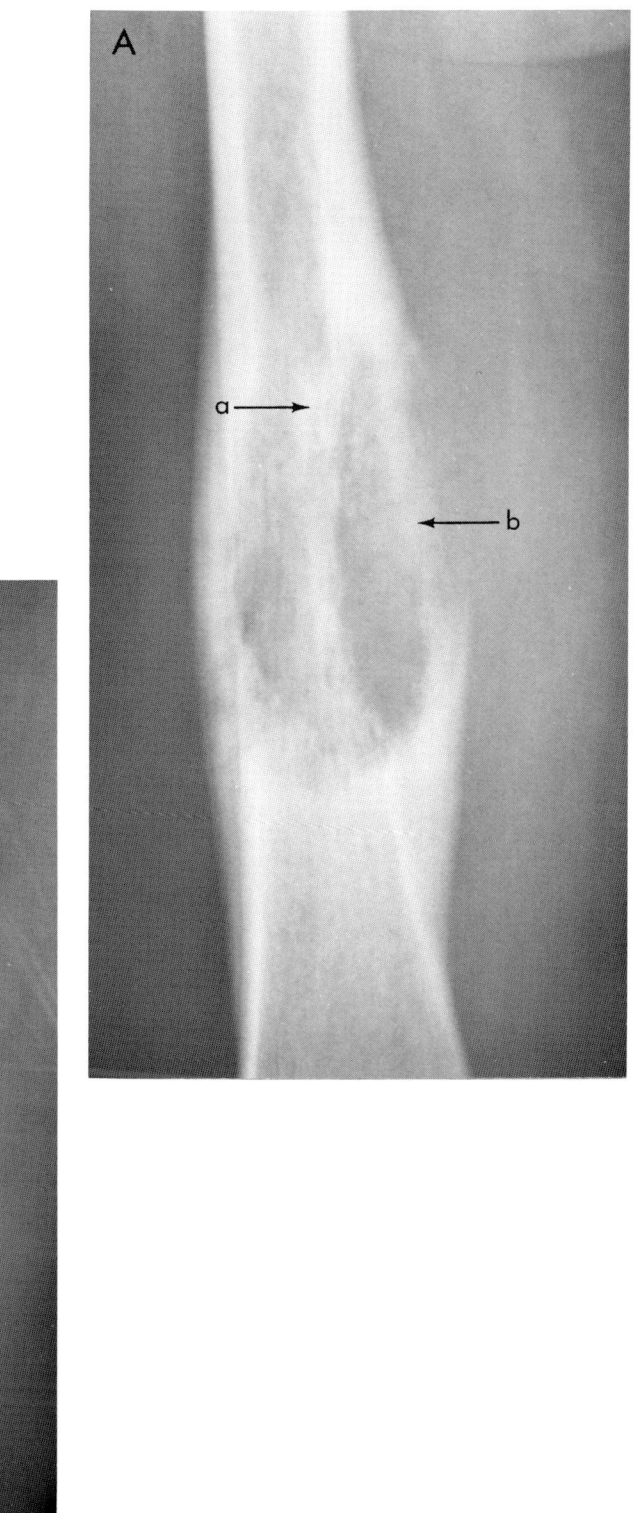
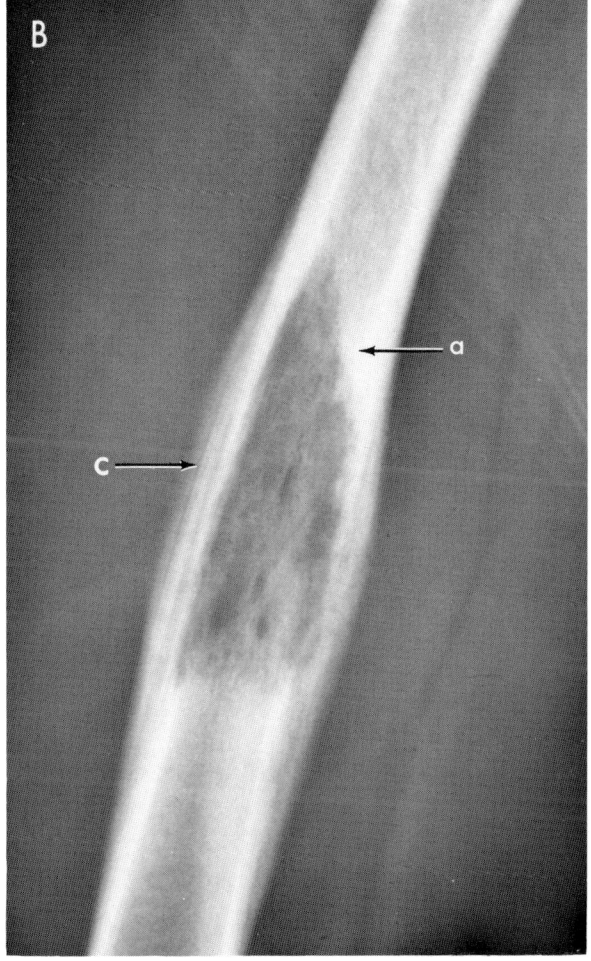

Figure 111 · Osteosarcoma of Femur / 277

Figure 112.—Parosteal sarcomas of the femur.

AFIP Case No. 1169622: **A,** anteroposterior, and **B,** lateral views.

DIAGNOSIS AND GRADE.—Parosteal sarcoma, femur; growth rate II.
LIFE INFORMATION.— Male, 32 years; well three years later.
LOCATION.—A circumscribed parosteal mass, centered on the middle third of the distal metaphysis, confined to the metaphysis.
SIZE.—6 × 5 × 3 cm.
MINERALIZATION OF TUMOR.—Mass of solid (**A, a**) and lumpy (**A, b**) tumor bone, with a number of radiolucent areas; ossified rim at superior margin.
DESTRUCTION.—Ill-defined moth-eaten pattern in cortex beneath the tumor.
PROLIFERATION.—Dense hyperostotic (**B, c**) and endostotic (**B, d**) new bone, increasing thickness of the cortex beneath the tumor.

DIFFERENTIAL DIAGNOSIS	PROBABILITY
Parosteal sarcoma	100

COMMENT: A typical parosteal sarcoma with peripheral soft tissue elements, and destruction of underlying bone which does not appear to penetrate cortex totally. The uncalcified portion usually consists of cartilage, fibrous tissue or unmineralized osteoid; when the tissue is fibrous, underlying tumor bone is often highly irregular, as here.

AFIP Case No. 962302: **C,** lateral projection.

DIAGNOSIS AND GRADE.—Parosteal sarcoma, femur; growth rate IC.
LIFE INFORMATION.—Female, 43 years; well seven years later.
LOCATION.—A circumscribed parosteal tumor on the posterior metaphysial cortex of the distal femur.
SIZE.—5 × 3 cm.
MINERALIZATION OF TUMOR.—Contiguous mass of tumor bone containing lumps, floccules and radiolucent cap (**arrows**); no cleavage plane.
DESTRUCTION.—None.
PROLIFERATION.—Endosteal proliferation of bone beneath the tumor.

DIFFERENTIAL DIAGNOSIS	PROBABILITY
Parosteal sarcoma	100

COMMENT: A garden variety of parosteal sarcoma. The flocculation indicates a surface cap of cartilage.

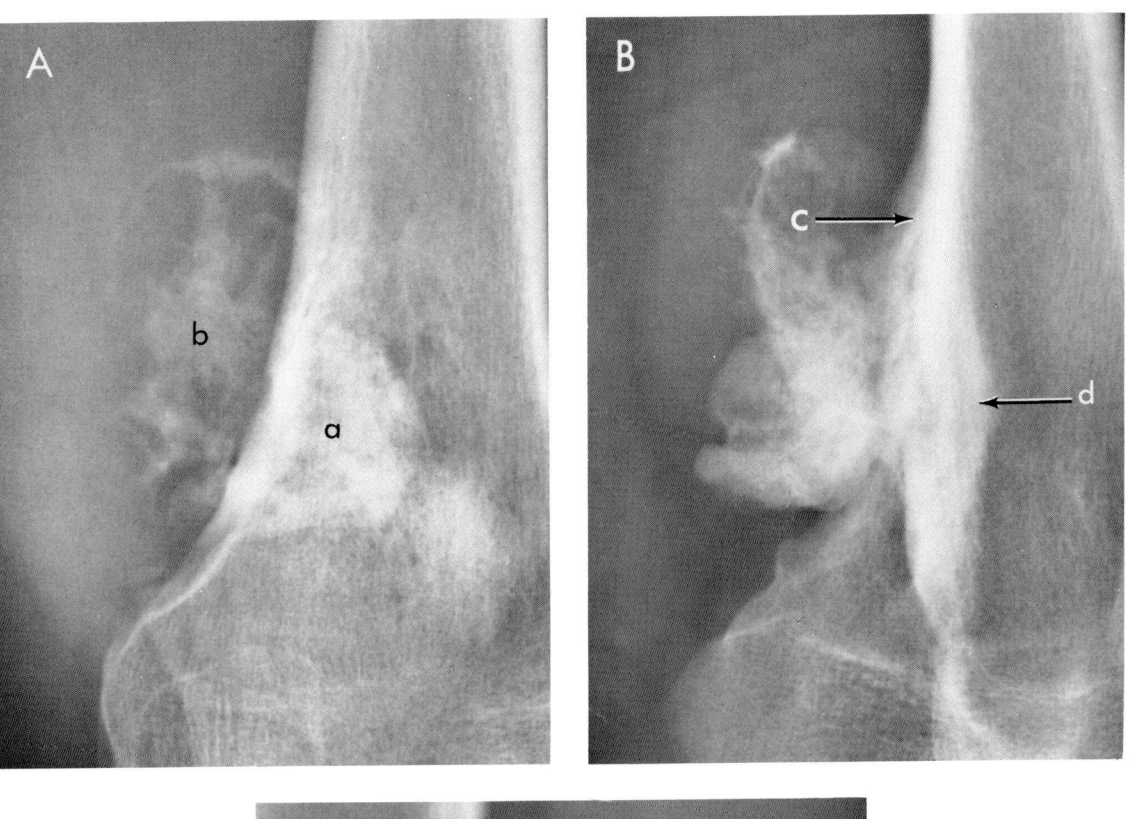
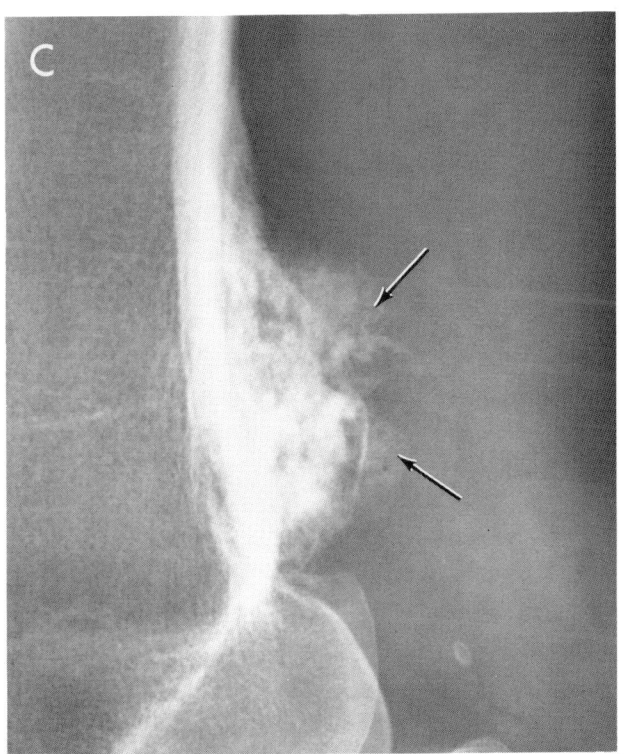

Figure 112 · Parosteal Sarcomas of Femur / 279

Figure 113.—Parosteal sarcoma of the femur.

AFIP Case No. 1011399: **A,** lateral, and **B,** anteroposterior views.

DIAGNOSIS AND GRADE.—Parosteal sarcoma, femur; growth rate II.
LIFE INFORMATION.—Male, 31 years; well five years after onset.
LOCATION.—Parosteal tumor on the posterior metaphysial cortex of the distal femur, extending down to the level of the epiphysis and up to the shaft.
SIZE.—8 × 5 × 3 cm.
MINERALIZATION OF TUMOR.—A lumpy mass of tumor bone, with several circumscribed radiolucent areas; no cleavage plane or ossified rim.
DESTRUCTION.—A moth-eaten pattern of holes, probably within the tumor rather than in the cortex.
PROLIFERATION.—None.

DIFFERENTIAL DIAGNOSIS	PROBABILITY
Parosteal sarcoma	.99
Osteochondroma	< .01

COMMENT: A low flat parosteal sarcoma with irregular surface.

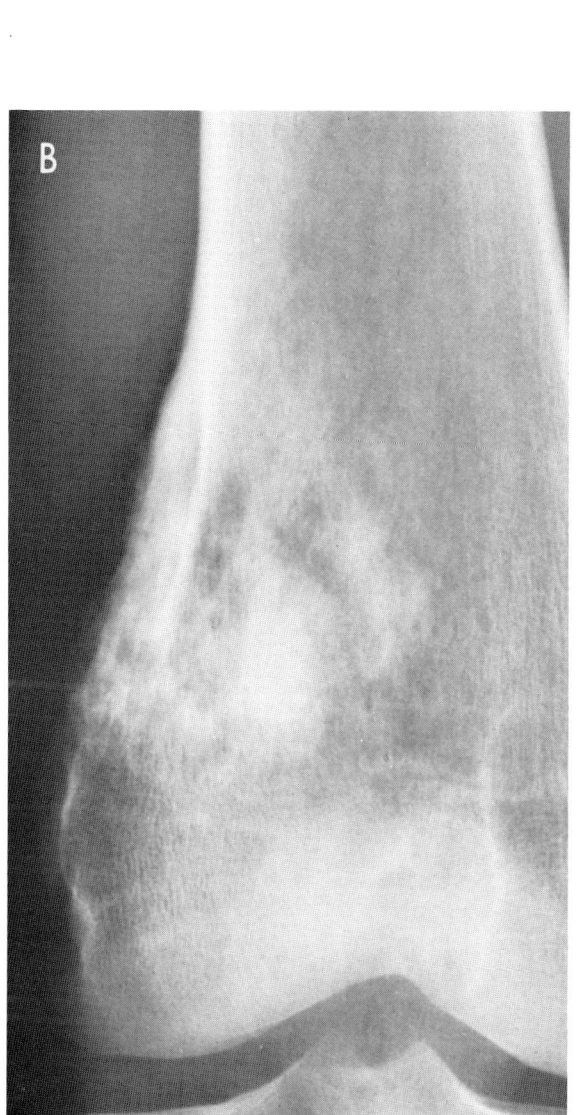
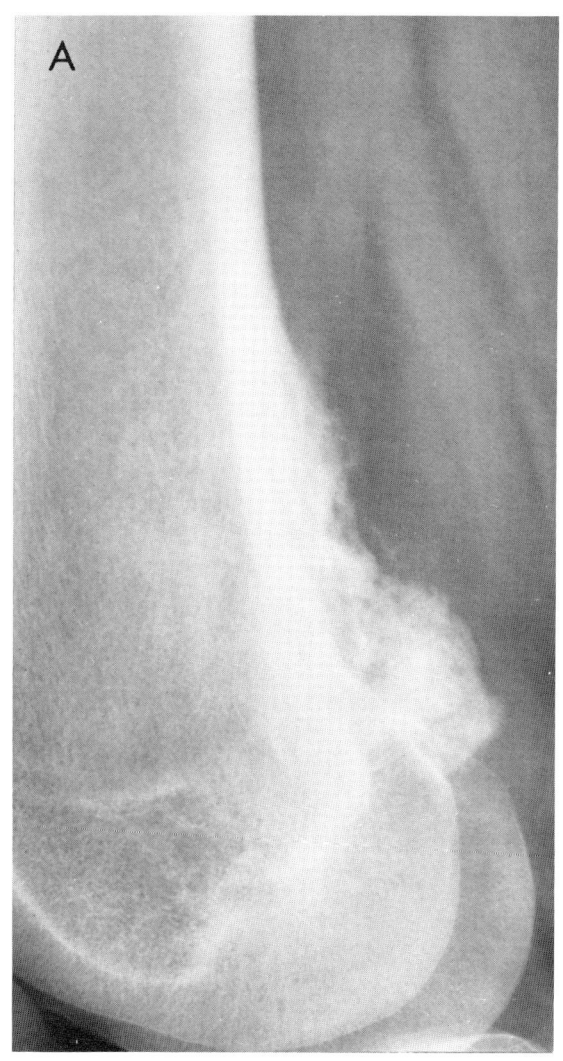

Figure 113 · Parosteal Sarcoma of Femur / 281

Figure 114.—Parosteal sarcoma of the femur.

AFIP Case No. 1200785: Anteroposterior views—**A**, initial study; **B**, 3 months later; **C**, 10 months later.

DIAGNOSIS AND GRADE.—Parosteal sarcoma, femur; growth rate II.
LIFE INFORMATION.—Male, 66 years; last known to be well.
LOCATION.—A circumscribed bony mass just above the lesser trochanter, on the medial surface of the femoral neck.
SIZE.—Initially 5 × 3 cm.
MINERALIZATION OF TUMOR.—In **A** the extraosseous lesion consists of a dense, sharply circumscribed mass of tumor bone attached to the underlying cortex, with an overlying radiolucent soft tissue mass of some magnitude.
DESTRUCTION.—Initially, vague rarefaction in the trochanter.

Three months later (**B**) the dense parosteal mass is breaking up, and there is now a clearly defined pattern of destruction in the base of the lesser trochanter.

Ten months later (**C**) the tumor, increased to 6 × 5 cm, shows an extensive moth-eaten pattern of destruction, with lumps and clouds of tumor bone in the extraosseous portion.
PROLIFERATION.—None.

	DIFFERENTIAL DIAGNOSIS	PROBABILITY
Exam. 1	Parosteal sarcoma	.97
	Myositis ossificans	.02
	Osteosarcoma	< .01
Exam. 2	Osteosarcoma	.96
	Fibrosarcoma	.02
	Chondrosarcoma	.01

COMMENT: A seemingly quiescent tumor which in 10 months appears to change its character entirely, a change clearly reflected in the computer differential diagnosis.

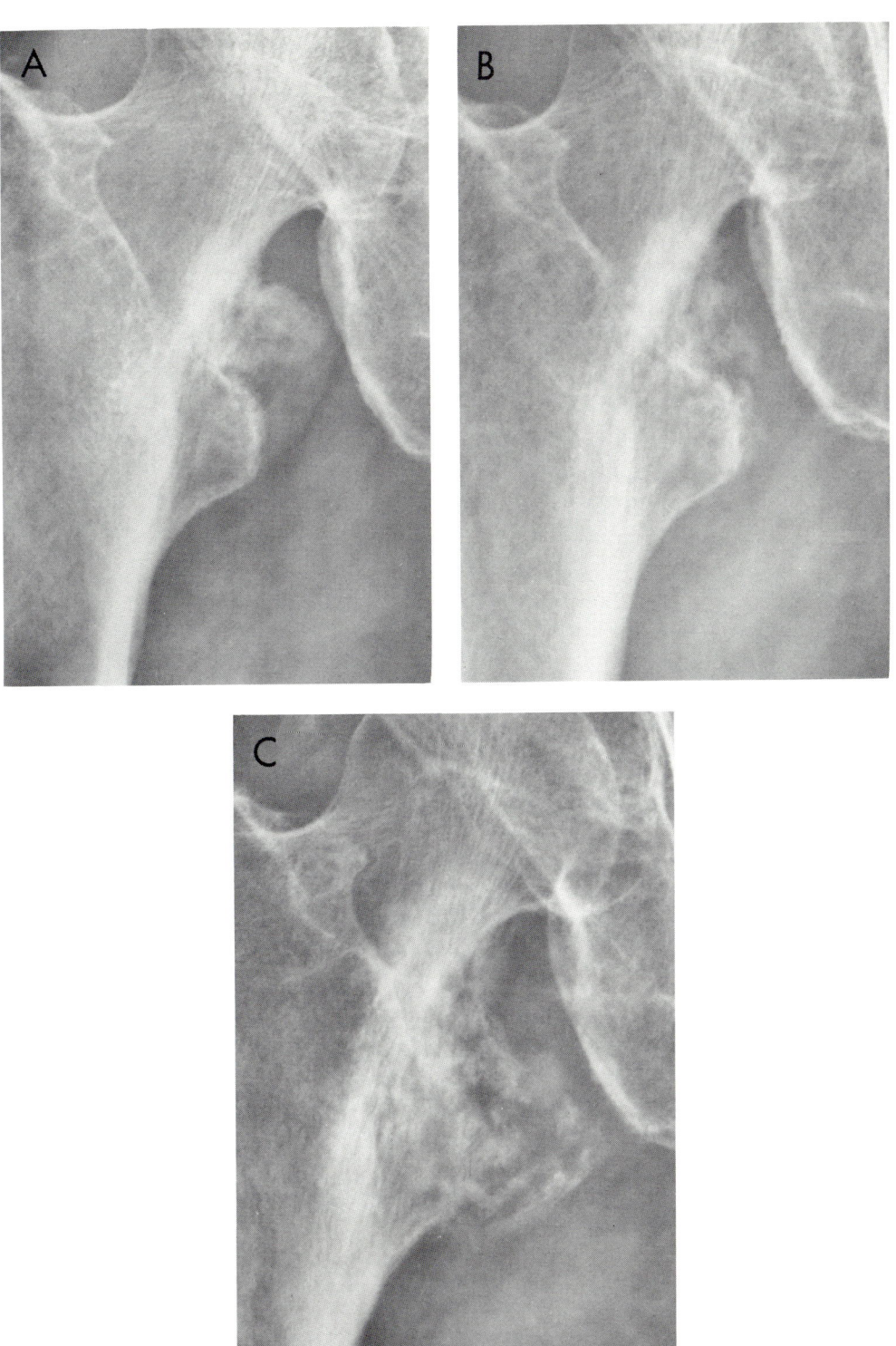

Figure 114 · Parosteal Sarcoma of Femur / 283

Figure 115.—Parosteal sarcoma of the femur.

AFIP Case No. 1166130: **A,** anteroposterior, and **B,** lateral views.

DIAGNOSIS AND GRADE.—Parosteal sarcoma, femur; growth rate IC.
LIFE INFORMATION.—Male, 43 years; well two years after onset.
LOCATION.—A fairly circumscribed tumor centered on the cortex of the middle third of the distal metaphysis, involving three quadrants of the circumference and extending distally to the epiphysis and proximally to the shaft.

SIZE.—10 × 7 × 6 cm.
MINERALIZATION OF TUMOR.—Dense tumor bone comprising the bulk of the extraosseous mass, with overlying radiolucent tissue, and seeming to wrap around the shaft; well-developed cleavage plane (**A, arrow**); edge of the tumor bone quite irregular.
DESTRUCTION.—None; the cortex is intact everywhere.
PROLIFERATION.—None.

DIFFERENTIAL DIAGNOSIS	PROBABILITY
Parosteal sarcoma	.95
Osteosarcoma	.03
Osteochondroma	< .01
Myositis ossificans	< .01

COMMENT: While apparently a very mature bone-forming tumor, the location and enveloping pattern around the shaft present an appearance different from that in the preceding cases.

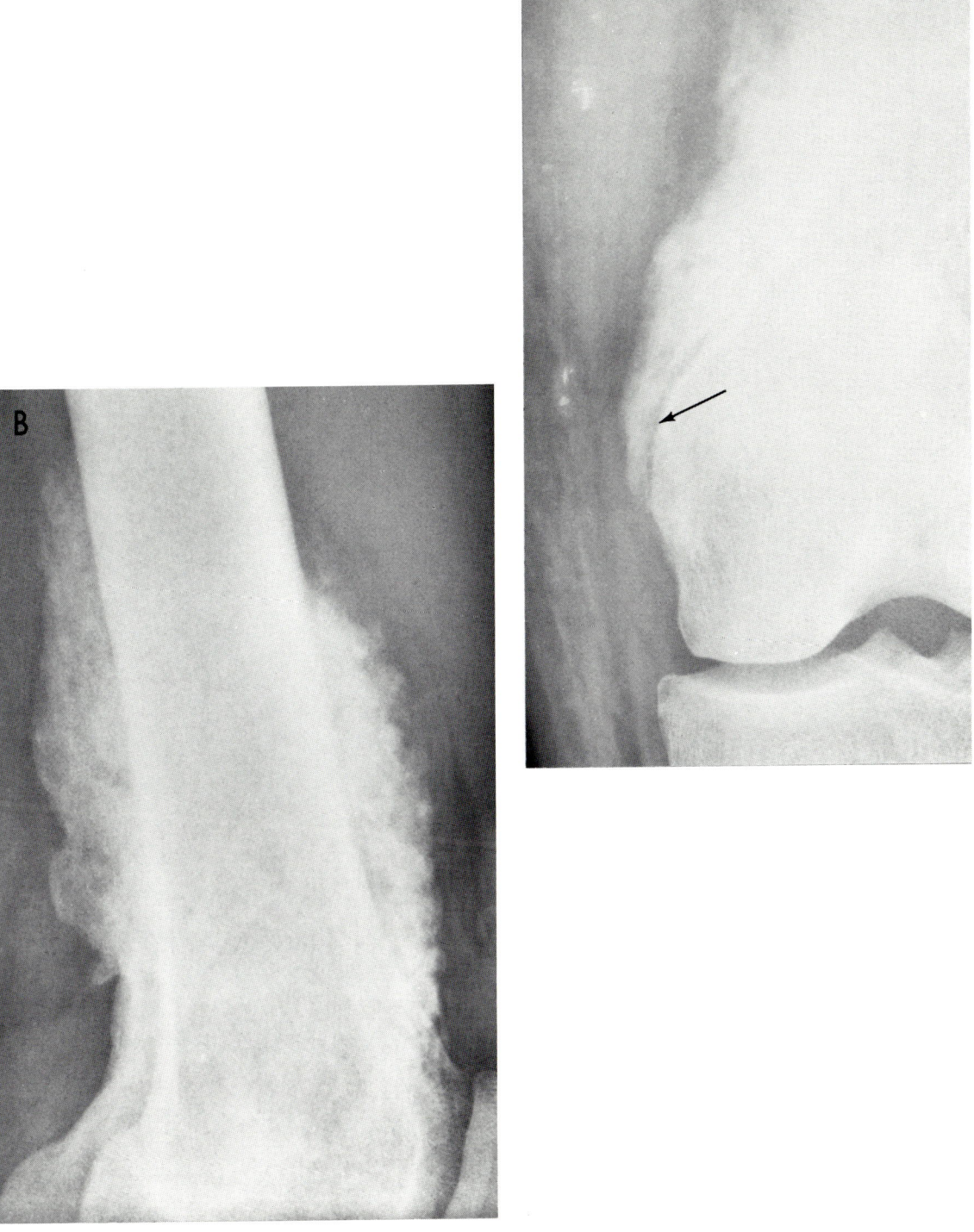

Figure 115 · Parosteal Sarcoma of Femur / 285

Figure 116.—Parosteal sarcoma of the femur.

AFIP Case No. 840231: **A,** anteroposterior, and **B,** lateral views.

DIAGNOSIS AND GRADE.—Parosteal sarcoma, femur; growth rate IC.

LIFE INFORMATION.—Male, 25 years; survival unknown.

LOCATION.—A large circumscribed mass parosteally centered at the level of the middle third of the distal femoral metaphysis, extending distally to involve the epiphysis and proximally to involve the shaft.

SIZE.—$14 \times 9 \times 7$ cm.

MINERALIZATION OF TUMOR.—Contiguous tumor bone based solidly on the posterior cortex, with endosteal thickening of cortex; several small radiolucencies in the mass and a small cleavage plane (**A, arrow**); edges of the tumor bone smooth and sharp, with the tumor seeming to wrap around the cortex.

DESTRUCTION.—None.

PROLIFERATION.—None.

DIFFERENTIAL DIAGNOSIS	PROBABILITY
Parosteal sarcoma	.92
Osteochondroma	.07
Osteosarcoma	< .01
Myositis ossificans	< .01

COMMENT: The tumor seems to be growing so slowly that it displays the same functions as mature bone, such as formation of buttresses and endosteal bone.

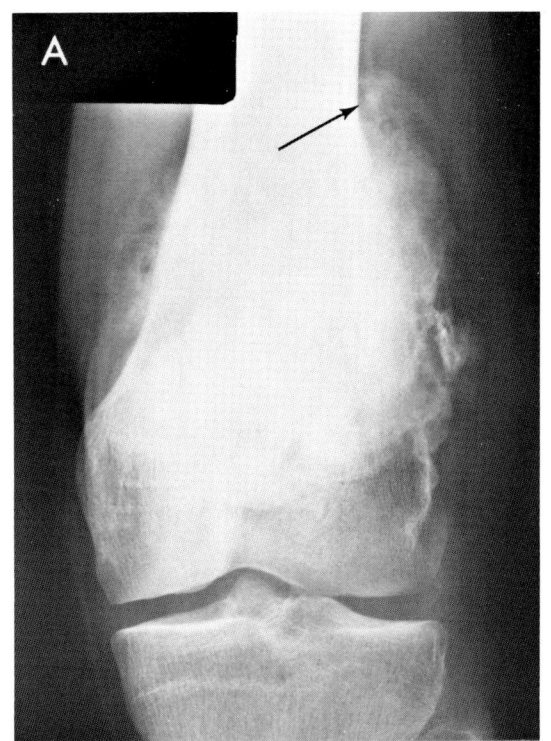
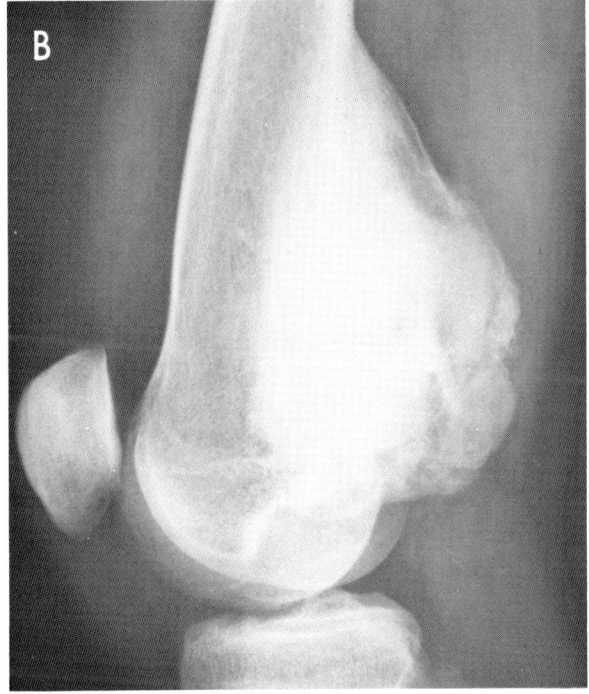

Figure 116 · Parosteal Sarcoma of Femur

Figure 117.—Parosteal sarcomas of the femur and tibia.

AFIP Case No. 1011792: **A,** anteroposterior, and **B,** lateral views.

DIAGNOSIS AND GRADE.—Parosteal sarcoma, femur; growth rate IC.
LIFE INFORMATION.—Female, 18 years; survival unknown.
LOCATION.—A parosteal circumscribed tumor centered on the posterior metaphysial cortex of the distal femur.
SIZE.—8 × 3 × 6 cm.
MINERALIZATION OF TUMOR.—Dense mass of contiguous tumor bone, with oval radiolucencies; one small cleavage plane (**B, arrow**).
DESTRUCTION.—At least one oval geographic area; regular contour.
PROLIFERATION.—Sclerotic rim around a small area of destruction; large buttress at upper margin, probably tumor bone.

DIFFERENTIAL DIAGNOSIS	PROBABILITY
Parosteal sarcoma	.89
Osteosarcoma	.10

COMMENT: A typical parosteal sarcoma. The posterior cortex is replaced by cancellous bone, much as in benign osteochondroma. Only a trace of the original cortex remains.

AFIP Case No. 1071994: **C,** anteroposterior view.

DIAGNOSIS AND GRADE.—Parosteal sarcoma, tibia; growth rate IC.
LIFE INFORMATION.—Male, 15 years; well five years later.
LOCATION.—A small, smooth circumscribed lump located parosteally on the medial shaft of the upper tibia.
SIZE.—2 × 1 cm.
MINERALIZATION OF TUMOR.—Dense tumor bone with cleavage plane (**arrow**).
DESTRUCTION.—None.
PROLIFERATION.—None.

DIFFERENTIAL DIAGNOSIS	PROBABILITY
Parosteal sarcoma	.82
Myositis ossificans	.11
Osteosarcoma	.06

COMMENT: Differentiation is between myositis ossificans and parosteal sarcoma. In this situation both radiologist and pathologist are often in trouble. The history is usually helpful, being long with parosteal sarcoma and brief with myositis.

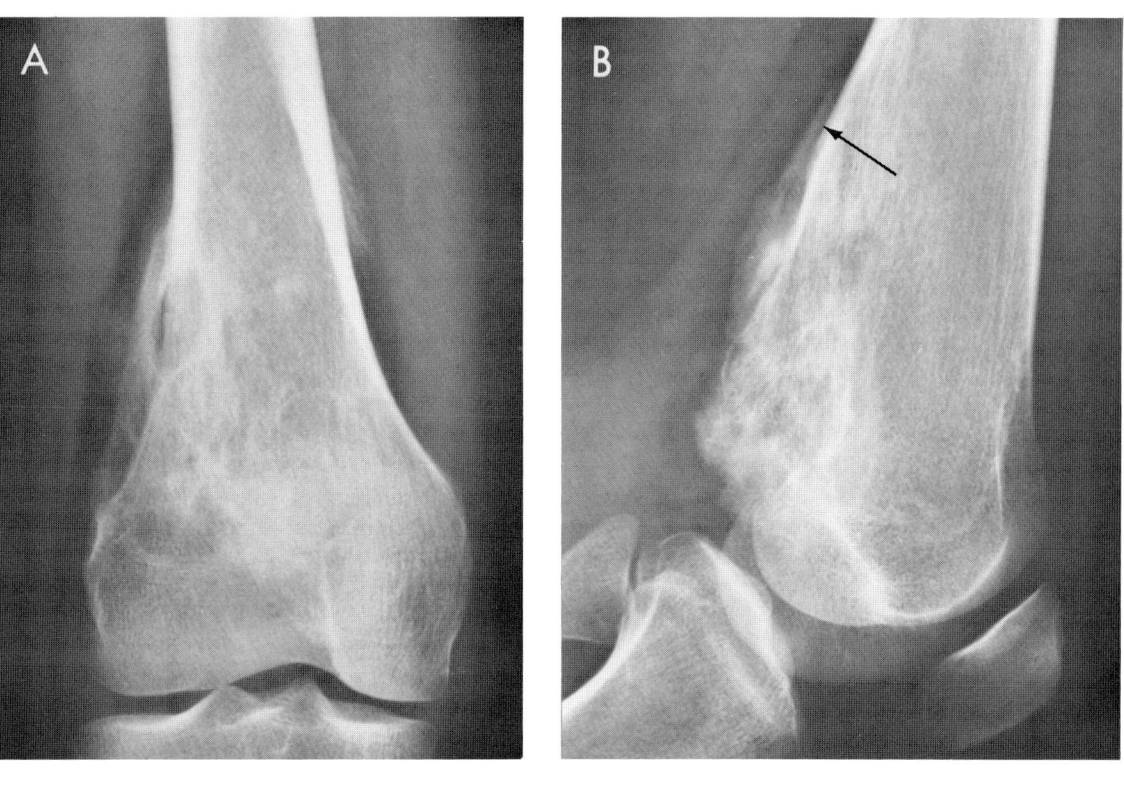
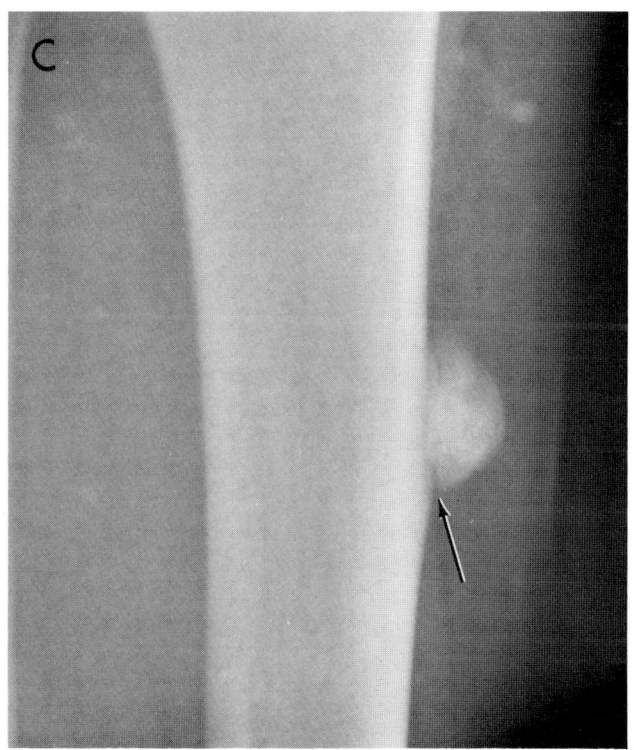

Figure 117 · Parosteal Sarcomas / 289

Figure 118.—Parosteal sarcoma of the fibula.

AFIP Case No. 1138854: **A,** anteroposterior, and **B,** lateral views.

DIAGNOSIS AND GRADE.—Parosteal sarcoma, fibula; growth rate IC.

LIFE INFORMATION.—Male, 12 years; survival unknown.

LOCATION.—A tumor centered parosteally over the proximal metaphysis, extending to the shaft and the level of the growth plate.

SIZE.—7 × 3 × 2 cm.

MINERALIZATION OF TUMOR.—A sharply circumscribed solid pattern of tumor bone, with inherent radiating spicular pattern; cleavage plane between tumor and cortex.

DESTRUCTION.—Well-defined geographic pattern within the medullary cavity beneath the tumor; lobulated contour.

PROLIFERATION.—Cortex beneath the tumor expanded about 5 mm, with overall tubular widening of the metaphysis.

DIFFERENTIAL DIAGNOSIS	PROBABILITY
Parosteal sarcoma	.54
Osteosarcoma	.45

COMMENT: A well-defined parosteal sarcoma which may have an underlying fibrous medullary lesion. This has the pattern of a double tumor or of a bone-forming lesion arising in a preexisting benign fibrous tumor.

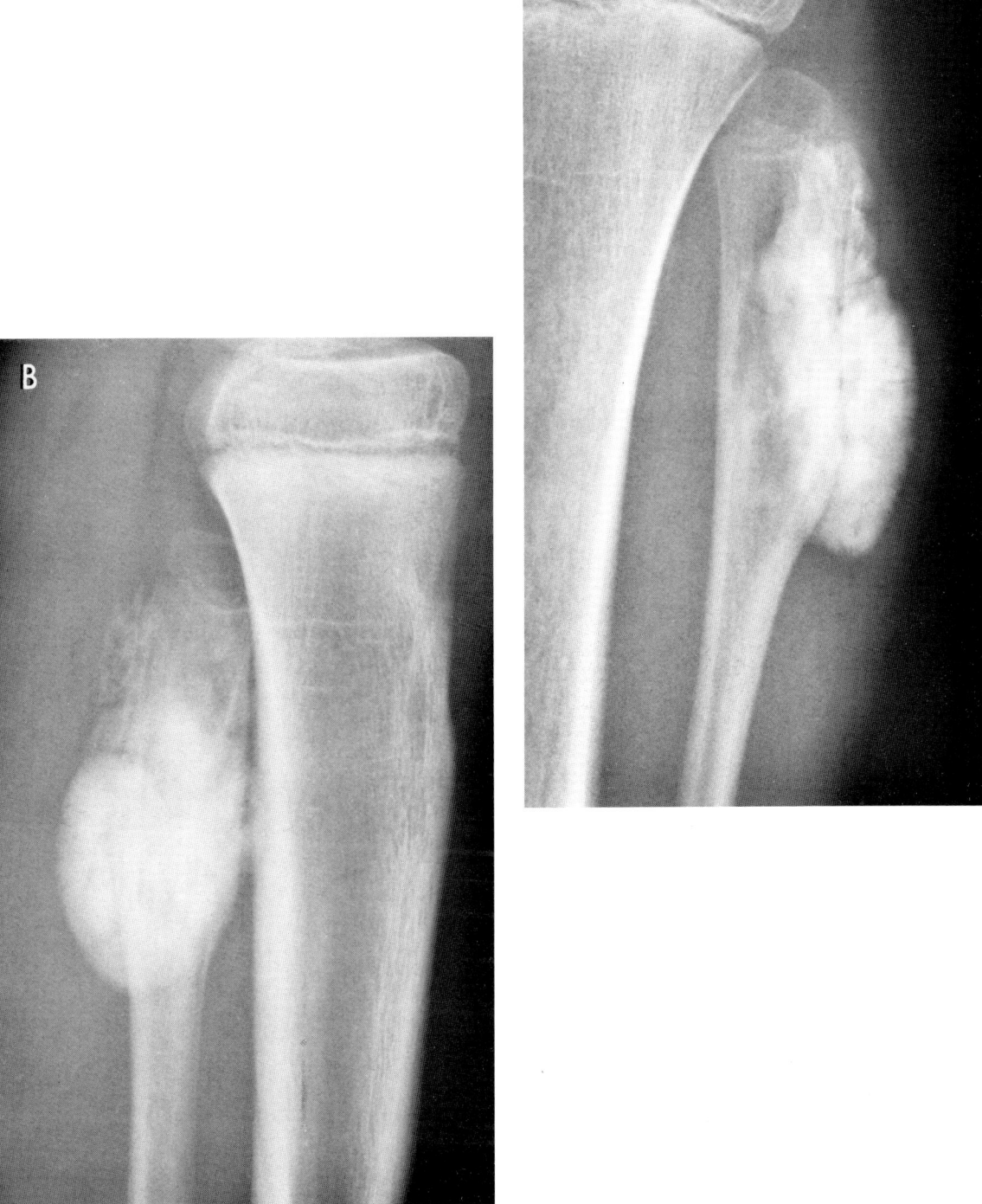

Figure 118 · Parosteal Sarcoma of Fibula / 291

Figure 119.—Parosteal sarcoma of the tibia.

AFIP Case No. 1027447: Anteroposterior views—**A,** initial examination; **B,** 17 months later.

DIAGNOSIS AND GRADE.—Parosteal sarcoma, tibia; growth rate IC.
LIFE INFORMATION.—Male, 29 years; well five years after onset.
LOCATION.—A parosteal mass of tumor bone attached to the cortex of the proximal tibial metaphysis between tibia and fibula, extending to the epiphysis and down onto the shaft.
SIZE.—11 × 4 × 3 cm.
MINERALIZATION OF TUMOR.—A veillike accumulation of tumor bone, with lamina of radiolucent substance; distinct cleavage plane between tumor and shaft (**B, arrow**).
DESTRUCTION.—None definite, although as viewed through tumor bone the cortex seems to be missing; also some spotty reduction of cancellous bone in the metaphysis beneath the lesion (**a**).
PROLIFERATION.—The cortex seems to have been remodeled outward beneath the tumor, as in osteochondroma.

DIFFERENTIAL DIAGNOSIS	PROBABILITY
Parosteal sarcoma	.42
Osteosarcoma	.36
Chondrosarcoma	.14
Myositis ossificans	.05

COMMENT: This is one of a variety of parosteal sarcomas which both radiologically and histologically resembles myositis ossificans. The patient had a diagnosis of myositis ossificans for five years before parosteal sarcoma was finally diagnosed.

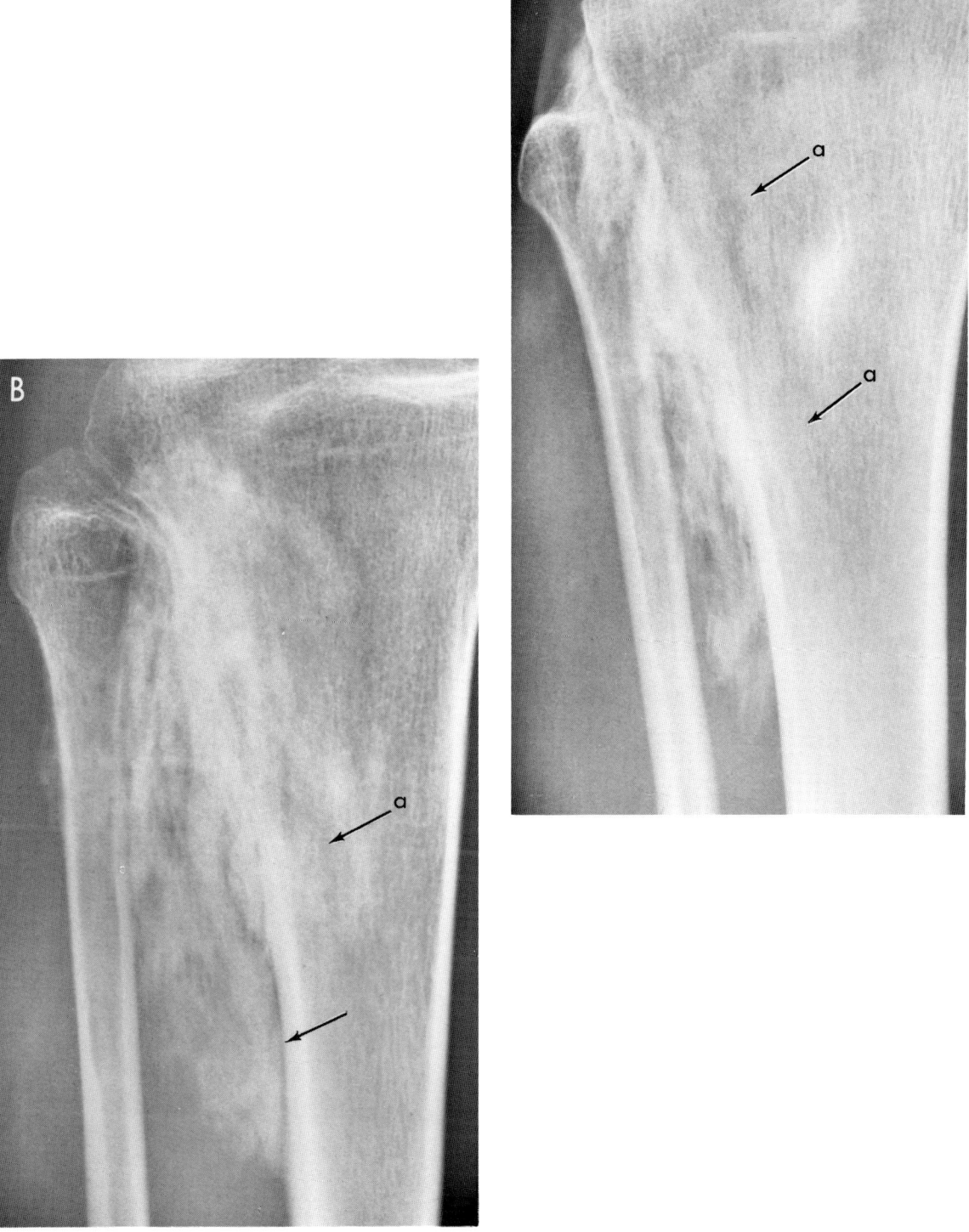

Figure 119 · Parosteal Sarcoma of Tibia / 293

Figure 120.—Parosteal sarcoma of the skull.

AFIP Case No. 740221: **A,** anteroposterior, and **B,** lateral views.

DIAGNOSIS AND GRADE.—Parosteal sarcoma, skull; growth rate IC.
LIFE INFORMATION.—Male, 32 years; survival unknown.
LOCATION.—A large circumscribed lesion of the occipital region which appears to lie in a greatly enlarged space between the inner and outer tables; no evidence of soft tissue extension. The location is intramedullary, not parosteal.

SIZE.—15 × 13 × 5 cm.
MINERALIZATION OF TUMOR.—Multiple lumps and floccules of tumor matrix mineralization in a radiolucent background.
DESTRUCTION.—Geographic; lobulated contour.
PROLIFERATION.—Both inner and outer tables are thinned and have been expanded more than 1 cm, with the result that this large tumor is encapsulated between the tables of the occiput.

DIFFERENTIAL DIAGNOSIS	PROBABILITY
Chondrosarcoma	.89
Fibrosarcoma	.10

COMMENT: Parosteal sarcoma has traditionally been identified by location. In this instance, the histologic characteristics were similar to those of parosteal sarcoma, but the location is not consistent with this classification.

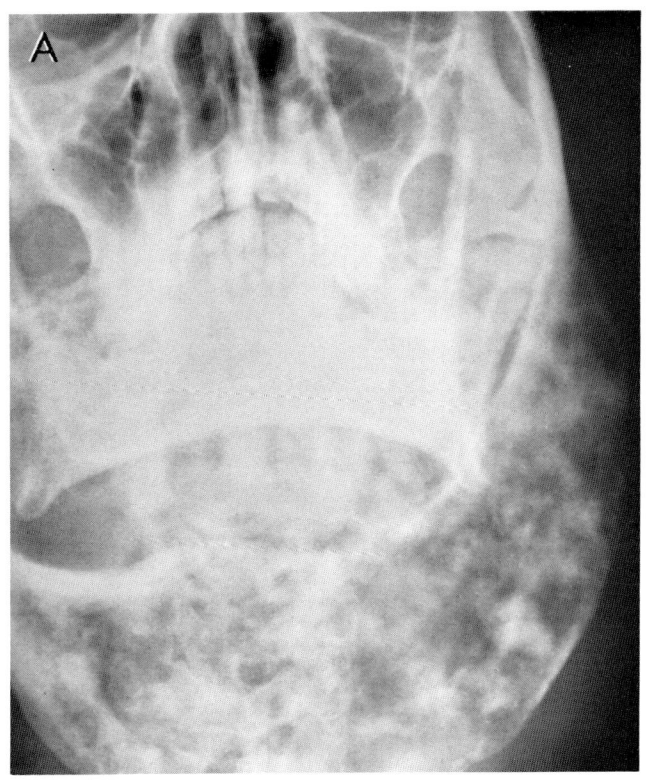
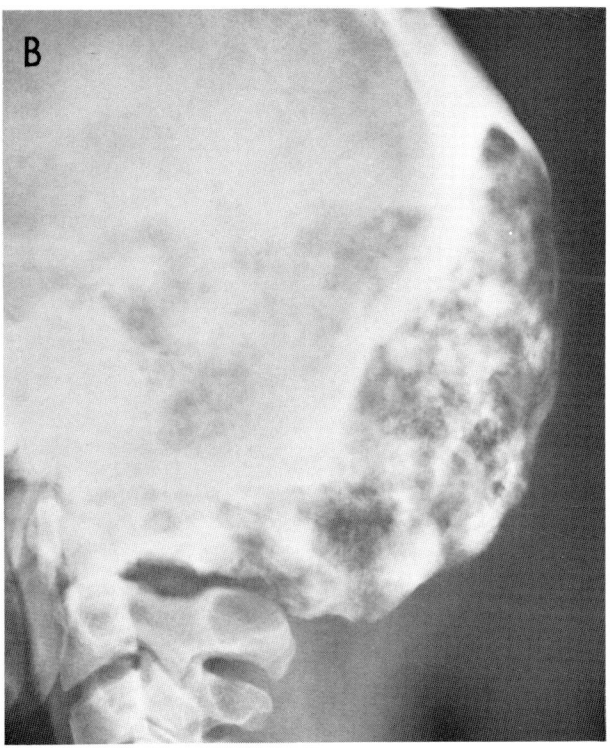

Figure 120 · Parosteal Sarcoma of Skull

Figure 121.—Myositis ossificans of the femur.

AFIP Case No. 1072072: Anteroposterior views—**A**, 18 days after injury; **B**, at 1 month.

DIAGNOSIS AND GRADE.—Myositis ossificans, femur; not graded.

LIFE INFORMATION.—Female, 8 years; well four years later.

LOCATION.—Initially, an ill-defined parosteal lesion in the posterolateral aspect of lower femoral shaft.

SIZE.—3 × 2 × 2 cm.

MINERALIZATION OF TUMOR.—Initially, none.

DESTRUCTION.—None.

PROLIFERATION.—A single delicate lamina of subperiosteal new bone (**A, a**).

One month later (**B**) the lamina of periosteal new bone has become thickened. There is now a circumscribed mass of cloudy tumor bone, with a faint mineralized rim at the margin (**x**). There is no cleavage plane.

DIFFERENTIAL DIAGNOSIS	PROBABILITY
Myositis ossificans	.61
Osteosarcoma	.35
Chondrosarcoma	.02
Parosteal sarcoma	< .01

COMMENT: The soft tissue mass and the periosteal lesion are two separate lesions reacting to trauma. With healing the two fuse, so that the lesion comes to look like an osteochondroma. With Figure 122, showing myositis ossificans at six months and four years, the sequence of developing patterns is well illustrated.

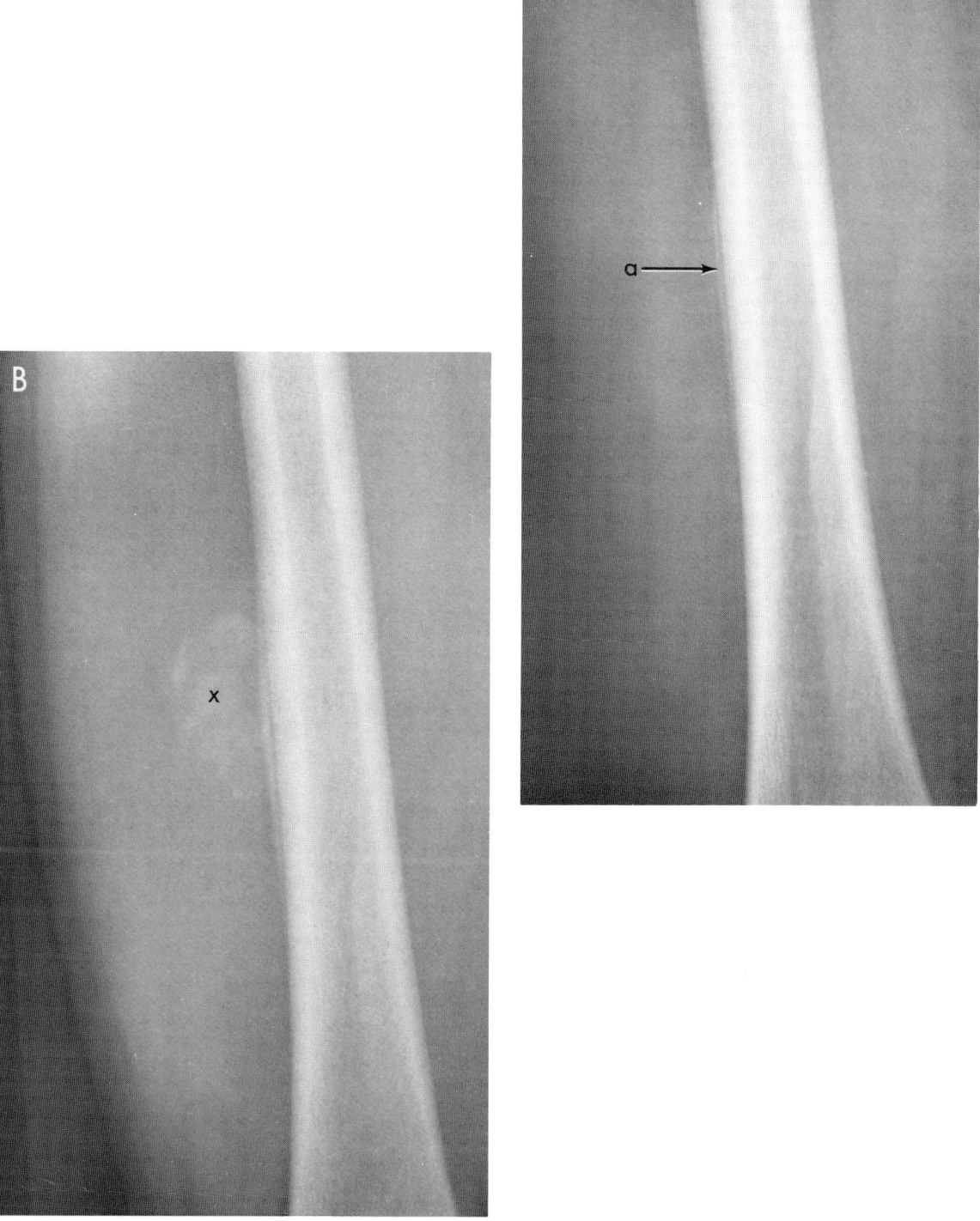

Figure 121 · Myositis Ossificans of Femur / 297

Figure 122.—Myositis ossificans of the femur.

AFIP Case No. 1100080: Anteroposterior views—**A,** six months after onset; **B,** four years later.

DIAGNOSIS AND GRADE.—Myositis ossificans, femur; not graded.
LIFE INFORMATION.—Male, 22 years; well six years after onset.
LOCATION.—A fairly well defined lesion located parosteally in the soft tissue posterior to the lower femoral shaft and based on the cortex.
SIZE.—First examination 7 × 1.5 cm.
MINERALIZATION OF TUMOR.—Veillike matrix mineralization at six months (**A, arrows**).
DESTRUCTION.—None.
PROLIFERATION.—None.

Four years after onset (**D**) size is diminished to 4 × 1 cm, and the lesion is now an almost solid hyperostosis.

DIFFERENTIAL DIAGNOSIS	PROBABILITY
Osteochondroma	.93
Parosteal sarcoma	.04
Osteosarcoma	.01
Myositis ossificans	< .01

COMMENT: The first symptom—pain of unknown cause—gradually increased. Biopsy, done about four months after onset, was interpreted as showing osteogenic sarcoma. The patient refused hip disarticulation. The veillike pattern of matrix mineralization is highly diagnostic of myositis ossificans.

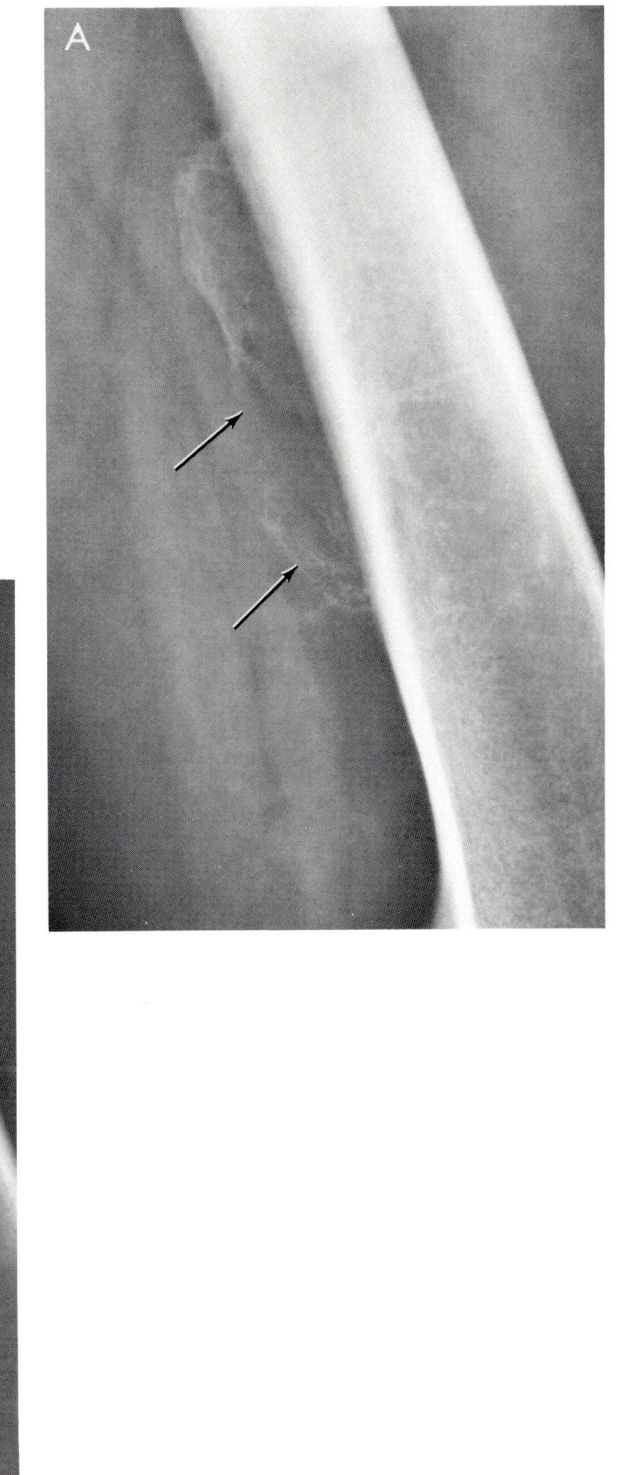
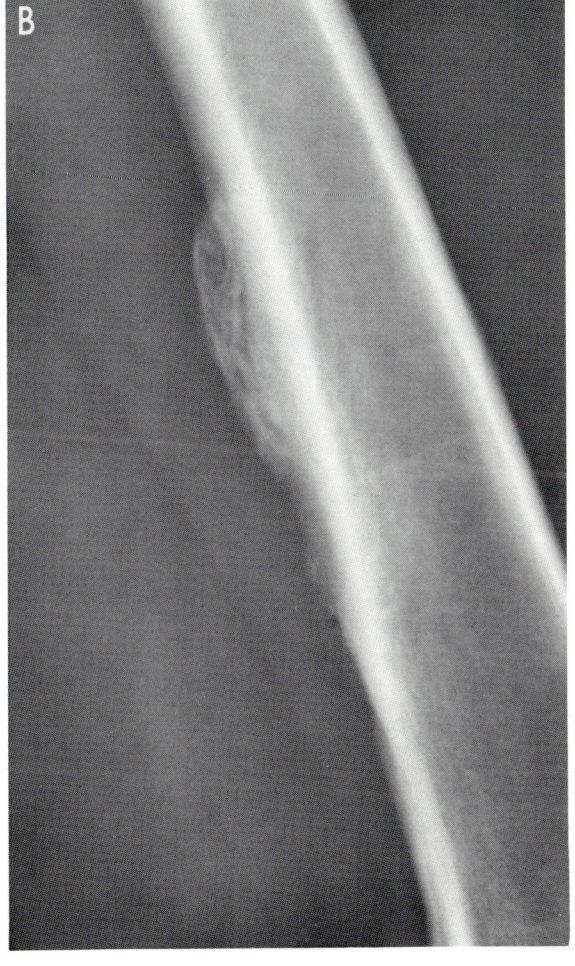

Figure 122 · Myositis Ossificans of Femur / 299

Figure 123.—Myositis ossificans of the radius.

AFIP Case No. 1084305: Anteroposterior views—**A,** one month after injury; **B,** four years later.

DIAGNOSIS AND GRADE.—Myositis ossificans, radius; ungraded.

LIFE INFORMATION.—Male, 48 years; well four years after onset.

LOCATION.—A circumscribed parosteal mass on the proximal radial shaft.

SIZE.—4 × 2 × 1.5 cm.

MINERALIZATION OF TUMOR.—At one month (**A**), a large contiguous mass of tumor bone and several smaller satellite nodules, fairly sharply circumscribed, with intrinsic radiating spiculation.

DESTRUCTION.—None.

PROLIFERATION.—None, beyond that described above.

Four years after onset (**B**) the mass has evolved into a dense mass of cortical and trabecular bone.

DIFFERENTIAL DIAGNOSIS	PROBABILITY
Myositis ossificans	.99
Osteosarcoma	< .01

COMMENT: This case demonstrates the difficulty in distinguishing between early myositis ossificans and a parosteal sarcoma (see Fig. 118).

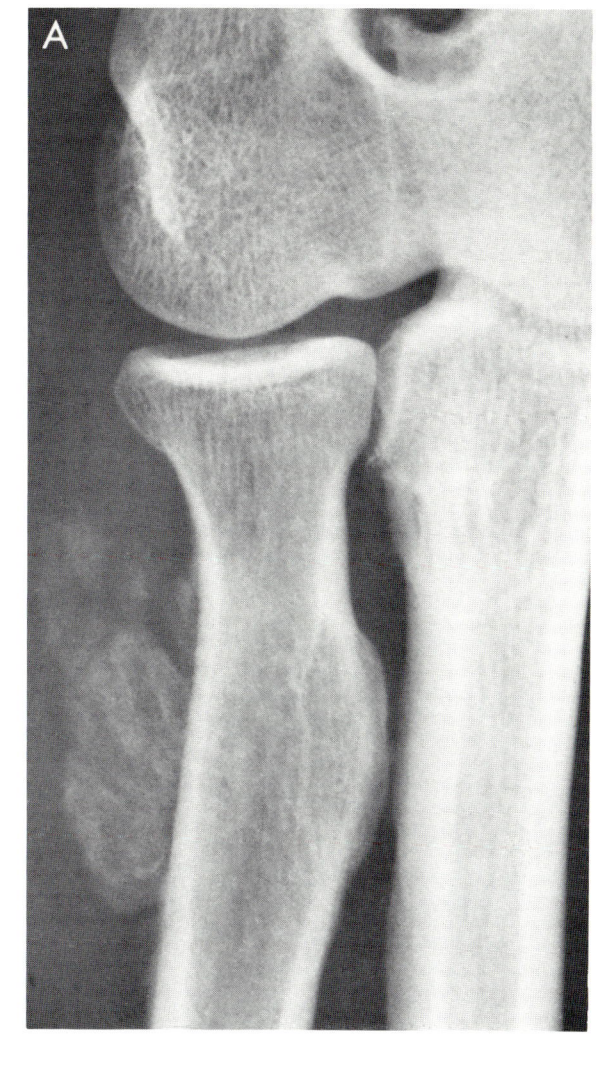
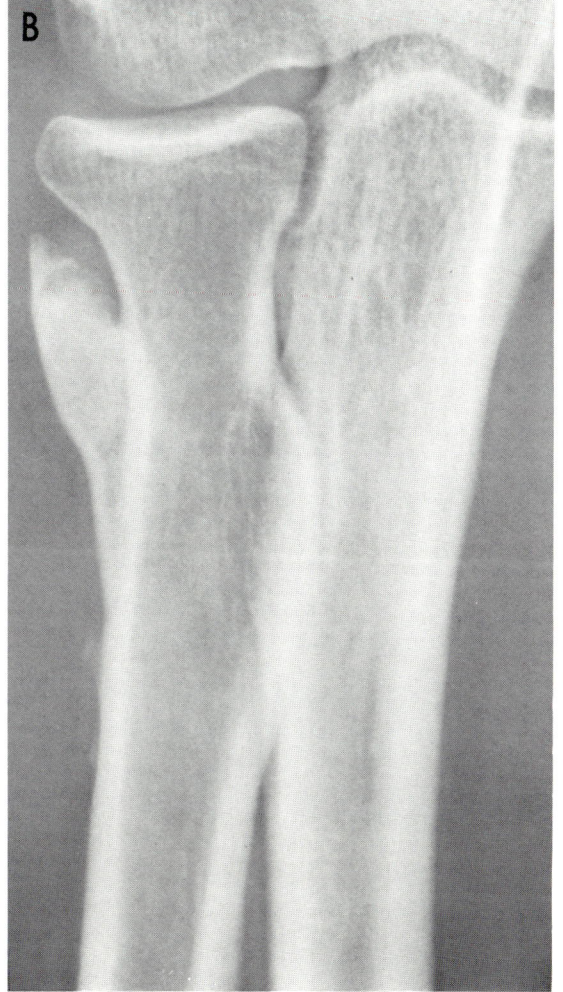

Figure 123 · Myositis Ossificans of Radius / 301

Figure 124.—Myositis ossificans of the ulna.

AFIP Case No. 1174968: Anteroposterior views—**A**, five weeks after onset; **B**, two years later.

DIAGNOSIS AND GRADE.—Myositis ossificans, ulna; ungraded.

LIFE INFORMATION.—Female, 16 years; well two years after onset.

LOCATION.—A parosteal lesion on the distal metaphysis.

SIZE.—20 × 8 mm.

MINERALIZATION OF TUMOR.—It is difficult to distinguish between the periosteal reparative response and the mineralization which occurs within myositis ossificans. Beyond the clearly defined periosteal reaction are clouds of calcific density which may not be periosteal in origin (**A, arrow**).

DESTRUCTION.—None.

PROLIFERATION.—A single thick lamina of periosteal new bone comprising a substantial part of the lesion.

DIFFERENTIAL DIAGNOSIS	PROBABILITY
Myositis ossificans	.99
Osteosarcoma	< .01
Chondrosarcoma	< .01

COMMENT: At first, the pattern resembles the periosteal reaction which develops over an early malignant tumor. Two years later the lesion has consolidated into a dense mass of normal appearing bone.

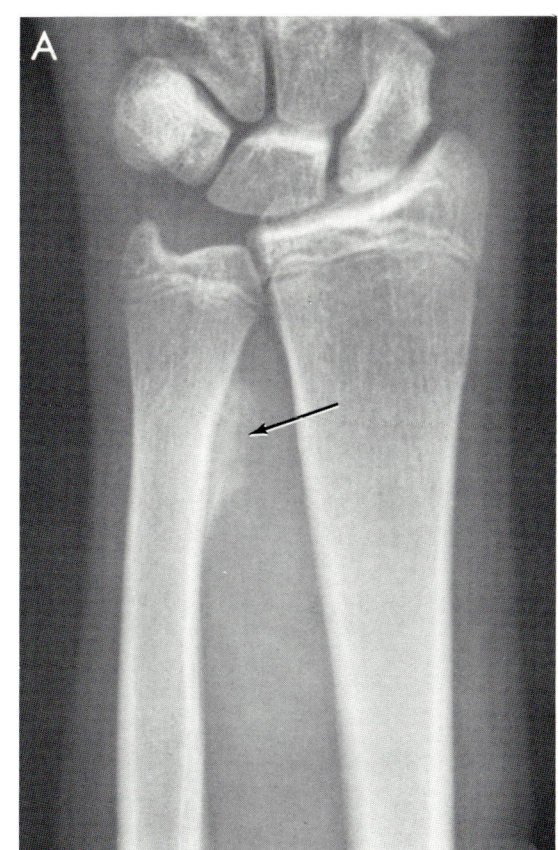
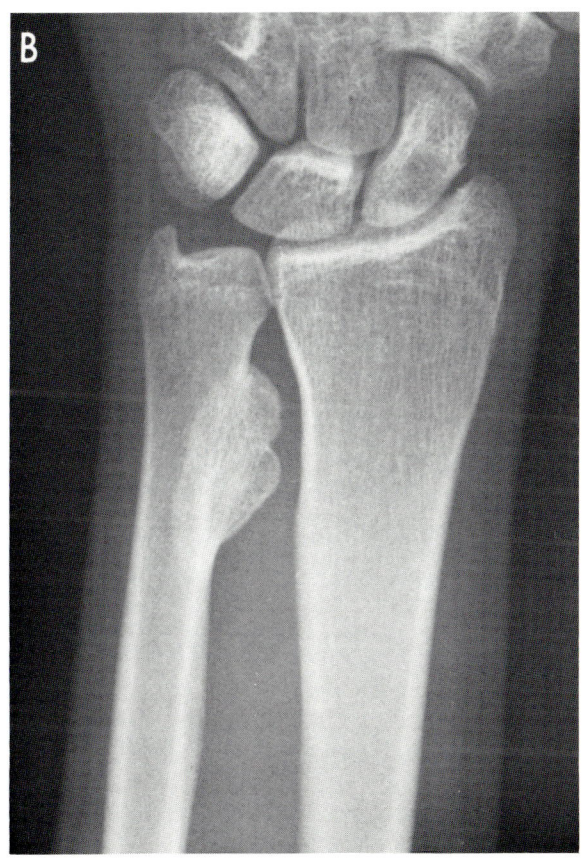

Figure 124 · Myositis Ossificans of Ulna / 303

Figure 125.—Myositis ossificans of the index finger.

AFIP Case No. 1024980: Posteroanterior views—**A,** initial examination; **B,** at 3 months.

DIAGNOSIS AND GRADE.—Myositis ossificans, index finger; not graded.

LIFE INFORMATION.—Male, 33 years; well five years later.

LOCATION.—An ill-defined parosteal lesion centered over the proximal shaft of the metacarpal of the index finger.

SIZE.—Initially 15 × 15 mm; at three months, 4 × 1 cm.

MINERALIZATION OF TUMOR.—None initially.

DESTRUCTION.—Shallow geographic erosion of cortex (**A, arrow**).

PROLIFERATION.—Initially, none. At three months (**B**) ill-defined flecks of calcific density in soft tissue mass; saucerized erosion enlarged; ill-defined Codman triangle.

DIFFERENTIAL DIAGNOSIS	PROBABILITY
Myositis ossificans	100

COMMENT: Surprisingly large component of destruction. The computer's unequivocal diagnosis is an interesting reflection on probability matrices. Its only experience with this exact pattern is with this lesion; therefore the absolute identification.

AFIP Case No. 1209621: Posteroanterior views—**C,** 1 week after onset; **D,** at 4 weeks; **E,** at 10 weeks.

DIAGNOSIS AND GRADE.—Myositis ossificans, index finger; ungraded.

LIFE INFORMATION.—Female, 53 years; well three years later.

LOCATION.—A parosteal soft tissue swelling medial to the shaft of the proximal phalanx.

SIZE.—Gradual enlargement to 4 × 1 cm at 10 weeks.

MINERALIZATION OF TUMOR.—None at 4 weeks; at 10 weeks, indistinct clouds of matrix mineralization; no cleavage plane.

DESTRUCTION.—None at 4 weeks; at 10 weeks, a diffuse permeative pattern.

PROLIFERATION.—None at 4 weeks; at 10 weeks, shaft enveloped in a single lamina of new bone, which is thick and irregular on the side of maximal involvement.

DIFFERENTIAL DIAGNOSIS	PROBABILITY
Myositis ossificans	.99
Osteosarcoma	< .01

COMMENT: Relatively quiescent at first, by 10 weeks a massive reactive response has developed, manifested by subperiosteal new bone and diffuse permeative response probably related to hyperemia. As in **B**, maximum reaction has occurred by 10 weeks. Amputation was through the metacarpophalangeal joint. (See Comment on preceding case.)

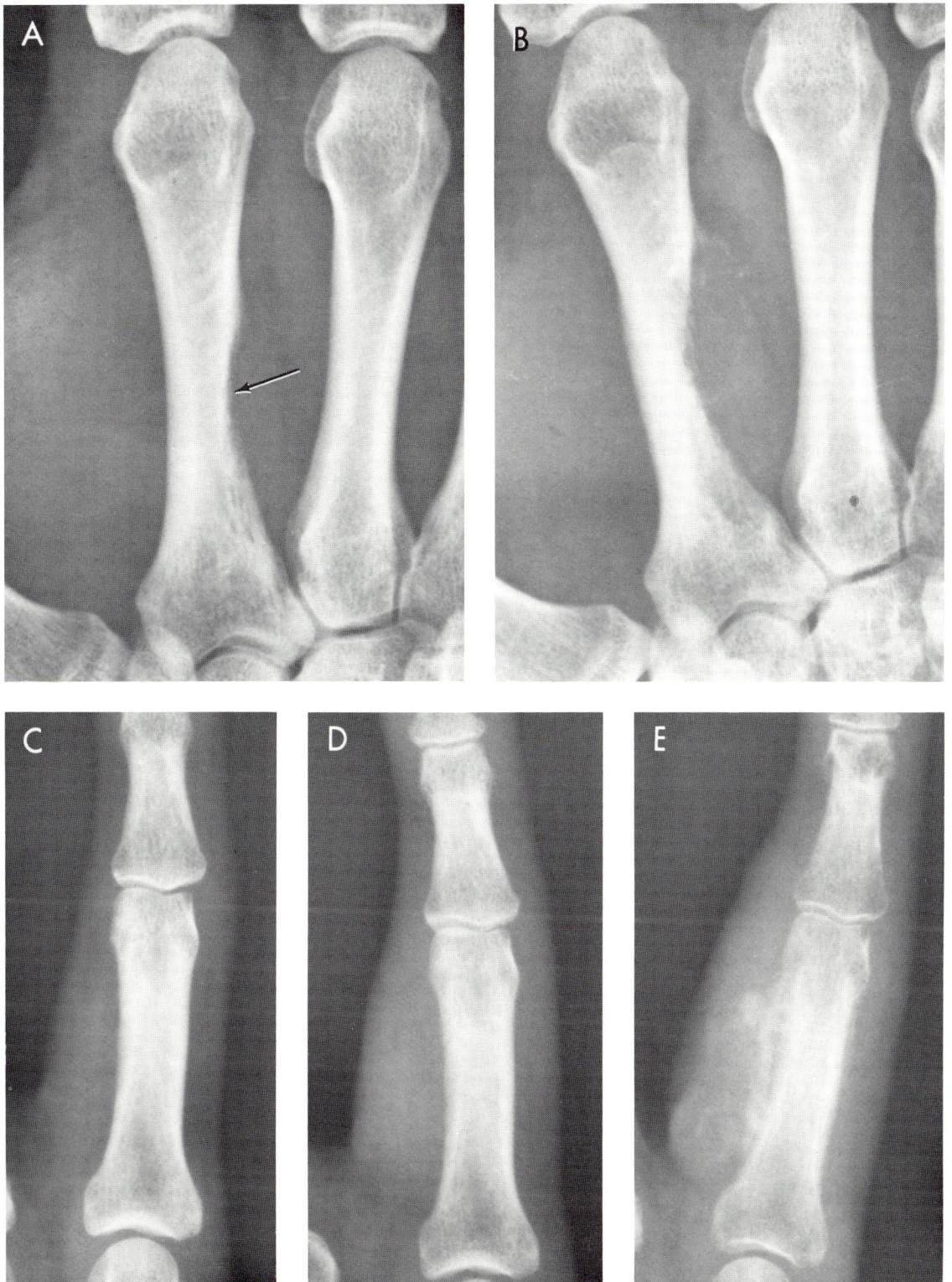

Figure 125 · Myositis Ossificans of Finger

Figure 126.—Myositis ossificans of the ring finger.

AFIP Case No. 1172087: Posteroanterior projections—**A,** initial study one week after onset; **B,** three weeks later.

DIAGNOSIS AND GRADE.—Myositis ossificans, ring finger; ungraded.

LIFE INFORMATION.—Female, 30 years; survival unknown.

LOCATION.—An oval parosteal soft tissue mass lateral to the shaft of the proximal phalanx.

SIZE.—Initially 2 × 1 cm.

MINERALIZATION OF TUMOR.—None initially.

DESTRUCTION.—A local area of rarefaction beneath the tumor.

PROLIFERATION.—Initially only a tiny subperiosteal fleck of new bone (**A, arrow**).

Three weeks later (**B**) the lesion, enlarged to 4 × 2 cm, shows a poorly defined crescentic pattern of calcific density near the periphery (**arrow**), increased local rarefaction and general permeative response. A lamina of thick irregular periosteal new bone has formed over the center of the phalanx.

DIFFERENTIAL DIAGNOSIS	PROBABILITY
Myositis ossificans	.99
Chondrosarcoma	< .01

COMMENT: Based on the time required for development of visible destruction or proliferation of bone, one would estimate that the picture in **A** is of an order of three weeks after injury. The developing pattern in **B** is typical of myositis.

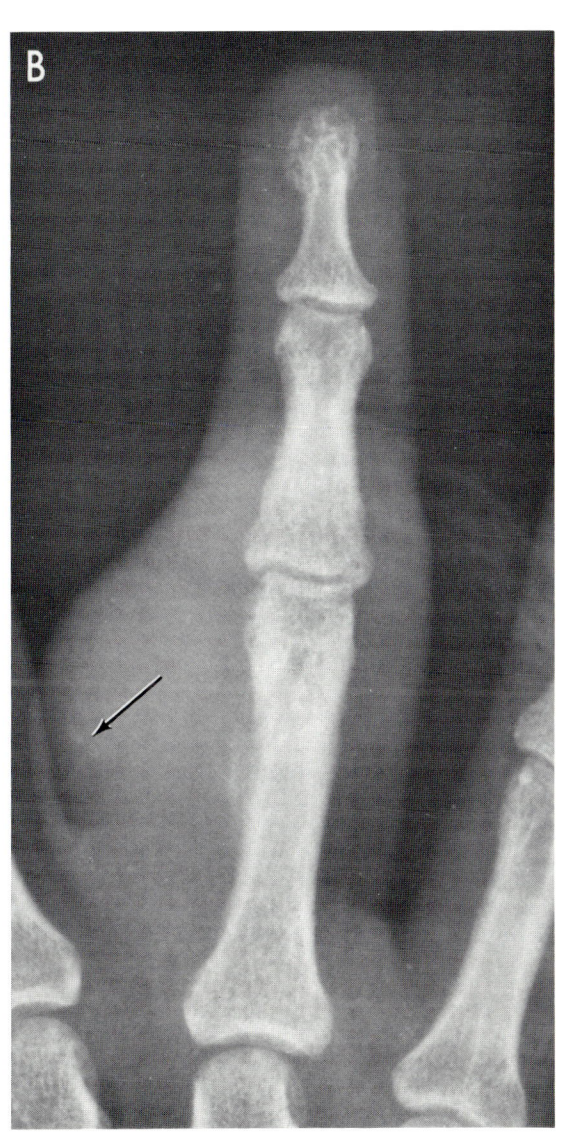
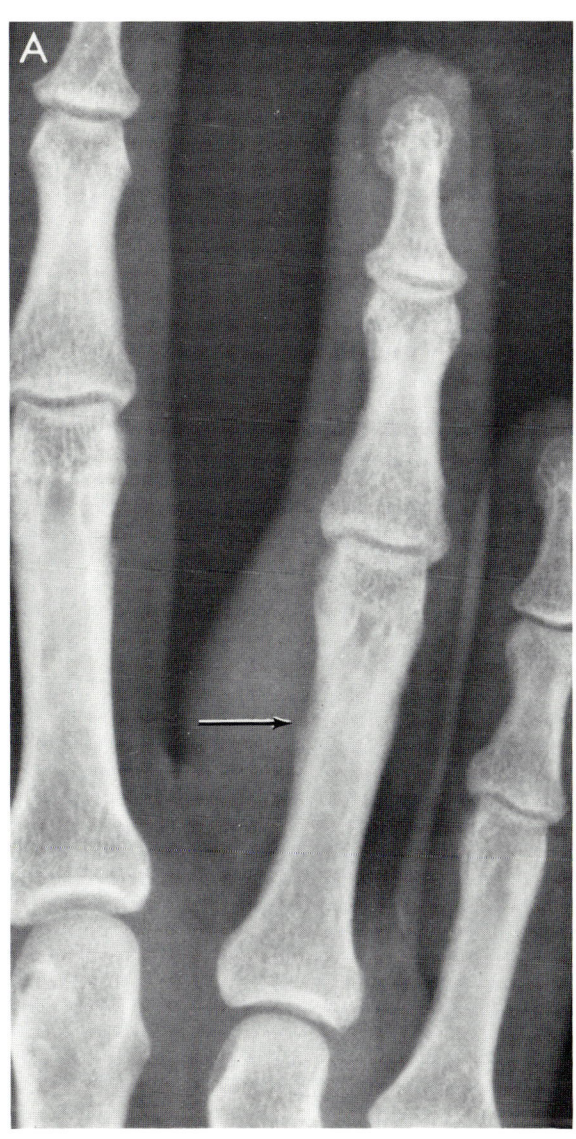

Figure 126 · Myositis Ossificans of Finger / 307

Figure 127.—Myositis ossificans of the index finger.

AFIP Case No. 1171688: Posteroanterior views—**A,** 10 days after onset; **B,** at 6 weeks; **C,** 15 months later.

DIAGNOSIS AND GRADE.—Myositis ossificans, index finger; not graded.

LIFE INFORMATION.—Female, 25 years; last known to be well.

LOCATION.—A parosteal soft tissue mass just medial to the shaft of the middle phalanx of the index finger.

SIZE.—3 × 1 cm.

MINERALIZATION OF TUMOR.—None in early stage.

DESTRUCTION.—None at any stage.

PROLIFERATION.—In **A** a small plaque of subperiosteal new bone on the shaft of the middle phalanx beneath the soft tissue mass suggests that the lesion was at least two weeks, and more probably three or four weeks, old at this time. In **B,** the fleck of new bone is considerably thicker, and at 15 months (**C**) it has developed into a small exostosis with several small flecks of calcific density near its apex.

DIFFERENTIAL DIAGNOSIS	PROBABILITY
Synovial sarcoma	.55
Myositis ossificans	.30
Soft tissue sarcoma	.13

COMMENT: An example of myositis ossificans of the finger without the permeative reaction observed in Figures 125 and 126.

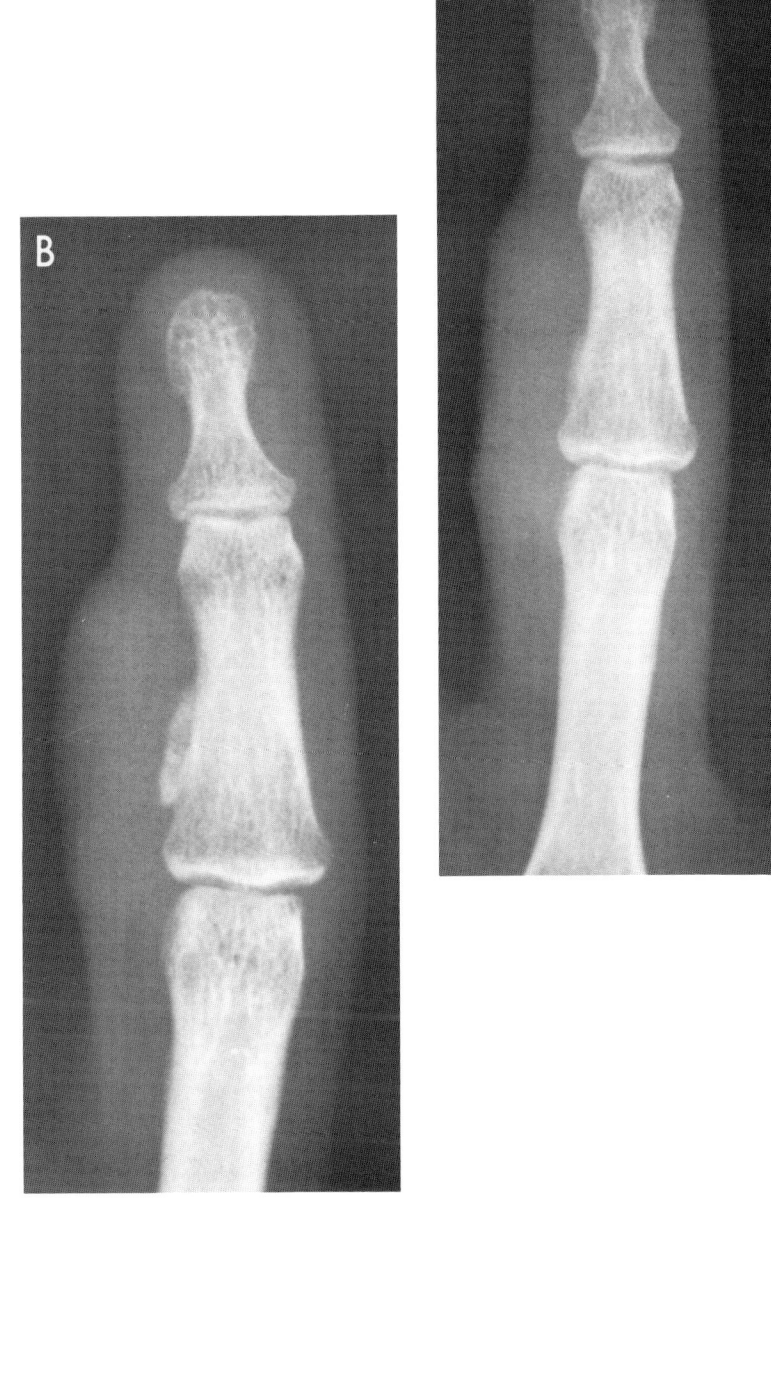

Figure 127 · Myositis Ossificans of Finger

Figure 128.—Myositis ossificans of the middle finger.

AFIP Case No. 1139372: Posteroanterior views—**A,** 5 weeks after injury; **B,** at 10 weeks; **C** and **D** 7 months later.

DIAGNOSIS AND GRADE.—Myositis ossificans, middle finger; ungraded.

LIFE INFORMATION.—Female, 41 years; last known to be well.

LOCATION.—An ill-defined lesion in the soft tissues lateral to the shaft and distal joint of the proximal phalanx.

SIZE.—Initially, 3 × 1 cm.

MINERALIZATION OF TUMOR.—None.

DESTRUCTION.—At five weeks, a focal permeative rarefaction beneath the extraosseous lesion (**A, arrow**).

PROLIFERATION.—A single thick regular lamina of periosteal new bone beneath the soft tissue mass and over the rarefied area (**A, a**).

At 10 weeks (**B**) the soft tissue mass is smaller, the permeated destructive pattern extends throughout the bones of the finger and a diffuse irregular enveloping periosteal response surrounds the shaft of the proximal phalanx.

At 7 months (**C** and **D**) the soft tissue lesion is no longer present, the permeated pattern is gone, and the bone is restored to normal appearance. There is a small dense residual hyperostosis (**D, arrow**).

DIFFERENTIAL DIAGNOSIS	PROBABILITY
Synovial sarcoma	.65
Myositis ossificans	.19
Soft tissue sarcoma	.15

COMMENT: The development of diffuse permeative destruction beneath the injury suggests a rapidly spreading tumor rather than a totally reactive response. This kind of reactive response must be watched for and evaluated when myositis ossificans is suspected.

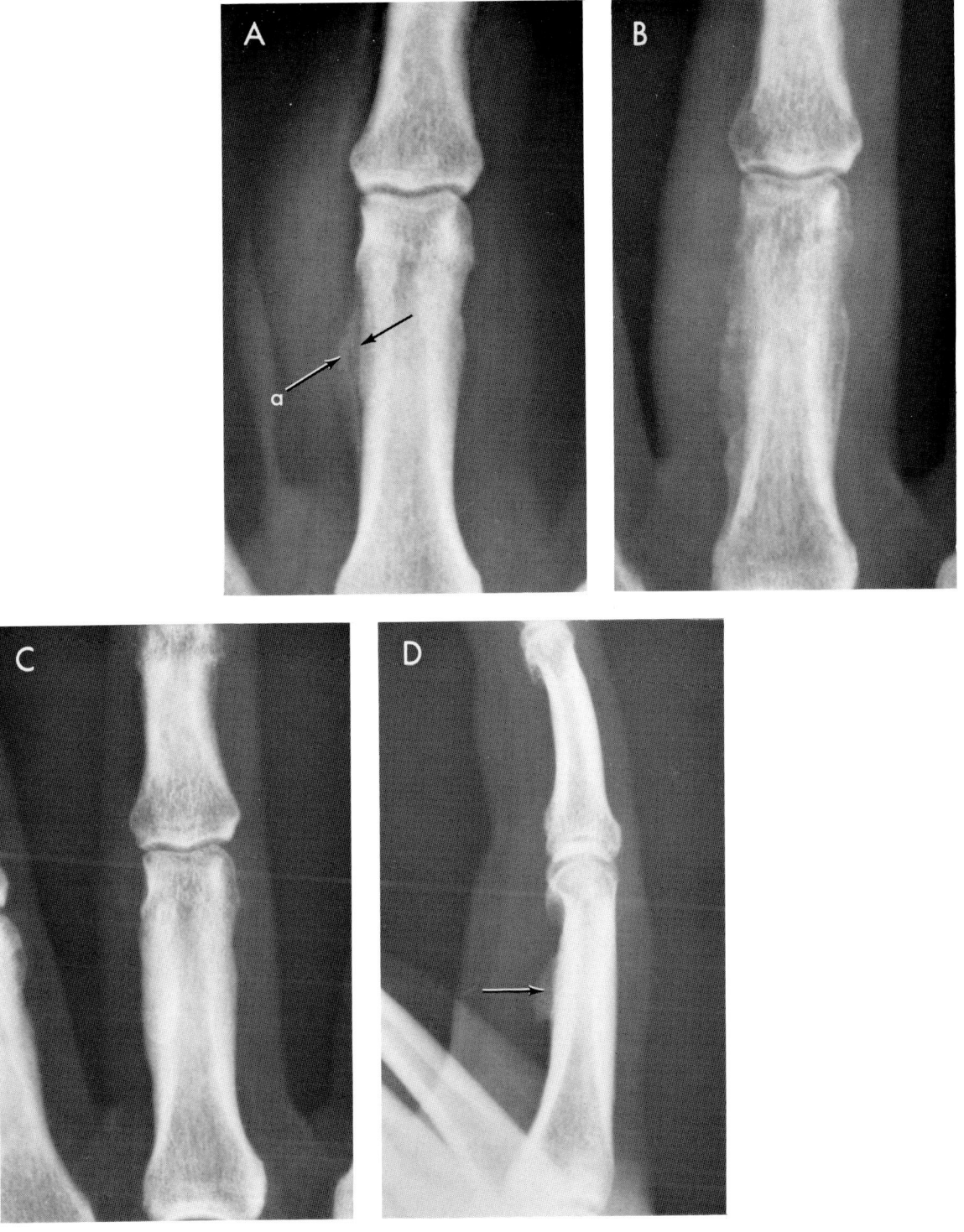

Figure 128 · Myositis Ossificans of Finger

Figure 129.—Myositis ossificans of the femur.

AFIP Case No. 1159474: Anteroposterior projection.

DIAGNOSIS AND GRADE.—Myositis ossificans, femur; not graded.

LIFE INFORMATION.—Male, 40 years; onset four months before examination; survival unknown.

LOCATION.—A large circumscribed parosteal lesion on the medial surface of the right upper femoral shaft.

SIZE.—14 × 25 cm.

MINERALIZATION OF TUMOR.—In the lesion, a network of floccules, clouds and lumps of matrix mineralization; a fairly well defined rim of matrix mineralization between lesion and shaft.

DESTRUCTION.—A 10 cm smooth excavation of the medial cortex from without; geographic pattern.

PROLIFERATION.—None.

DIFFERENTIAL DIAGNOSIS	PROBABILITY
Osteosarcoma	.53
Parosteal sarcoma	.31
Chondrosarcoma	.12
Fibrosarcoma	.01
Myositis ossificans	< .01

COMMENT: This case demonstrates the unusual degree of cortical erosion which may develop beneath myositis ossificans.

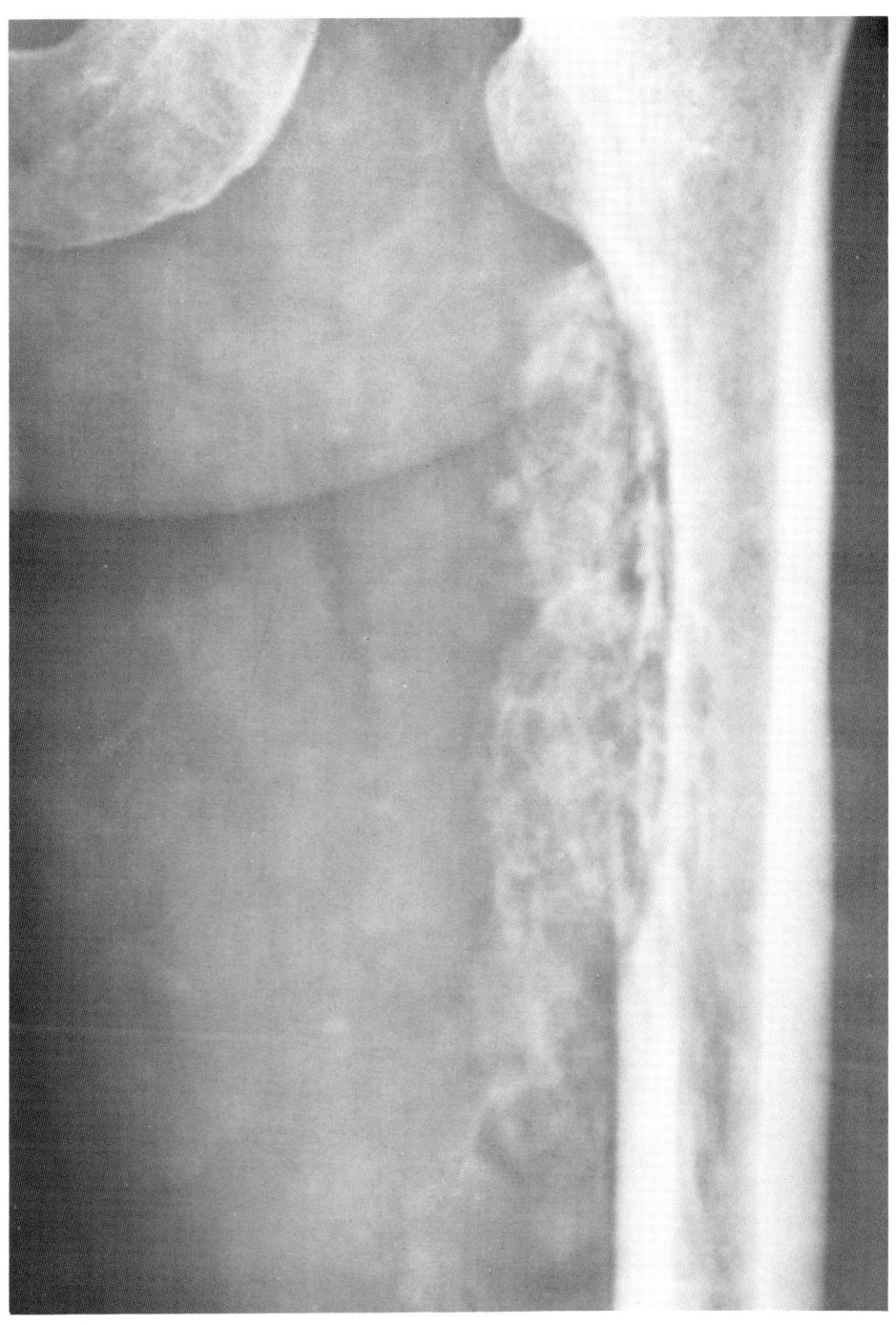

Figure 129 · Myositis Ossificans of Femur

Figure 130.—Myositis ossificans of the ischium.

AFIP Case No. 1087799: Anteroposterior views—**A,** 3 weeks after injury; **B,** 18 months later.

DIAGNOSIS AND GRADE.—Myositis ossificans, ischium; not graded.

LIFE INFORMATION.—Male, 15 years; well three years after onset.

LOCATION.—An ill-defined parosteal soft tissue lesion lateral to the ischium just below the acetabulum.

SIZE.—3 × 1 cm.

MINERALIZATION OF TUMOR.—Barely visible cloudy matrix mineralization occupying the portion of the soft tissue lesion based directly on bone (**A, arrows**).

DESTRUCTION.—Erosion of cortex underlying the lesion.

PROLIFERATION.—None.

Eighteen months later (**B**) the ischium has healed smoothly. There are several smooth islands of bone in the area formerly occupied by the mass (**arrows**).

DIFFERENTIAL DIAGNOSIS	PROBABILITY
Osteosarcoma	.99
Chondrosarcoma	< .01
Fibrosarcoma	< .01
Ewing's sarcoma	< .01

COMMENT: Initially the combination of cloudy matrix mineralization and vague erosion of bone suggests a malignant process, but in 18 months there are smooth healing and consolidation of the parosteal mass into a number of small islands of bone.

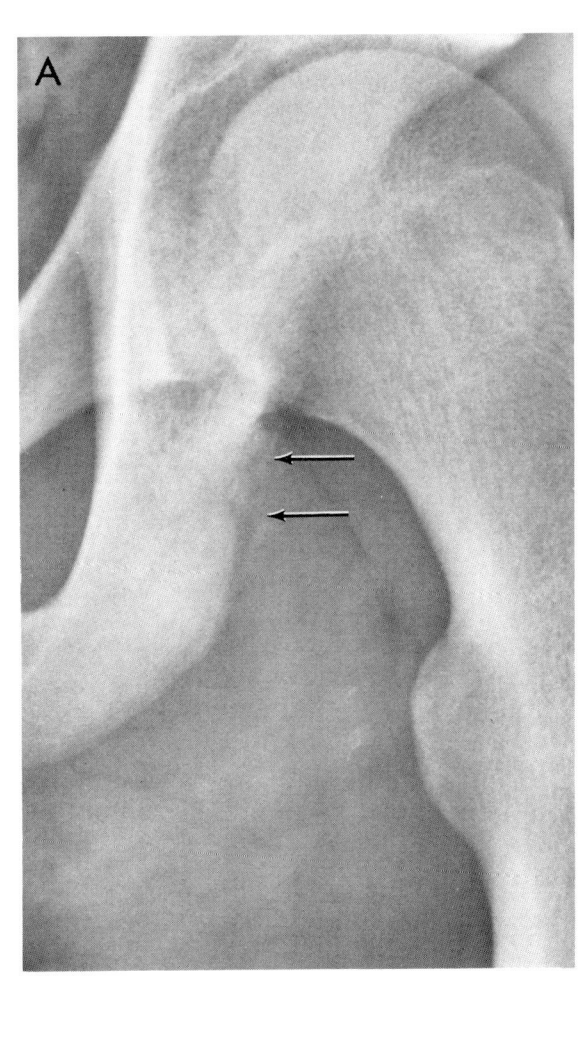
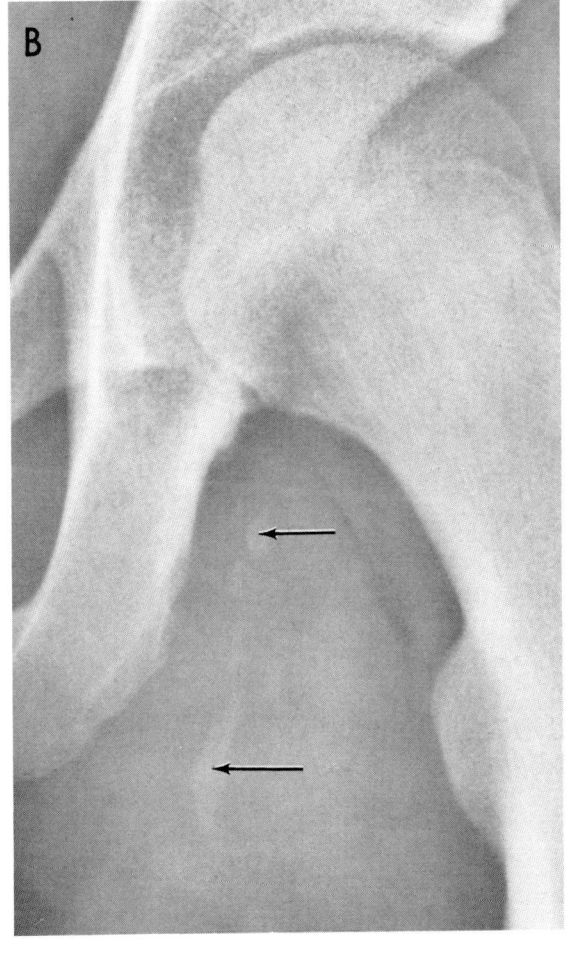

Figure 130 · Myositis Ossificans of Ischium

Figure 131.—Osteoblastomas of the cervical vertebrae and occiput.

AFIP Case No. 1162291: **A**, anteroposterior, and **B**, lateral views.

DIAGNOSIS AND GRADE.—Typical osteoblastoma, C6; not graded.

LIFE INFORMATION.—Male, 21 years; survival unknown.

LOCATION.—A well-circumscribed mass on the anterolateral aspect of the bodies of C5 to C7, C6 seeming most involved.

SIZE.—4 × 3 × 3 cm.

MINERALIZATION OF TUMOR.—A dense solid contiguous mass of tumor bone with some radiolucent central areas; at lower margin a narrow rim of tumor bone separated from the major mass by a radiolucent zone (**A, arrows**).

DESTRUCTION.—None.

PROLIFERATION.—None.

DIFFERENTIAL DIAGNOSIS	PROBABILITY
Osteoblastoma	100

COMMENT: An obviously bone-forming tumor with narrow rim of ossified matrix which seems to be characteristic.

AFIP Case No. 1141563: Lateral views—**C**, initially, and **D**, after radiation therapy.

DIAGNOSIS AND GRADE.— Osteoblastoma, occiput; not graded (see Comment).

LIFE INFORMATION.—Male, 22 years; died in two years of local extension.

LOCATION.—A poorly circumscribed posterior mass (**C, x**) in upper cervical region, based on the occipital cortex.

SIZE.—3 × 3 cm.

MINERALIZATION OF TUMOR.—Initially (**C**) clouds and flocculent tumor bone. After radiation therapy an ossified rim developed (**D, arrow**).

DESTRUCTION.—None apparent.

PROLIFERATION.—None apparent.

DIFFERENTIAL DIAGNOSIS	PROBABILITY
Osteoblastoma	.99
Chondrosarcoma	< .01
Osteosarcoma	< .01

COMMENT: A poorly circumscribed tumor clearly forming tumor bone. Impossible to grade because of absence of bone involvement.

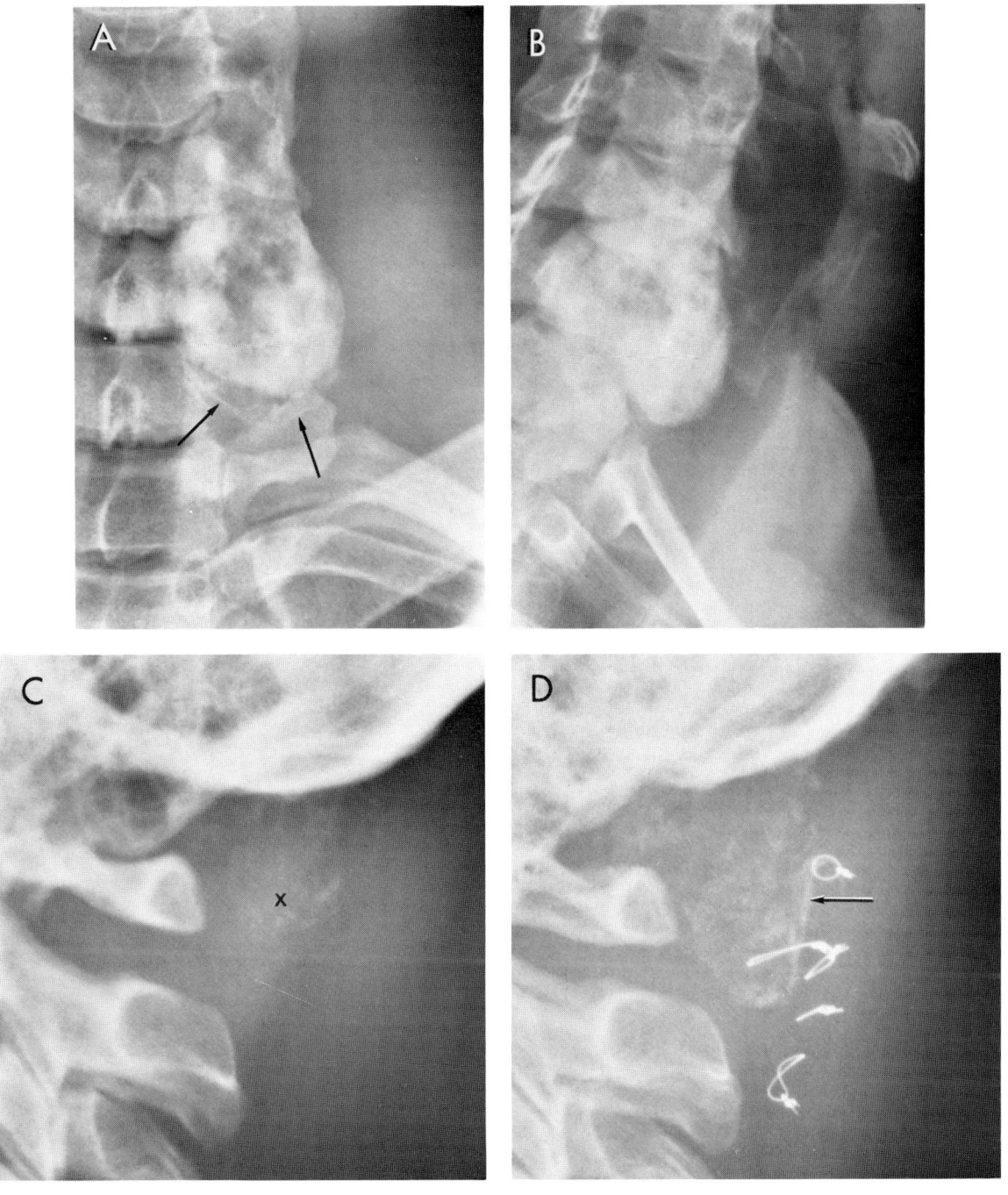

Figure 131 · Osteoblastomas of Cervical Region / 317

Figure 132.—Osteoblastoma of the inner table of the skull.

AFIP Case No. 1194334: **A,** lateral, and **B,** posteroanterior projections.

DIAGNOSIS OF GRADE.—Osteoblastoma, inner table of skull; not graded.

LIFE INFORMATION.—Male, 21 years; last known to be well.

LOCATION.—A large circumscribed tumor attached to the inner table of the frontal region of the skull.

SIZE.—9 × 7 × 6 cm.

MINERALIZATION OF TUMOR.—Lumps and clouds of tumor matrix mineralization, the edge of the tumor sharply circumscribed by a rim of dense mineralization (**arrows**).

DESTRUCTION.—None.

PROLIFERATION.—None.

DIFFERENTIAL DIAGNOSIS	PROBABILITY
Osteoblastoma	.99
Osteosarcoma	< .01
Chondrosarcoma	< .01

COMMENT: This tumor resembles in every detail the two examples of osteoblastoma in Figure 131. In this particular location a meningioma must be considered in differential diagnosis.

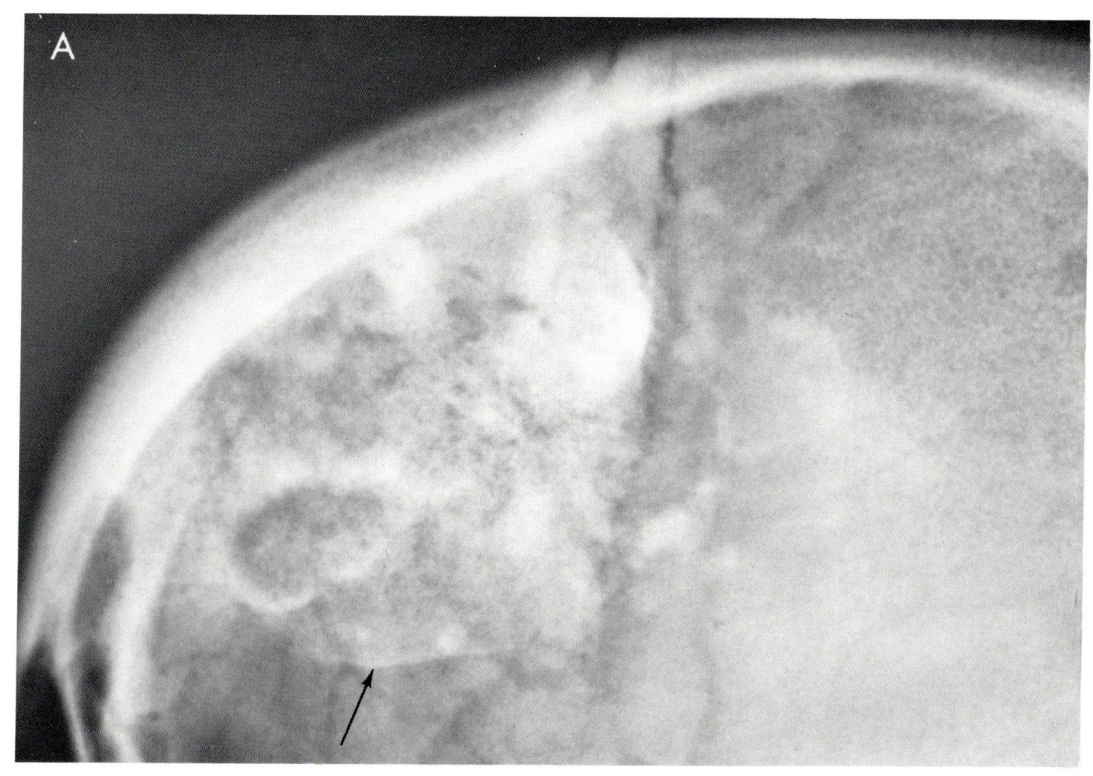
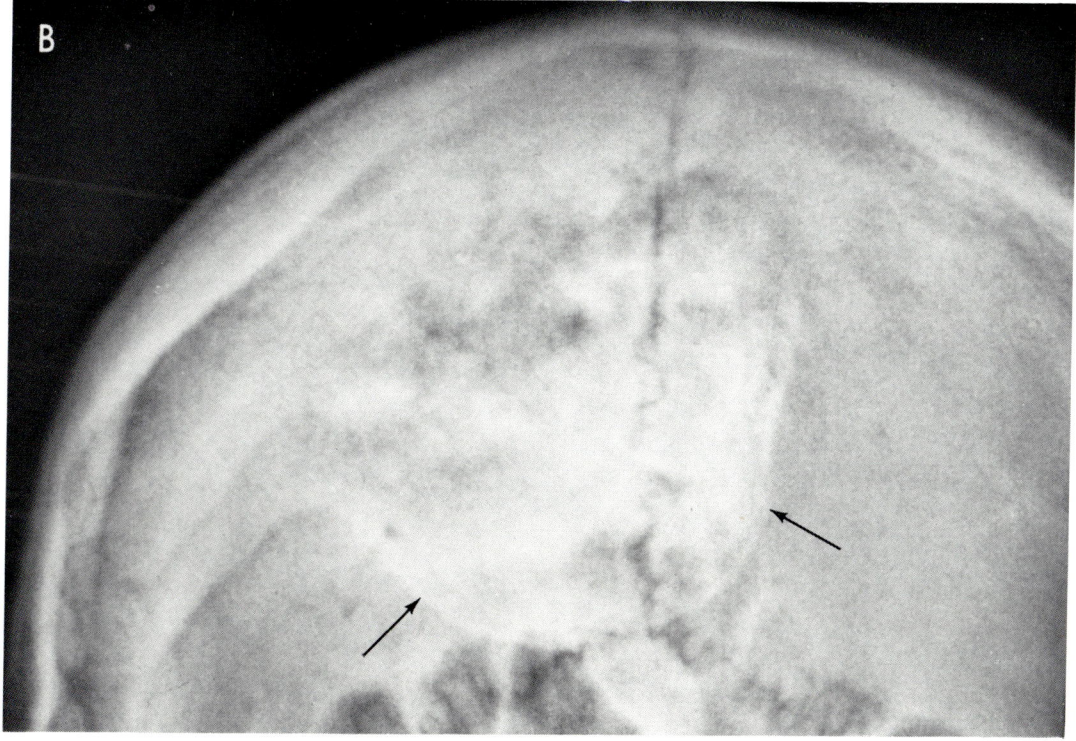

Figure 132 · Osteoblastoma of Skull / 319

Figure 133.—Osteoblastoma of the sacrum.

AFIP Case No. 1097658: **A,** anteroposterior, and **B,** lateral projections.

DIAGNOSIS AND GRADE.—Typical osteoblastoma, sacrum; see Comment.

LIFE INFORMATION.—Male, 19 years; survival unknown.

LOCATION.—A large well-circumscribed mass attached to the middle and lateral aspect, of the anterior surface of the sacrum.

SIZE.—8 × 7 × 3 cm.

MINERALIZATION OF TUMOR.—Scattered ground-glass and flocculent tumor matrix mineralization, (**a**) with a well-defined marginal rim of tumor bone (**arrows**).

DESTRUCTION.—None apparent.

PROLIFERATION.—None apparent.

DIFFERENTIAL DIAGNOSIS	PROBABILITY
Chondrosarcoma	.06
Osteoblastoma	.94

COMMENT: This large extraosseous tumor produces abundant poorly calcified tumor bone which, at the margin, sharply defines the tumor. Evaluation of growth rate is not practical, since the principal tools for such are destructive and proliferative changes, neither of which is present.

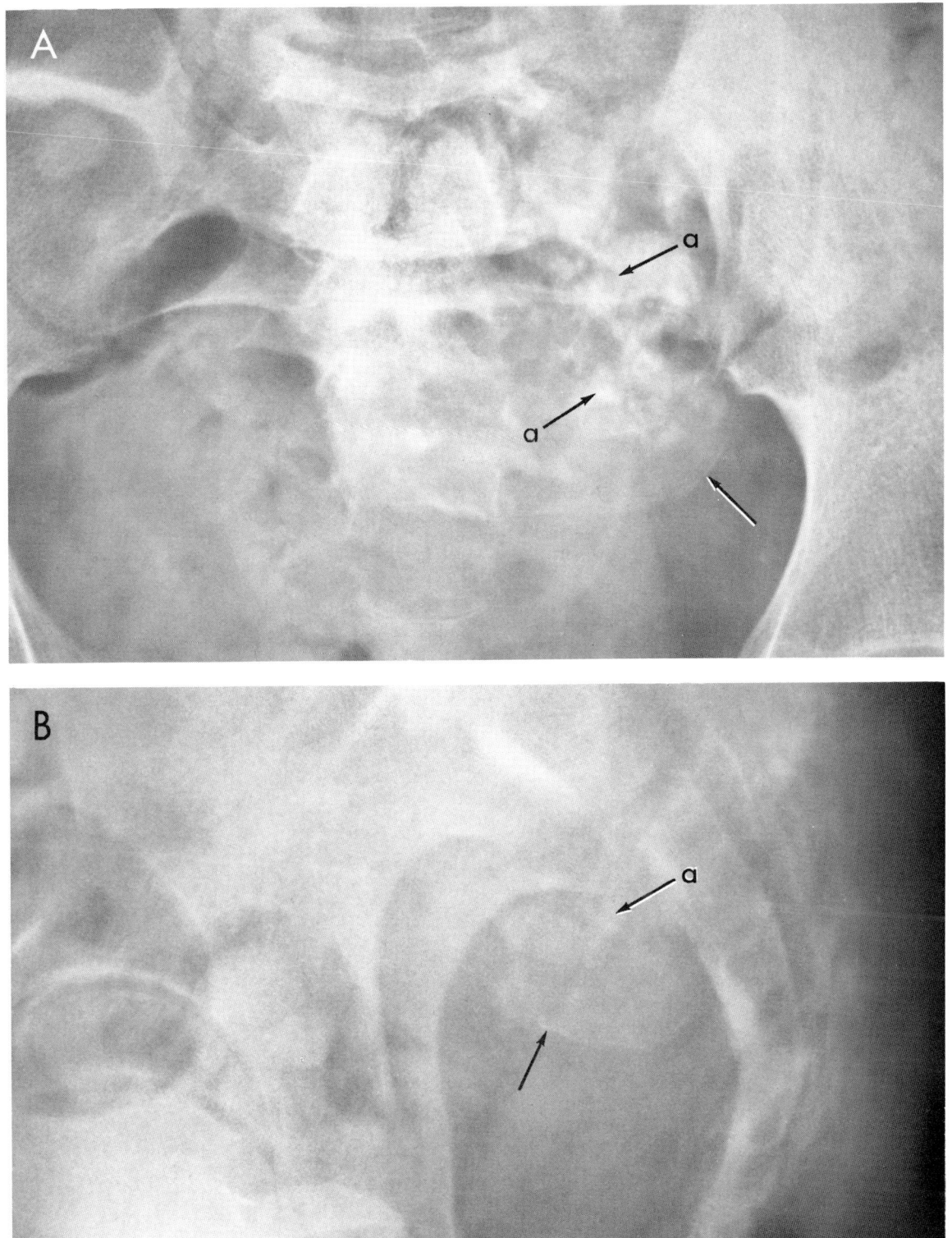

Figure 133 · Osteoblastoma of Sacrum

Figure 134.—Osteoblastoma of the cervical spine.

AFIP Case No. 1127146: **A,** slight oblique, and **B,** full oblique views.

DIAGNOSIS AND GRADE.—Osteoblastoma, C4; growth rate IC.
LIFE INFORMATION.—Male, 16 years; survival unknown.
LOCATION.—An ill-defined lesion centered laterally between C3 and C4.

SIZE.—3 × 2 × 2 cm, estimated.
MINERALIZATION OF TUMOR.—None.
DESTRUCTION.—Geographic, with bone loss principally in the region of the posterior pedicle and neural arch of C4.
PROLIFERATION.—None definite; perhaps very slight sclerosis (**arrows**).

DIFFERENTIAL DIAGNOSIS	PROBABILITY
Osteoblastoma	.92
Cyst	.06
Giant cell tumor	< .01
Fibrosarcoma	< .01

COMMENT: There seems to be nothing specific here for osteoblastoma, there being only four positive signs: the patient's age, location of the lesion, size, and geographic destruction—hardly sufficient for diagnosis.

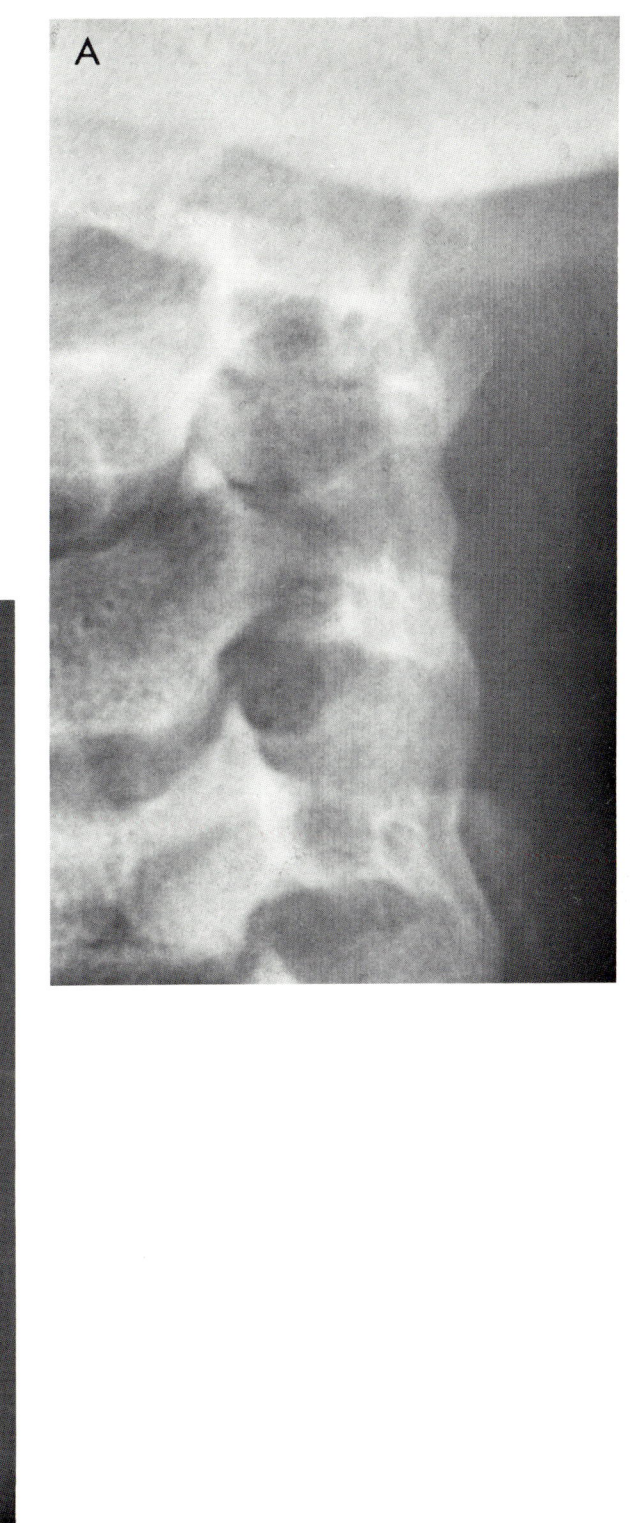
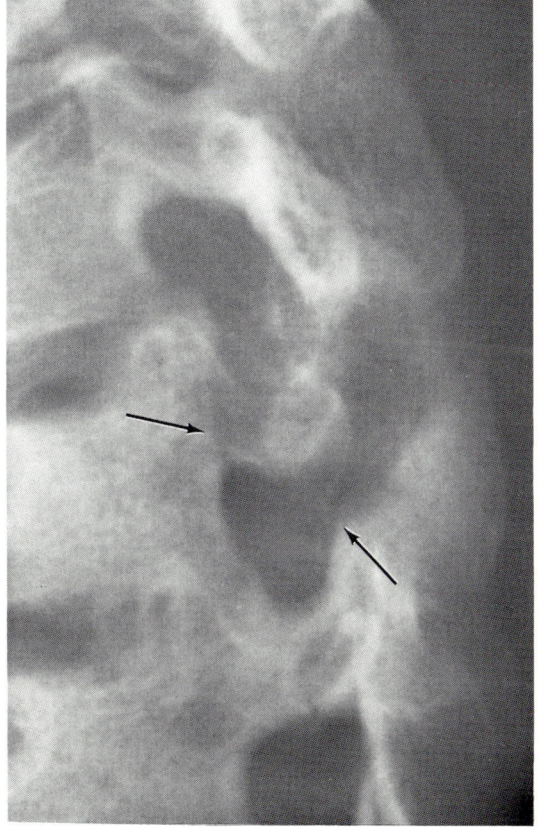

Figure 134 · Osteoblastoma of Cervical Spine / 323

Figure 135.—Osteoblastoma of a metacarpal and radius.

AFIP Case No. 1164270: **A,** oblique projection.

DIAGNOSIS AND GRADE.—Osteoblastoma, fifth metacarpal; growth rate IA.
LIFE INFORMATION.—Female, about 25 years; survival unknown.
LOCATION.—A circumscribed lesion in the shaft, extending into the metaphysis, proximally involving more than half the shaft; no soft tissue extension.
SIZE.—2.5 × 2 × 2 cm.
MINERALIZATION OF TUMOR.—None.
DESTRUCTION.—Geographic; regular contour.
PROLIFERATION.—About 8 mm of symmetrical new periosteal shell, whose inner surface has a reticulate pattern (see Fig. 32).

DIFFERENTIAL DIAGNOSIS	PROBABILITY
Osteoblastoma	.52
Cartilaginous tumor	.34
Giant cell tumor	< .01
Fibrosarcoma	< .01

COMMENT: No specific signs. Note incomplete destruction of the shaft, whose eroded stub projects into the tumor.

AFIP Case No. 1111241: **B,** anteroposterior projection.

DIAGNOSIS AND GRADE.—Osteoblastoma, radius; growth rate IA.
LIFE INFORMATION.—Female, 8 years; survival unknown.
LOCATION.—A circumscribed eccentric lesion in the distal metaphysis, extending distally to the growth plate and proximally to the shaft; no soft tissue extension.
SIZE.—3 × 2 cm.
MINERALIZATION OF TUMOR.—None.
DESTRUCTION.—Geographic; regular contour; incomplete penetration of cortex.
PROLIFERATION.—Faint zone of broad marginal sclerosis with 5 mm cortical expansion which encapsulates the tumor.

DIFFERENTIAL DIAGNOSIS	PROBABILITY
Cyst	.84
Chondromyxoid fibroma	.13
Osteoblastoma	.02
Giant cell tumor	< .01

COMMENT: A common nonspecific pattern.

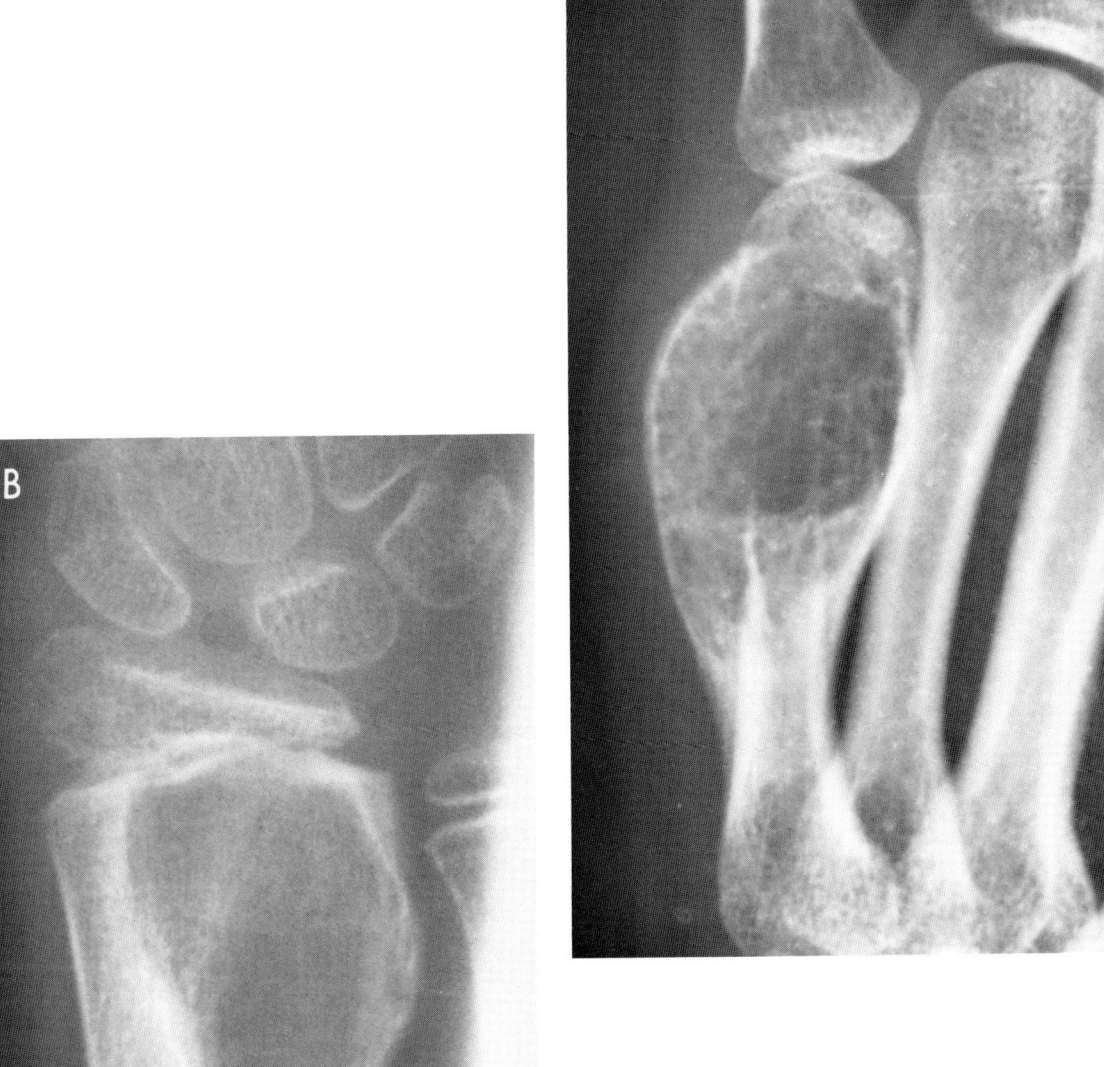

Figure 135 · Osteoblastomas / 325

Figure 136.—Osteoblastoma of the tibia.

AFIP Case No. 1189453: **A,** anteroposterior, and **B,** lateral views.

DIAGNOSIS AND GRADE.—Osteoblastoma, tibia; growth rate IB.

LIFE INFORMATION.—Female, 25 years; last known to be alive.

LOCATION.—A circumscribed lesion centered in the middle of the proximal tibial metaphysis, extending down to the shaft and up to the subarticular cortex of the knee.

SIZE.—8 × 7 × 5 cm.

MINERALIZATION OF TUMOR.—The lower half of the lesion contains a solid mass of ground-glass matrix mineralization of rather low density (**x**), becoming even less dense toward the margin of the tumor. The upper half is largely radiolucent, with lumps of tumor matrix (**A, arrows**).

DESTRUCTION.—Geographic; regular contour; incomplete penetration of cortex.

PROLIFERATION.—None definite.

DIFFERENTIAL DIAGNOSIS	PROBABILITY
Fibrosarcoma	.77
Osteoblastoma	.10
Osteosarcoma	.09
Chondrosarcoma	.02
Chondromyxoid fibroma	< .01

COMMENT: The diminishing ground-glass density of tumor matrix mineralization toward the edge of the tumor is most unusual. The absence of proliferative change of any sort is characteristic of most of the osteoblastomas in this series. The relative frequency of fibrosarcoma as compared with osteoblastoma in this location proved overpowering for the computer.

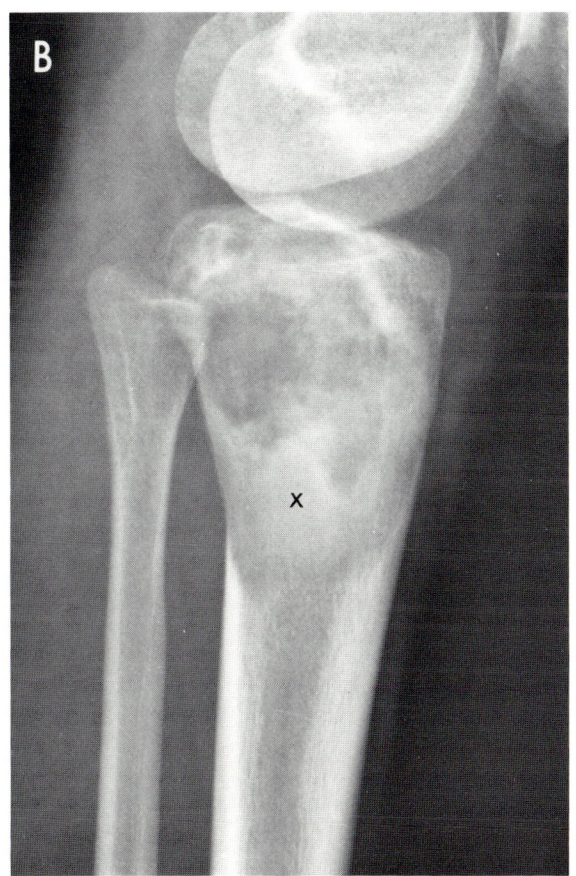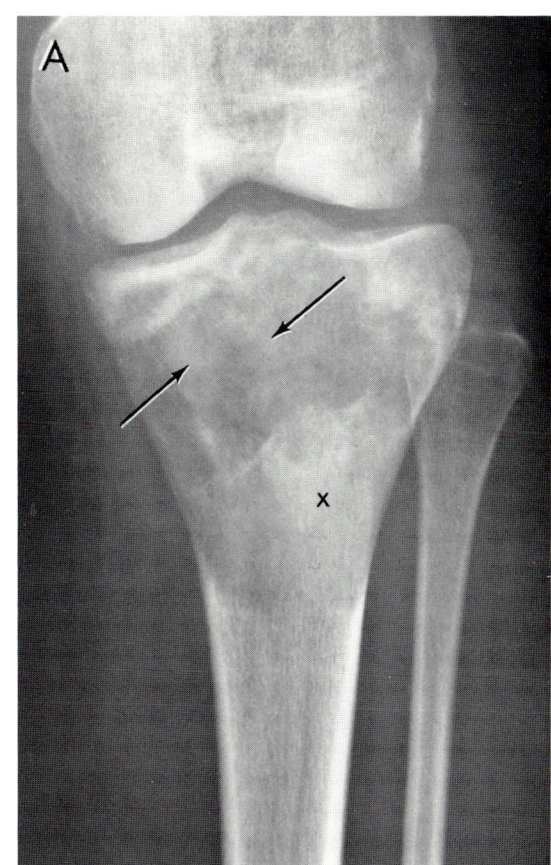

Figure 136 · Osteoblastoma of Tibia / 327

Figure 137.—Osteoid osteomas of the femur and astragalus.

AFIP Case No. 708055: **A,** anteroposterior, and **B,** lateral views.

DIAGNOSIS AND GRADE.—Osteoid osteoma (cortical), femur; growth rate IA.

LIFE INFORMATION.—Male, 33 years; survival unknown.

LOCATION.—A small circumscribed lesion in the anteromedial cortex of the proximal femoral shaft.

SIZE.—10 × 6 mm.

MINERALIZATION OF TUMOR.—None.

DESTRUCTION.—Geographic; ragged contour.

PROLIFERATION.—The nidus (**B, arrow**) lies in a dense hyperostosis of proliferative bone, with an opposing thinner endostosis.

DIFFERENTIAL DIAGNOSIS	PROBABILITY
Osteoid osteoma	100

COMMENT: A nearly typical osteoid osteoma.

AFIP Case No. 1163873: **C,** anteroposterior, and **D,** lateral views.

DIAGNOSIS AND GRADE.—Osteoid osteoma (subperiosteal) astragalus; growth rate IC.

LIFE INFORMATION.—Male, 30 years; survival unknown.

LOCATION.—A small ill-defined lesion on the superior surface of the astragalus at the junction of the body and neck, extending into soft tissues.

SIZE.—14 × 10 mm.

MINERALIZATION OF TUMOR.—A number of flecks of tumor bone (**a**) comprise a central density, some obscured by overlying bone.

DESTRUCTION.—Geographic; indistinct outline (**D, arrows**); total penetration of cortex.

PROLIFERATION.—None.

DIFFERENTIAL DIAGNOSIS	PROBABILITY
Osteoid osteoma	100

COMMENT: This osteoid osteoma is typical of those located subperiosteally near a joint.

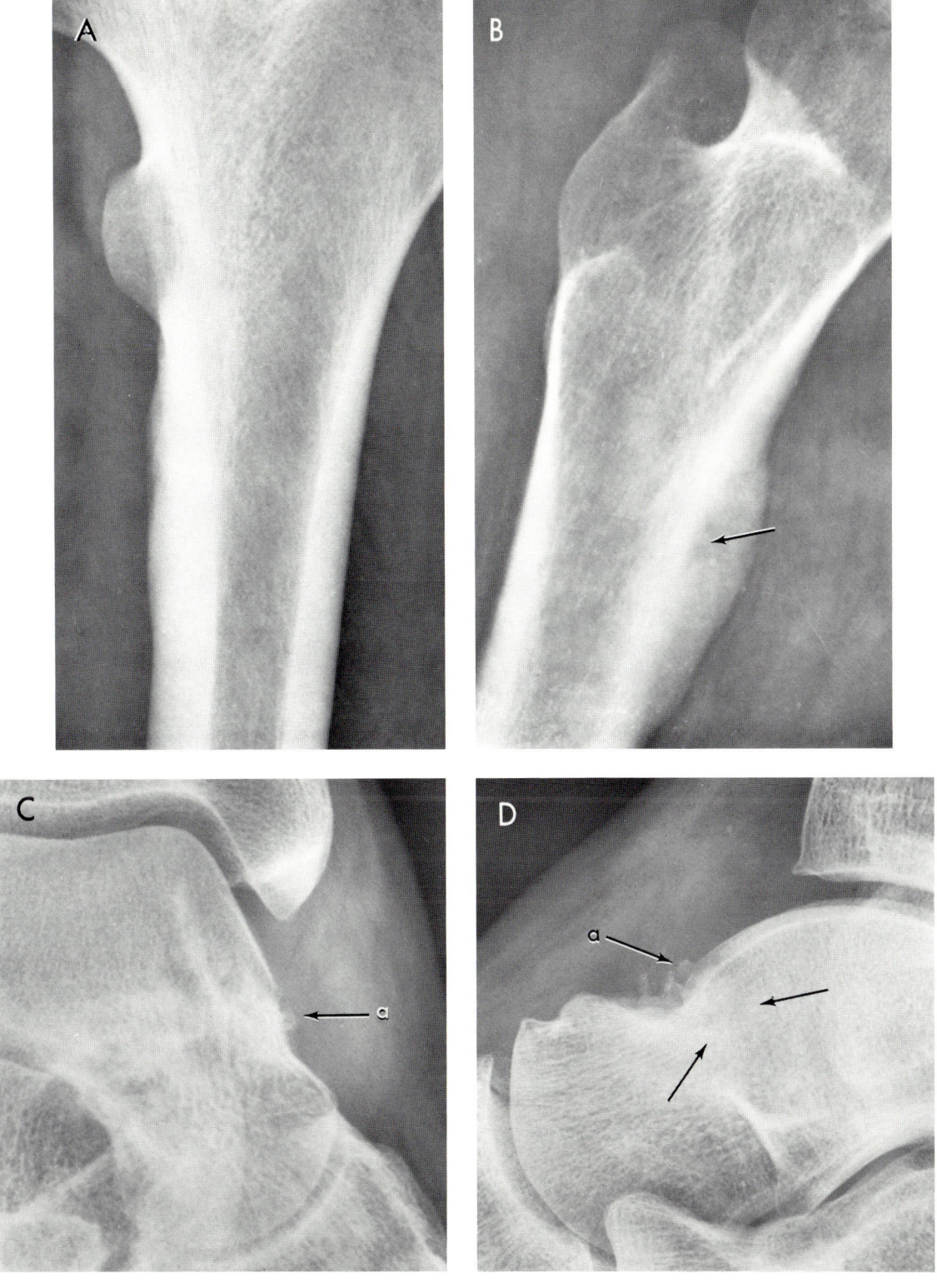

Figure 137 · Osteoid Osteomas

Figure 138.—Osteoid osteomas of the tibia.

AFIP Case No. 111591: **A,** anteroposterior, and **B,** lateral views.

DIAGNOSIS AND GRADE.—Osteoid osteoma, tibia; growth rate IA.
LIFE INFORMATION.—Male, 14 years; well three years later.
LOCATION.—A small circumscribed lesion eccentrically located in the central third of the proximal tibial metaphysis; no soft tissue extension.
SIZE.—16 × 8 × 6 cm.
MINERALIZATION OF TUMOR.—One definite fleck at each end of the lesion (**B, arrows**).
DESTRUCTION.—Geographic; regular contour.
PROLIFERATION.—A broad fading zone of marginal sclerosis with dense hyperostotic new bone on the adjacent cortex.

DIFFERENTIAL DIAGNOSIS	PROBABILITY
Osteoid osteoma	100

COMMENT: An atypical osteoid osteoma, arising in cancellous bone, where there is usually abundant proliferative response.

AFIP Case No. 1143115: **C,** anteroposterior, and **D,** lateral views.

DIAGNOSIS AND GRADE.—Osteoid osteoma (cortical), tibia; growth rate IA.
LIFE INFORMATION.—Male, 5 years; well three years later.
LOCATION.—A small circumscribed lesion in the anterior cortex of the proximal tibial metaphysis.
SIZE.—18 × 6 × 5 mm.
MINERALIZATION OF TUMOR.—None.
DESTRUCTION.—Geographic; regular contour.
PROLIFERATION.—Faint marginal sclerosis; no overlying periosteal response.

DIFFERENTIAL DIAGNOSIS	PROBABILITY
Osteoid osteoma	100

COMMENT: The lesion is atypical in view of the relatively scant proliferative response. Also it lies near a joint and is in the cortex.

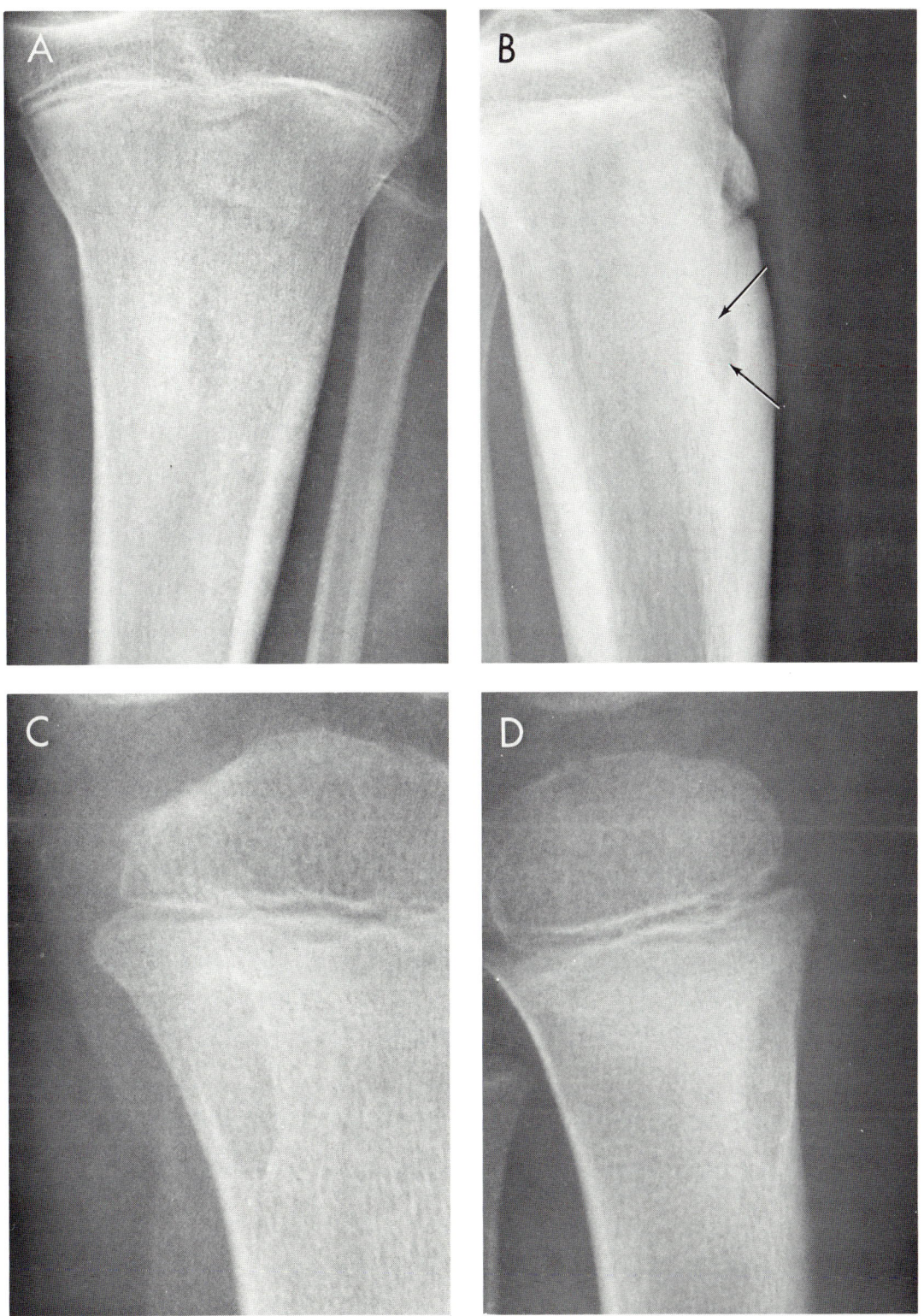

Figure 138 · Osteoid Osteomas of Tibia / 331

Figure 139.—Osteoid osteomas of the femur and tibia.

AFIP Case No. 1157466: **A,** anteroposterior, and **B,** lateral views.

DIAGNOSIS AND GRADE.—Osteoid osteoma, femur; growth rate IA.
LIFE INFORMATION.—Female, 38 years; survival unknown.
LOCATION.—An ill-defined subperiosteal lesion on the posteromedial surface of the upper femoral shaft.

SIZE.—Estimated 15 mm long and 3 mm thick.
MINERALIZATION OF TUMOR.—Presumably a central plaque of irregular new bone (**B, arrow**).
DESTRUCTION.—Slight geographic excavation of cortex surrounding the lesion; contour regular.
PROLIFERATION.—Periosteal hyperostosis proximally and distally.

DIFFERENTIAL DIAGNOSIS	PROBABILITY
Osteoid osteoma	.99
Cartilaginous tumor	< .01

COMMENT: A very ill-defined lesion characterized principally by the hyperostotic response.

AFIP Case No. 1179739: **C,** anteroposterior, and **D,** lateral views.

DIAGNOSIS AND GRADE.—Osteoid osteoma, tibia; growth rate IA.
LIFE INFORMATION.—Female, 19 years; well six years later.
LOCATION.—A small circumscribed eccentrically located lesion in the middle third of the proximal metaphysis.

SIZE.—Destroyed area about $1.5 \times 1.5 \times 1.5$ cm; the reactive area much larger.
MINERALIZATION OF TUMOR.—A questionable central fleck.
DESTRUCTION.—Geographic; regular contour.
PROLIFERATION.—A broad, dense zone of sclerosis surrounding the lesion; hyperostosis on the metaphysial surface remote from the lesion (**arrows**).

DIFFERENTIAL DIAGNOSIS	PROBABILITY
Osteoid osteoma	.99
Chondromyxoid fibroma	< .01

COMMENT: This pattern is characteristic of osteoid osteoma but not pathognomonic. The histologic diagnosis of the contributing pathologist was osteoblastoma.

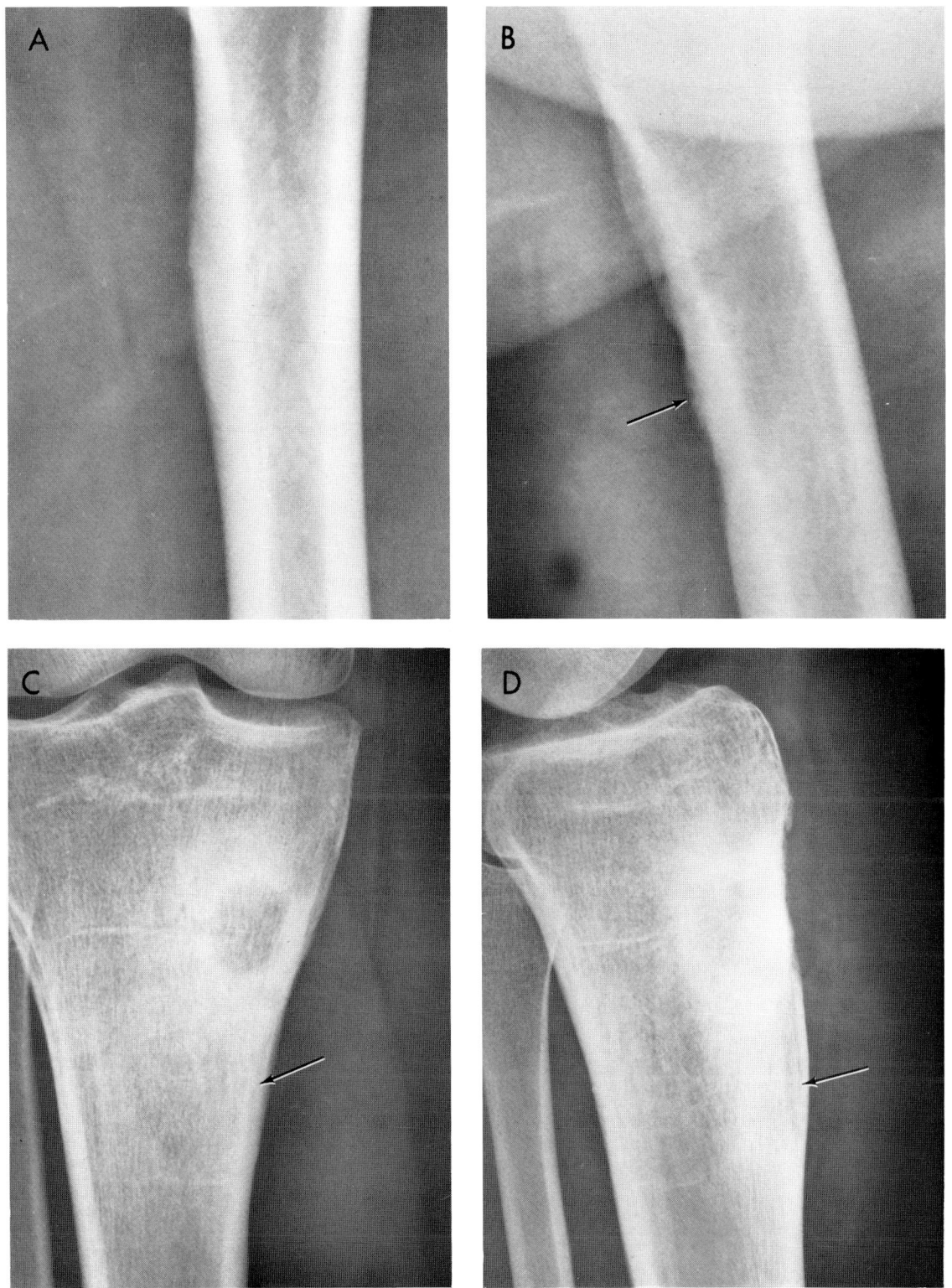

Figure 139 · Osteoid Osteomas

Figure 140.—Osteoid osteomas of a toe and finger.

AFIP Case No. 1177642: **A,** anteroposterior, and **B,** oblique views.

DIAGNOSIS AND GRADE.—Osteoid osteoma, toe; growth rate IA.
LIFE INFORMATION.—Female, 12 years; survival unknown.
LOCATION.—A lesion in the middle phalanx of the fourth toe.

SIZE.—Less than 1 cm.
MINERALIZATION OF TUMOR.—Dense central fleck (**arrows**).
DESTRUCTION.—A vague rarefied zone, probably geographic destruction around the dense nidus.
PROLIFERATION.—None.

DIFFERENTIAL DIAGNOSIS	PROBABILITY
Osteoid osteoma	.99
Osteosarcoma	< .01
Chondrosarcoma	< .01

COMMENT: A typical osteoid osteoma of the toe.

AFIP Case No. 1169564: **C,** posteroanterior, and **D,** lateral views.

DIAGNOSIS AND GRADE.—Osteoid osteoma, finger; growth rate IA.
LIFE INFORMATION.—Male, 15 years; last known to be well.
LOCATION.—A lesion centered eccentrically in the distal metaphysis of the middle phalanx, fourth finger; considerable soft tissue swelling.

SIZE.—Less than 1 cm.
MINERALIZATION OF TUMOR.—A round central fleck (**arrows**).
DESTRUCTION.—A vague halo of geographic pattern; indistinct contour.
PROLIFERATION.—None.

DIFFERENTIAL DIAGNOSIS	PROBABILITY
Osteoid osteoma	.56
Osteosarcoma	.42
Chondrosarcoma	< .01

COMMENT: This is typical of osteoid osteomas in the rays of the hands and feet. The hyperostotic area proximal to the lesion (**a**) is normal.

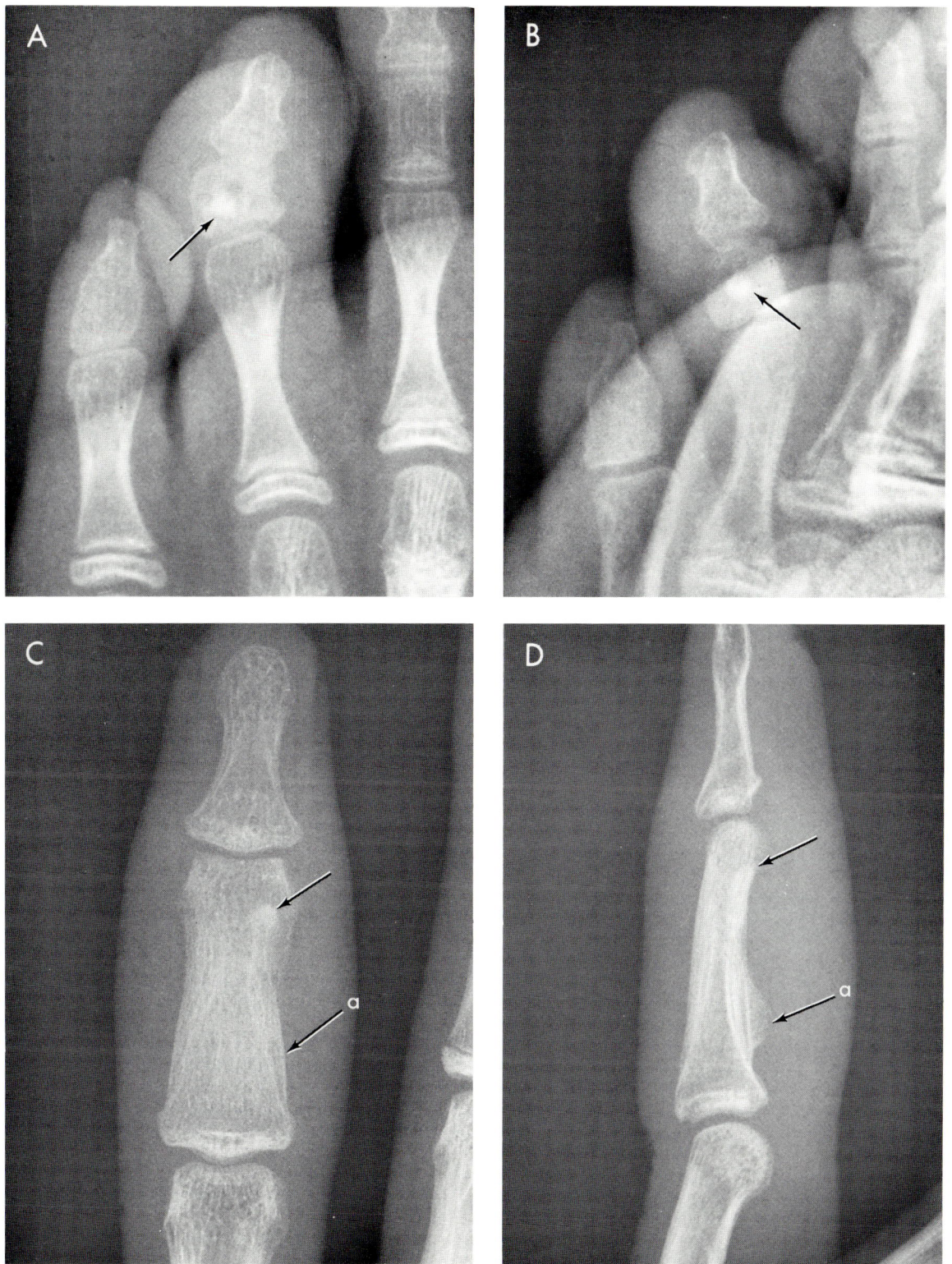

Figure 140 · Osteoid Osteomas of Digits / 335

PART 6

Round Cell Tumors

Figure 141.—Ewing's sarcoma of the femur.

AFIP Case No. 1130688: **A,** anteroposterior, and **B,** lateral views.

DIAGNOSIS AND GRADE.—Ewing's sarcoma, femur; growth rate III.

LIFE INFORMATION.—Male, 19 years; survived 2 years after onset, 20 months after diagnosis.

LOCATION.—A diffuse eccentrically located tumor in the upper third of the shaft.

SIZE.—$14 \times 5 \times 4$ cm.

MINERALIZATION OF TUMOR.—None.

DESTRUCTION.—Permeative pattern (**A, a**).

PROLIFERATION.—Irregular endosteal thickening of the cortex at the center of the tumor (**A, b**); on the outer surface, the cortex thickened due to deposition of at least five regular layers of periosteal new bone, some of them destroyed centrally, the residual segments at the edge of the tumor representing Codman triangles (**A, c**); posteriorly, hair-on-end spiculation (**B, d**).

DIFFERENTIAL DIAGNOSIS	PROBABILITY
Ewing's sarcoma	.99
Osteosarcoma	< .01

COMMENT: The five layers of periosteal new bone produce the classic onion-peel appearance. In time, and especially after radiation therapy, they fuse to produce dense hyperostosis. Such periosteal layering seems more regular and delicate in Ewing's sarcoma than in other tumors, particularly osteosarcoma.

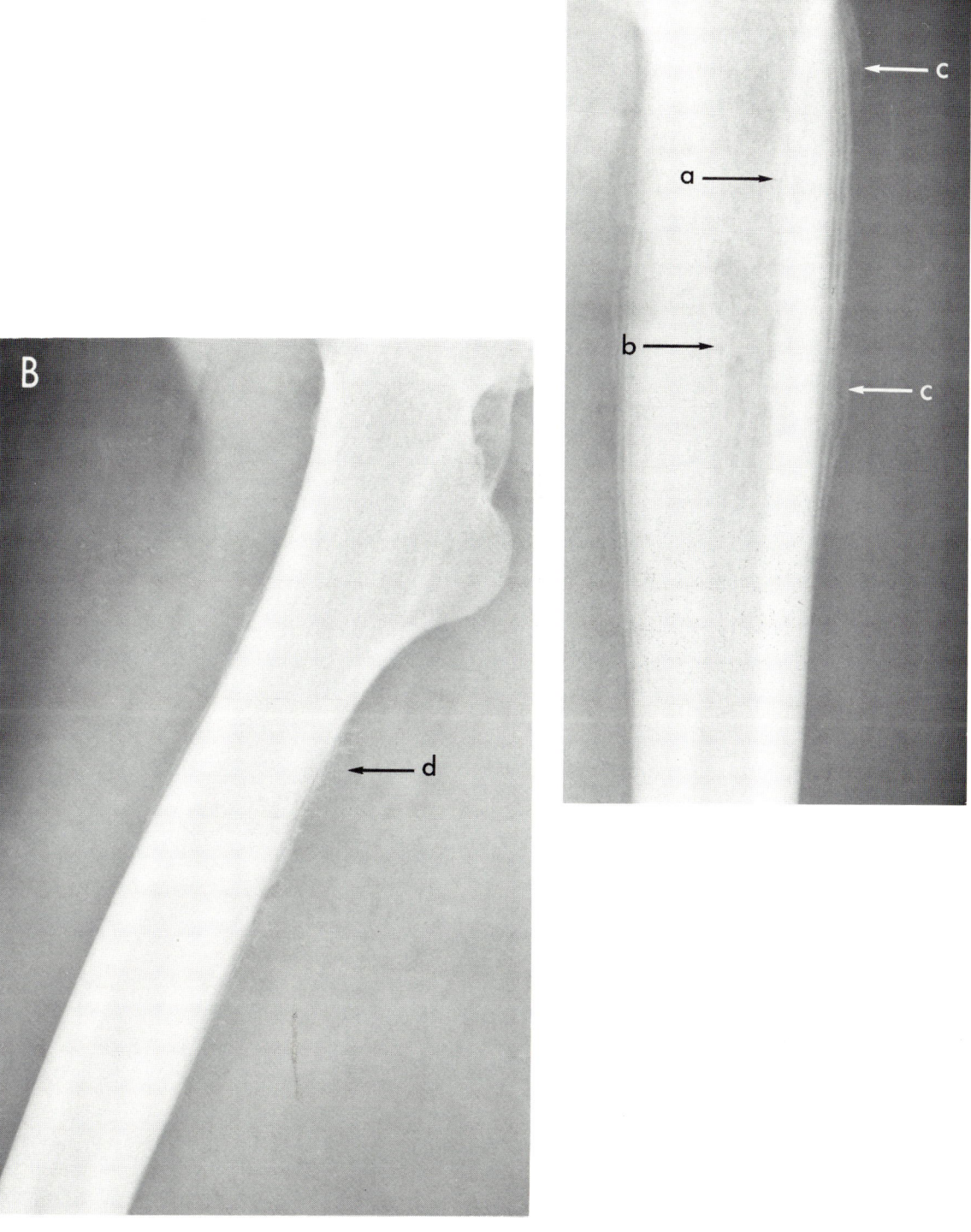

Figure 141 · Ewing's Sarcoma / 339

Figure 142.—Ewing's sarcomas of the fibula and tibia.

AFIP Case No. 1136657: **A,** anteroposterior projection.

DIAGNOSIS AND GRADE.—Ewing's sarcoma, fibula; growth rate III.
LIFE INFORMATION.—Female, 12 years; survival unknown.
LOCATION.—A diffuse lesion centered in the proximal shaft, extending into metaphysis to level of growth plate; large soft tissue extension.

SIZE.—10 × 4 × 4 cm.
MINERALIZATION OF TUMOR.—None.
DESTRUCTION.—Permeative; total penetration of cortex.
PROLIFERATION.—Mottled pattern accentuating normal trabecular pattern in the metaphysis; multiple laminae of subperiosteal new bone; two Codman triangles; hair-on-end spiculation.

DIFFERENTIAL DIAGNOSIS	PROBABILITY
Ewing's sarcoma	.99
Osteosarcoma	< .01

COMMENT: The delicate lamination and hair-on-end spiculation favor Ewing's sarcoma more than osteosarcoma.

AFIP Case No. 1154814: **B,** anteroposterior projection.

DIAGNOSIS AND GRADE.—Ewing's sarcoma, tibia; growth rate III.
LIFE INFORMATION.—Female, 11 years; survived a year.
LOCATION.—A diffuse tumor centered in the midshaft.

SIZE.—9 × 3.5 cm.
MINERALIZATION OF TUMOR.—None.
DESTRUCTION.—Permeative pattern (**a**).
PROLIFERATION.—Four Codman triangles (**arrows**); two laminae of periosteal new bone.

DIFFERENTIAL DIAGNOSIS	PROBABILITY
Ewing's sarcoma	.96
Osteosarcoma	.02
Reticulum cell sarcoma	< .01

COMMENT: It is unusual to see four Codman triangles in one projection. Four in two projections is a very ominous prognostic sign.

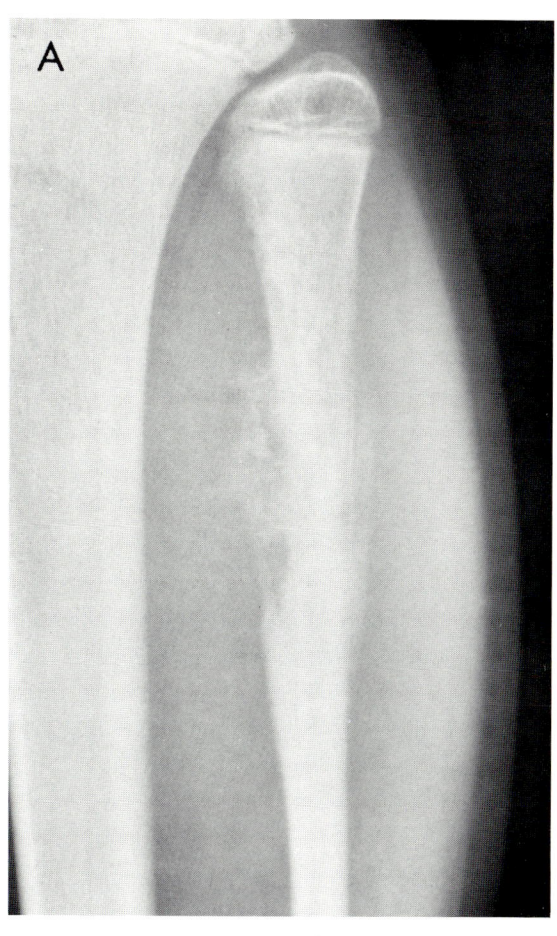

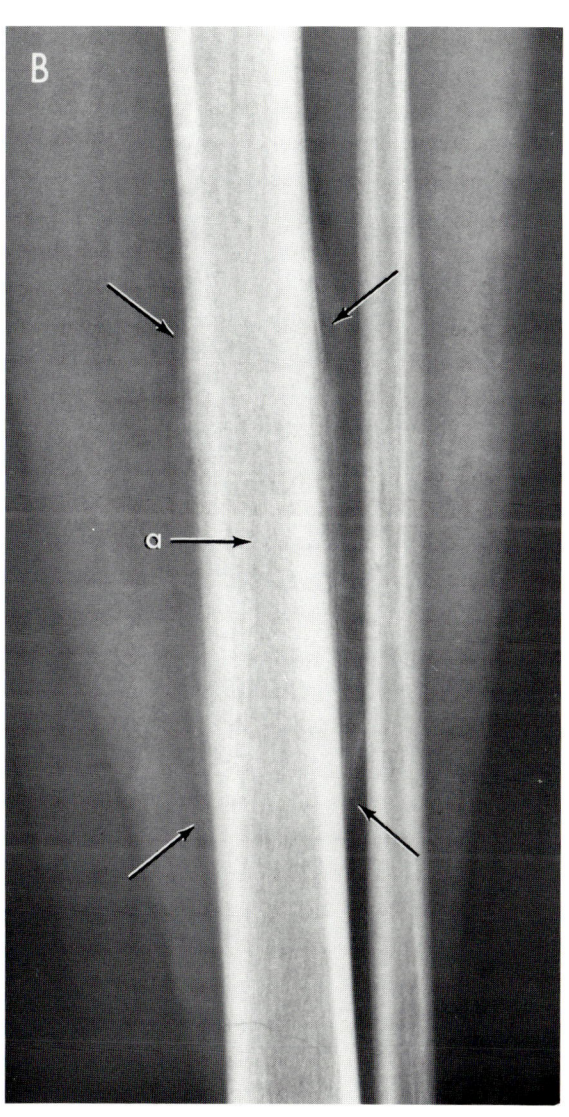

Figure 142 · Ewing's Sarcomas / 341

Figure 143.—Ewing's sarcoma of the fibula.

AFIP Case No. 704565: Anteroposterior projection.

DIAGNOSIS AND GRADE.—Ewing's sarcoma, fibula; growth rate IC. (See Comment.)

LIFE INFORMATION.—Female, 12 years; received radiation therapy to a neoplastic lesion in the body of T10 more than 11 years after original diagnosis; last known to be alive.

LOCATION.—A lesion centered in the midshaft of the fibula involving the proximal and distal portions of the shaft.

SIZE.—14 × 4 × 4 cm.

MINERALIZATION OF TUMOR.—None.

DESTRUCTION.—Nearly all of the original cortex has been destroyed. At the lower end of the lesion, the pattern is clearly geographic bone destruction with a sharp line of demarcation between destroyed and normal bone. The pattern at the upper end is less well defined, with ragged contour.

PROLIFERATION.—Nearly all of the bone in the center of the tumor is periosteal new bone of mildly expanded character. The pattern could be described as septate, reticulate or honey-combed. There are some radiating spicules.

DIFFERENTIAL DIAGNOSIS	PROBABILITY
Ewing's sarcoma	.99
Fibrosarcoma	< .01

COMMENT: Interpretation of this lesion is more difficult because of some inconsistencies. Undoubtedly there is geographic bone destruction at the lower edge of the tumor. Also there is expanded cortex, with a peculiar reticulate pattern involving it. I have seen this combination of findings principally within a slowly growing round cell tumor. The closest match to this is the fibrosarcoma in Figure 50, *A* and *B*, where the resemblance is startlingly similar.

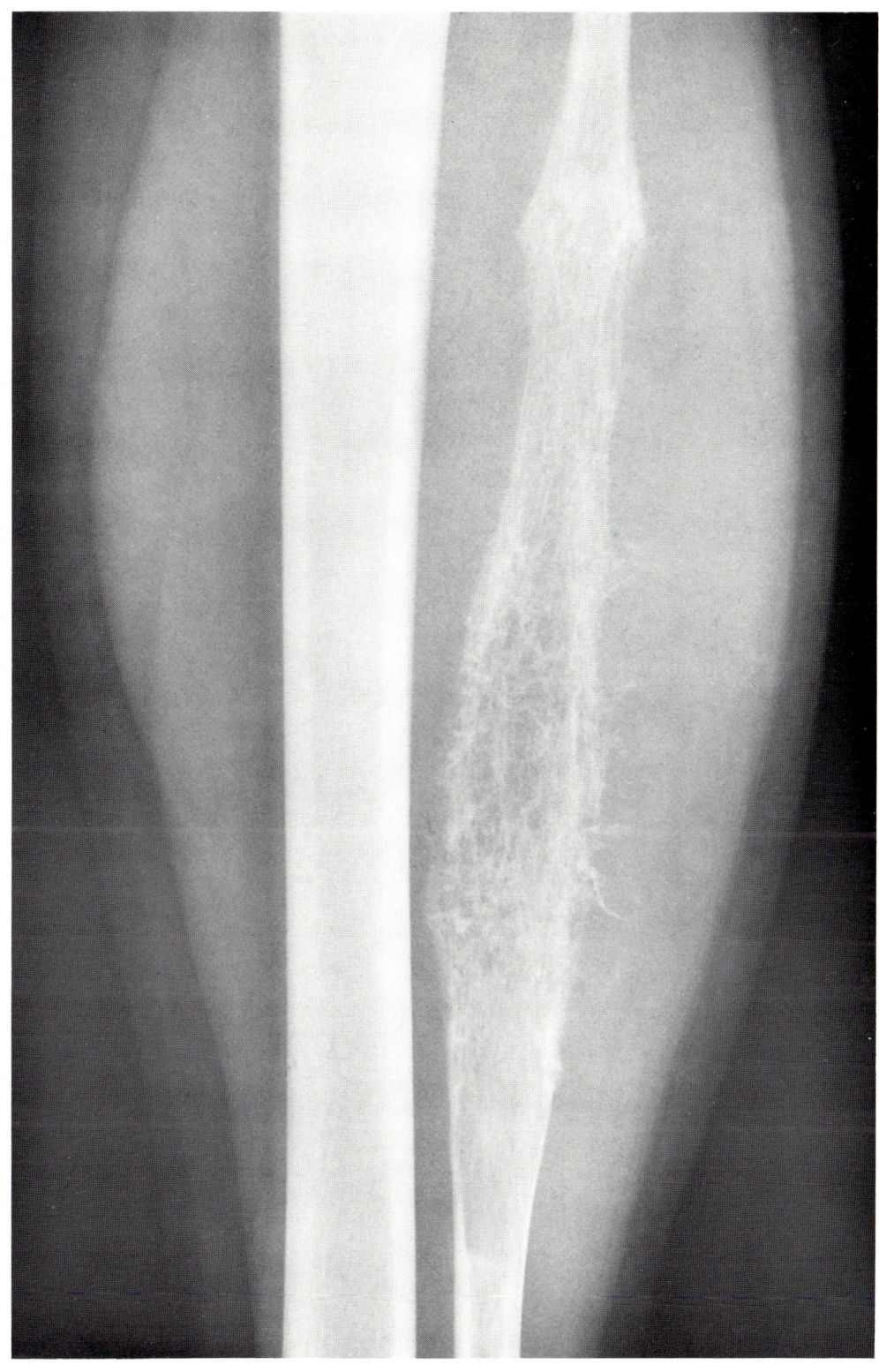

Figure 143 · Ewing's Sarcoma of Fibula / 343

Figure 144.—Ewing's sarcoma of a metatarsal.

AFIP Case No. 1136228: Anteroposterior views—**A,** initial study; **B,** 11 months, and **C,** 13 months later.

DIAGNOSIS AND GRADE.—Ewing's sarcoma, metatarsal; growth rate III.

LIFE INFORMATION.—Male, 8 years; survived 19 months after onset, 7 months after tissue diagnosis.

LOCATION.—A lesion in the shaft and base of the third metatarsal.

SIZE.—5 × 1.5 cm.

MINERALIZATION OF TUMOR.—None.

DESTRUCTION.—Initially (**A**) no conclusive alteration of density or structure, although there is a suggestion of permeation. A degree of unsharpness to the outer cortex is ascribed to proliferative change (see below). At 11 months (**B**) the cortex of the shaft has faded nearly to invisibility because of permeative destruction, even more pronounced in **C**.

PROLIFERATION.—Initially (**A**) each metatarsal shows at least a single regular lamina of periosteal new bone, a normal finding. In the metatarsal which ultimately displays the tumor is an extra softer lamina which produces an appearance of unsharpness (**a**). At 11 months (**B**) multiple consolidating layers of periosteal new bone seem to have taken up supportive function in an expanded position. At 13 months (**C**) they are being destroyed by the rapidly expanding tumor and new layers are appearing farther out. Definite hair-on-end spiculation is now present (**b**).

DIFFERENTIAL DIAGNOSIS	PROBABILITY
Ewing's sarcoma	.95
Fibrosarcoma	.03
Osteosarcoma	.01
Chondrosarcoma	< .01

COMMENT: In retrospect, in **A** there is clearly an extra lamina of subperiosteal new bone on the diseased metatarsal. Even if this elusive finding were recognized, is it a significant early sign of tumor? We believe that it is. In **B,** the presence of tumor is indisputable. The computer run is for this second examination.

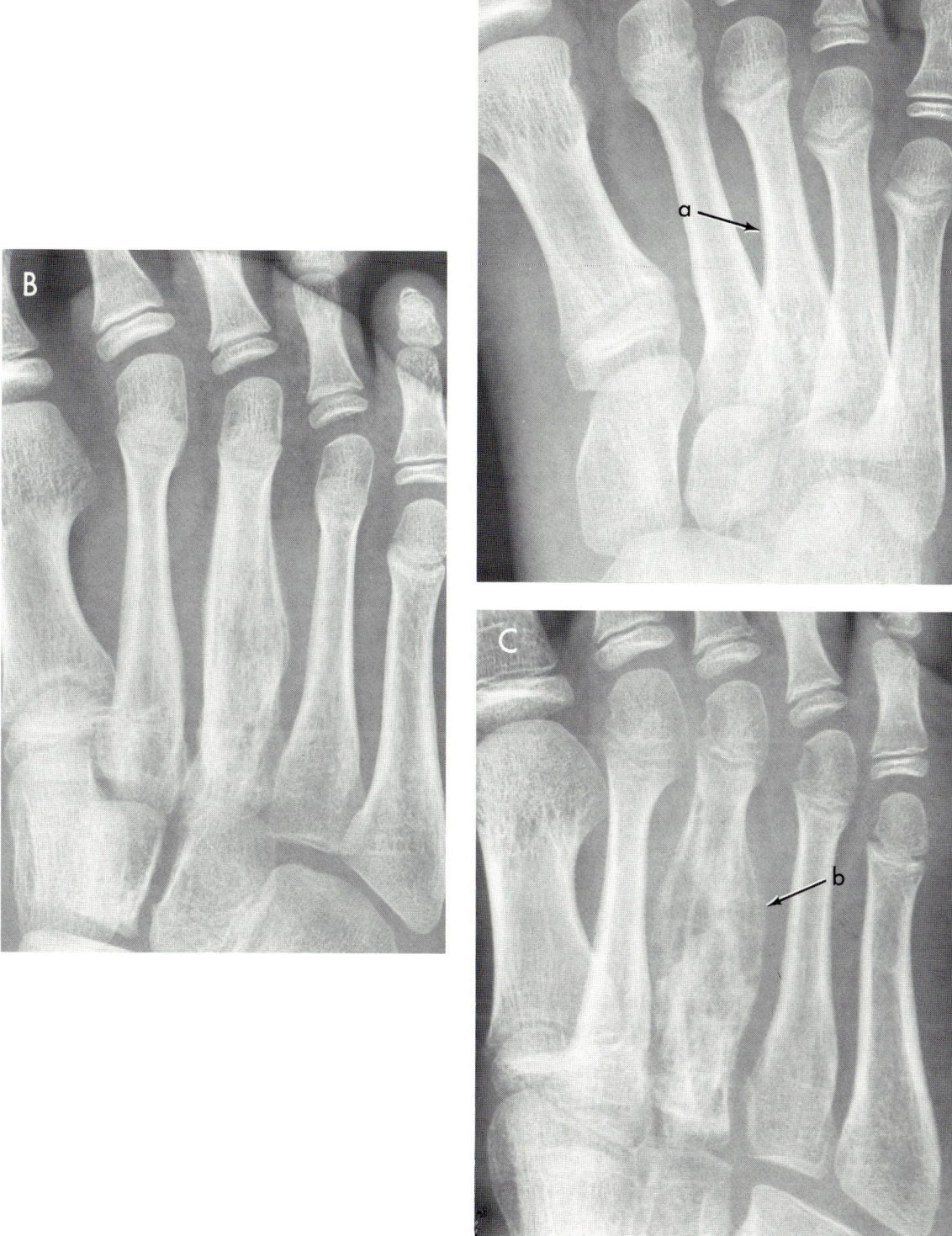

Figure 144 · Ewing's Sarcoma of Metatarsal / 345

Figure 145.—Ewing's sarcoma of the humerus.

AFIP Case No. 1163189: Anteroposterior views—**A,** abnormal right humerus, compared with normal left (**B**); right humerus at 3 weeks (**C**), 10 weeks (**D**), 20 weeks (**E**), and 30 weeks (**F**).

DIAGNOSIS AND GRADE.—Ewing's sarcoma, humerus; growth rate III.
LIFE INFORMATION.—Male, 4 years; survived 30 months after onset.
LOCATION.—A lesion centered on the shaft, extending into the metaphysis.

SIZE.—Initially 6 × 3 cm; ultimately involving the entire shaft.
MINERALIZATION OF TUMOR.—None.
DESTRUCTION.—In **A,** most obvious destruction is a geographic lesion at the junction of metaphysis and shaft (**arrows**). However, careful comparison with the normal counterpart (**B**) shows distinct loss of sharpness and density of the cortex throughout the metaphysis and upper shaft, produced by permeative pattern. This is increasingly distinct on each subsequent exposure.
PROLIFERATION.—In **A,** especially when compared with **B,** there is diffuse increase of density in the upper metaphysis. In the proximal shaft is distinct endostosis due to deposition of reactive bone on the medullary network of spongy bone and on the inner surface of the cortex, becoming more apparent in each subsequent film. At 10 weeks (**C**) a single lamina of subperiosteal new bone has appeared; at 20 weeks (**E**) there are three, and at 30 weeks (**F**) at least five, and hair-on-end spiculation is present (**arrow**).

DIFFERENTIAL DIAGNOSIS	PROBABILITY
Ewing's sarcoma	.87
Osteosarcoma	.09
Fibrosarcoma	.02

COMMENT: This valuable case demonstrates the progressive development of radiologic signs over 30 weeks in a rapidly advancing malignant tumor. In retrospect one can detect several definite signs of disease in **A,** made about a month after onset of symptoms. We are accustomed to seeing the full-blown pattern in **F,** at 30 weeks, recognizing this tumor only in its advanced form.

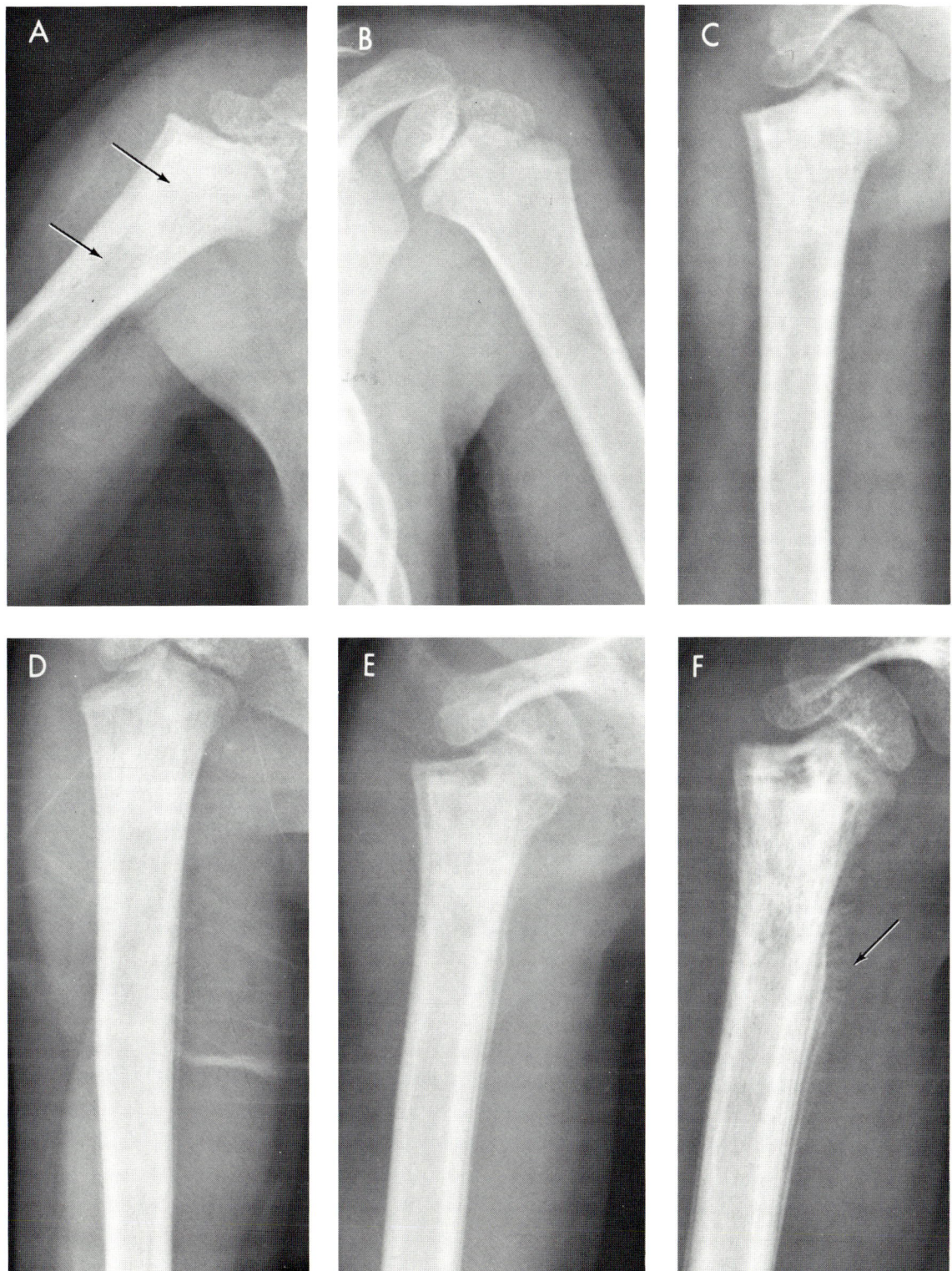

Figure 145 · Ewing's Sarcoma of Humerus

Figure 146.—Ewing's sarcoma of the pelvis.

AFIP Case No. 1042686: Anteroposterior projection.

DIAGNOSIS AND GRADE.—Ewing's sarcoma, pelvis; growth rate III.

LIFE INFORMATION.—Male, 17 years; survived 38 months.

LOCATION.—A tumor diffusely involving nearly the entire ilium, with large soft tissue tumor extending into the abdomen.

SIZE.—14 × 13 cm.

MINERALIZATION OF TUMOR.—Some linear branching patterns of calcific density in the soft tissue mass medially (**arrows;** see Comment); elsewhere the tumor is radiolucent.

DESTRUCTION.—Permeative; note rarefaction beneath growth plate of crest (**x**).

PROLIFERATION.—Mottled pattern of increased density throughout the tumor involving bone, consolidating to become quite dense laterally and conforming to normal trabecular pattern.

DIFFERENTIAL DIAGNOSIS	PROBABILITY
Ewing's sarcoma	.82
Reticulum cell sarcoma	.11
Osteosarcoma	.05
Fibrosarcoma	< .01

COMMENT: The mottled pattern of proliferative change is expected where Ewing's sarcoma involves spongy bone. The branching calcific densities in soft tissue are troublesome because of at least three possible causes. (1) The most likely is new bone arising from periosteum displaced and fragmented by tumor. The linear branching suggests this origin. (2) Tumor matrix mineralization is possible but unlikely since Ewing's is not known to produce such mineralization and the pattern of densities is unlike any known to arise from tumor bone. (3) There may be calcification in necrotic tumor, usually less structured in appearance than this. It is important to identify this calcification correctly since one's diagnosis of histologic type depends on it. Regardless of diagnosis, the radiographic evidence is of an aggressive, highly malignant tumor. For another round cell tumor displaying soft tissue mineralization, see Figure 159.

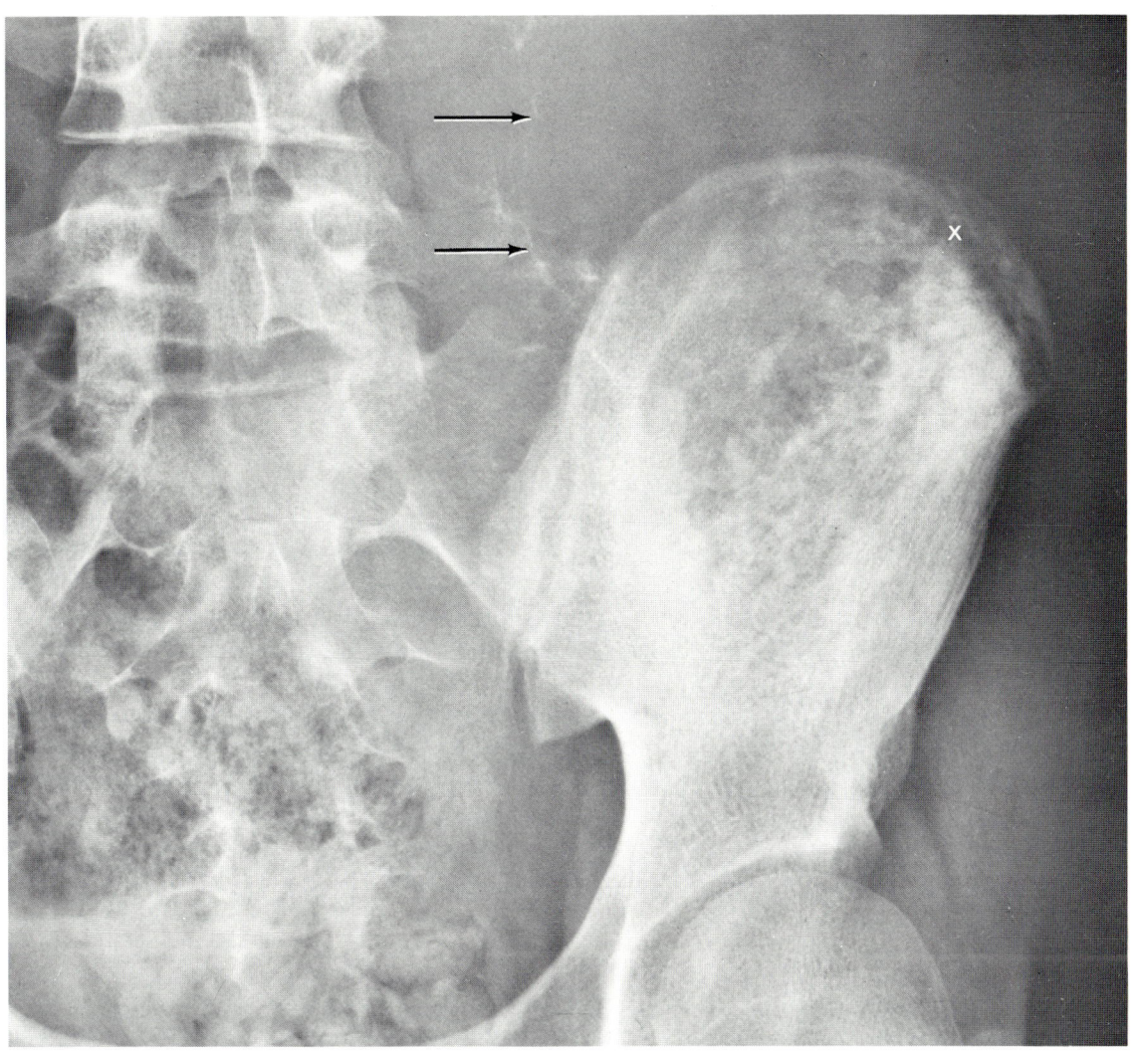

Figure 146 · Ewing's Sarcoma of Pelvis / 349

Figure 147.—Ewing's sarcoma of the humerus.

AFIP Case No. 1062430: Anteroposterior projection.

DIAGNOSIS AND GRADE.—Ewing's sarcoma, humerus; growth rate III.
LIFE INFORMATION.—Male, 20 years; survived 10 months after onset.
LOCATION.—A diffuse tumor centered in the midshaft, extending proximally, distally and subperiosteally.

SIZE.—15 × 3 cm.
MINERALIZATION OF TUMOR.—None.
DESTRUCTION.—Classic demonstration of permeative pattern.
PROLIFERATION.—Two delicate laminae of periosteal new bone.

DIFFERENTIAL DIAGNOSIS	PROBABILITY
Ewing's sarcoma	.77
Reticulum cell sarcoma	.22
Osteosarcoma	< .01
Chondrosarcoma	< .01

COMMENT: In reference to the laminated new bone, "delicate" signifies that the layers of new bone are thinner than the radiolucent spaces between them. In this expanded program of computer diagnosis, Ewing's sarcoma does not seem to have the high level of diagnosability that it had earlier in less complex programs.

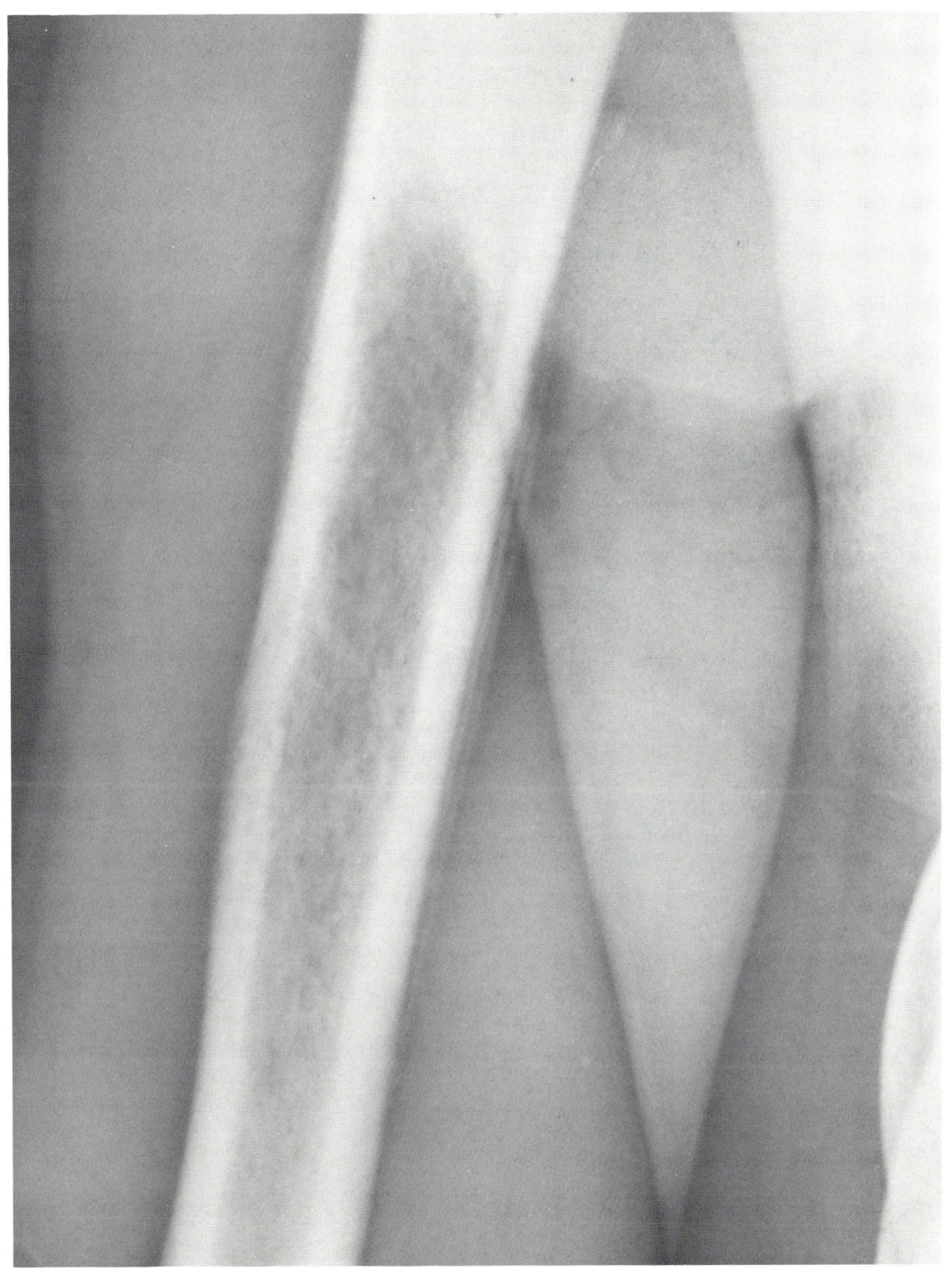

Figure 147 · Ewing's Sarcoma of Humerus / 351

Figure 148.—Ewing's sarcoma of a rib.

AFIP Case No. 1154958: Anteroposterior projection.

DIAGNOSIS AND GRADE.—Ewing's sarcoma, rib; growth rate III.

LIFE INFORMATION.—Male, 16 years; survived six months after onset.

LOCATION.—A tumor in the middle and anterior thirds of the left rib, with huge extraosseous mass.

SIZE.—16×10 cm.

MINERALIZATION OF TUMOR.—None.

DESTRUCTION.—Permeative pattern (**arrow**).

PROLIFERATION.—None definite.

DIFFERENTIAL DIAGNOSIS	PROBABILITY
Ewing's sarcoma	.75
Reticulum cell sarcoma	.16
Osteosarcoma	.06
Chondrosarcoma	.01
Fibrosarcoma	< .01

COMMENT: Ewing's sarcoma of the rib is usually characterized by a large extraosseous tumor.

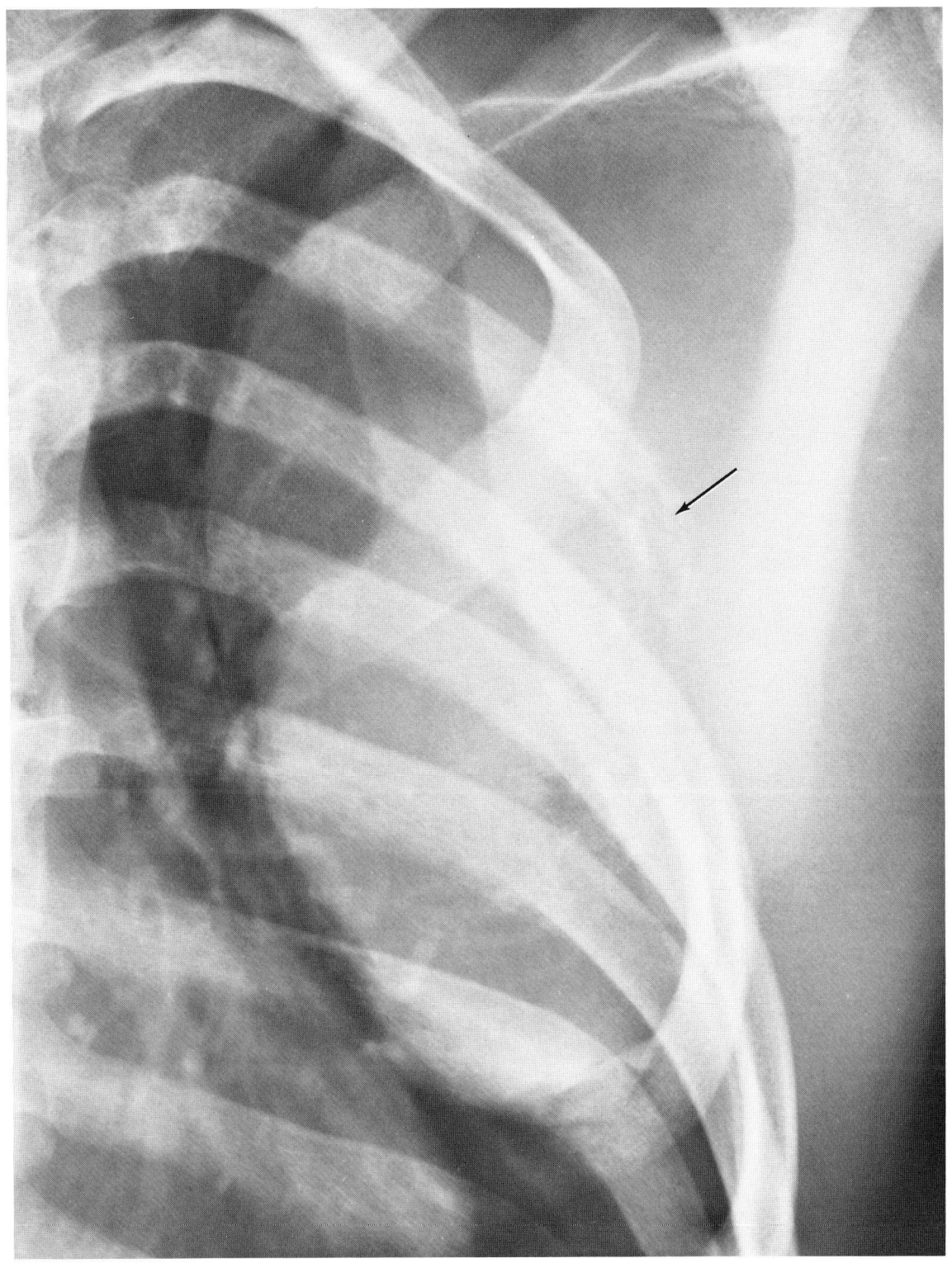

Figure 148 · Ewing's Sarcoma of Rib / 353

Figure 149.—Ewing's sarcomas of the ischium and ilium.

AFIP Case No. 933964: **A,** anteroposterior projection.

DIAGNOSIS AND GRADE.—Ewing's sarcoma, ischium; growth rate III.
LIFE INFORMATION.—Male, 20 years; survival unknown.
LOCATION.—A diffuse tumor involving the entire ischium.
SIZE.—8 × 4 cm.
MINERALIZATION OF TUMOR.—None.
DESTRUCTION.—Permeative pattern (**a**).
PROLIFERATION.—Diffuse mottled increased density (**b**); a single regular lamina of new bone below—the epiphysial center.

DIFFERENTIAL DIAGNOSIS	PROBABILITY
Reticulum cell sarcoma	.55
Ewing's sarcoma	.43
Osteosarcoma	< .01
Fibrosarcoma	< .01

COMMENT: Mottled proliferation, again critical to identification of histologic type. The basic pattern is of a highly aggressive malignant tumor, regardless of histology.

AFIP Case No. 1080037: **B,** anteroposterior projection.

DIAGNOSIS AND GRADE.—Ewing's sarcoma, pelvis; growth rate III.
LIFE INFORMATION.—Male, 15 years; survived 18 months.
LOCATION.—A diffuse tumor in the medial half of the ilium.
SIZE.—9 × 6 cm.
MINERALIZATION OF TUMOR.—None.
DESTRUCTION.—Moth-eaten pattern.
PROLIFERATION.—Dense mottling throughout a major segment (**x**).

DIFFERENTIAL DIAGNOSIS	PROBABILITY
Ewing's sarcoma	.71
Reticulum cell sarcoma	.23
Osteosarcoma	.04
Fibrosarcoma	.01
Chondrosarcoma	< .01

COMMENT: Again, identification of histologic type depends on interpretation of the increased density. The mottling near the edge of the tumor is an accentuation of normal trabecular pattern due to apposition of new bone on the surface of existing spongy bone, especially inferiorly. Its interpretation as tumor density rather than proliferative density would lead to diagnosis of osteosarcoma or chondrosarcoma.

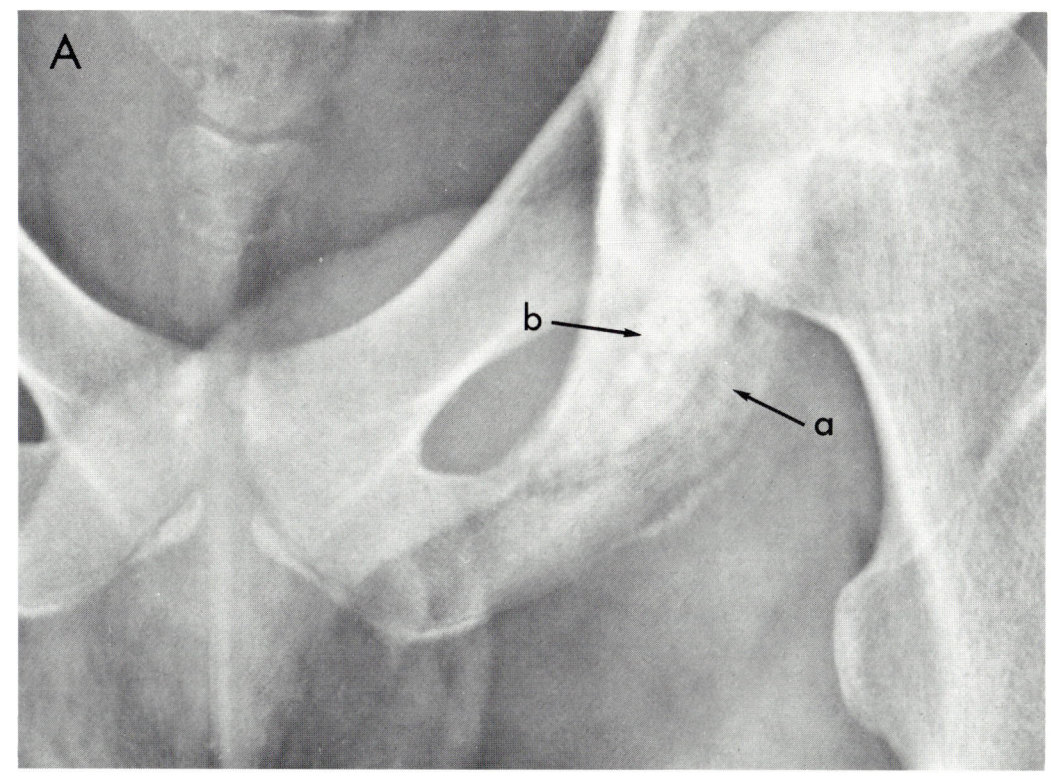
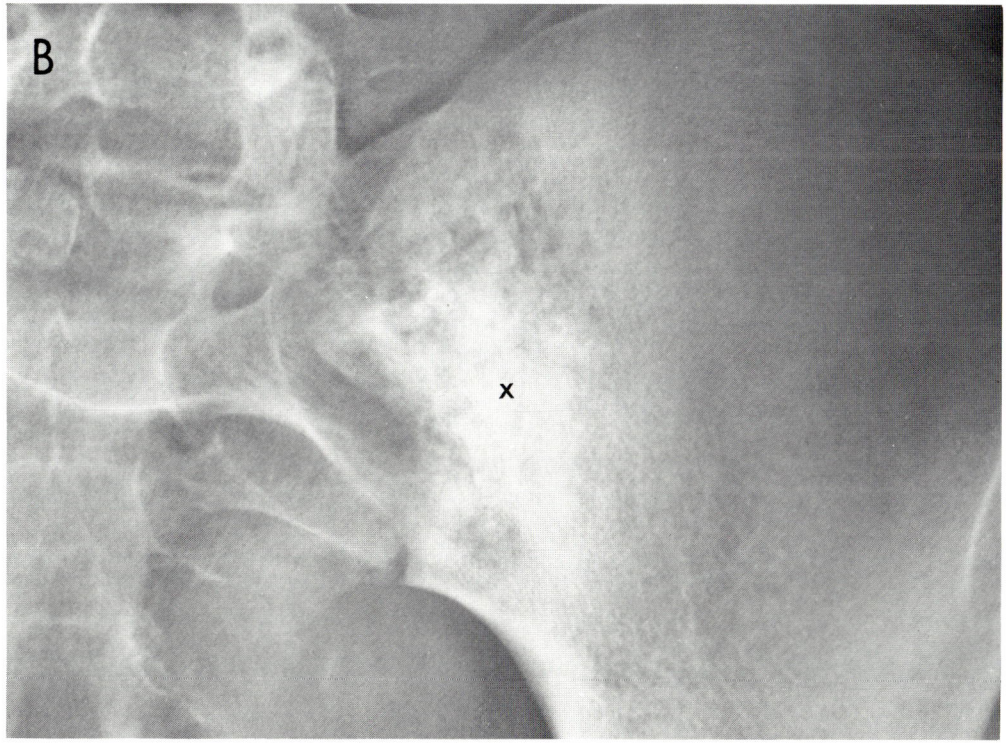

Figure 149 · Ewing's Sarcomas of Pelvis

Figure 150.—Ewing's sarcomas of the pubis and femur.

AFIP Case No. 957122: **A,** anteroposterior projection.

DIAGNOSIS AND GRADE.—Ewing's sarcoma, pubis; growth rate IC.
LIFE INFORMATION.—Male, 19 years; well five years later.
LOCATION.—A circumscribed lesion involving the entire pubis.

SIZE.—9 × 6 cm.
MINERALIZATION OF TUMOR.—None.
DESTRUCTION.—Geographic; total penetration of cortex; ragged contour.
PROLIFERATION.—Faint sclerosis in the residual bone at the lower margin of the tumor (**x**).

DIFFERENTIAL DIAGNOSIS	PROBABILITY
Fibrosarcoma	.40
Ewing's sarcoma	.27
Chondrosarcoma	.25
Giant cell tumor	.04
Cyst	.01
Chondromyxoid fibroma	.01

COMMENT: Behavior is consistent with the radiologic estimate of growth rate.

AFIP Case No. 1208176: **B,** lateral projection.

DIAGNOSIS AND GRADE.—Ewing's sarcoma, femur; growth rate III.
LIFE INFORMATION.—Male, 24 years; survived seven months.
LOCATION.—A diffuse tumor centered on the posterior cortex of the midshaft; large extraosseous component.

SIZE.—15 × 9 cm.
MINERALIZATION OF TUMOR.—None.
DESTRUCTION.—Permeative pattern.
PROLIFERATION.—A single amorphous lamina of periosteal new bone, with two irregular Codman triangles (**arrows**).

DIFFERENTIAL DIAGNOSIS	PROBABILITY
Osteosarcoma	.58
Ewing's sarcoma	.20
Fibrosarcoma	.12
Reticulum cell sarcoma	.06
Chondrosarcoma	.02

COMMENT: Apparent centering on the cortex or parosteally is unusual for Ewing's sarcoma.

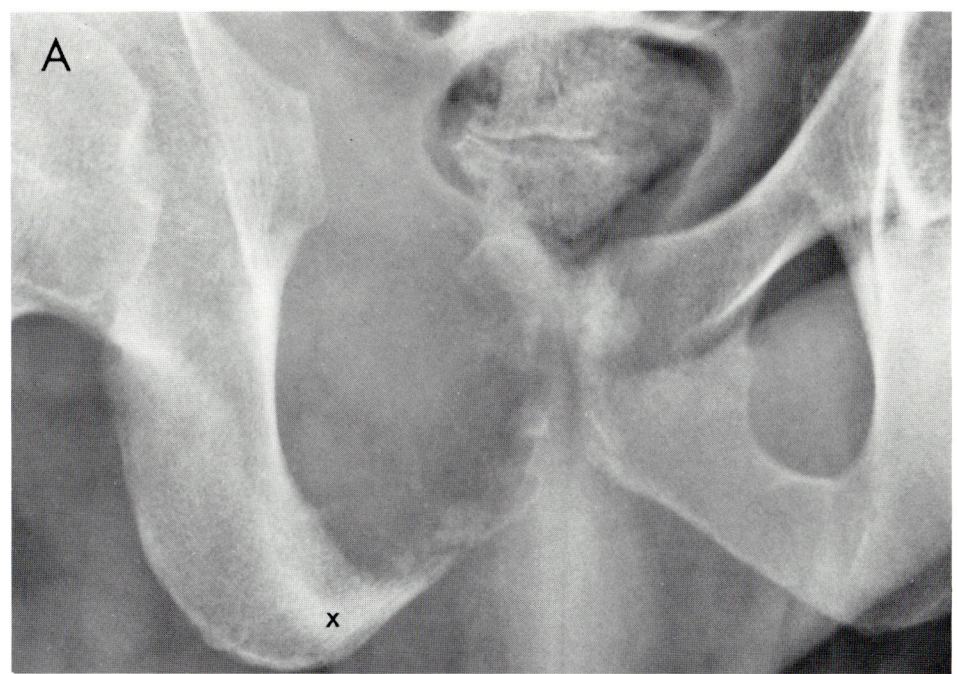
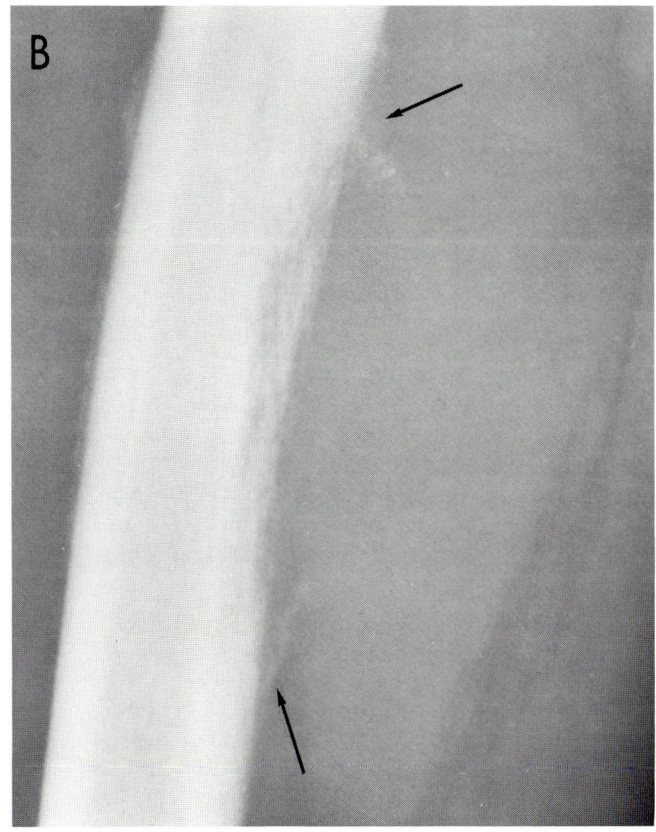

Figure 150 · Ewing's Sarcomas

Figure 151.—Ewing's sarcoma of the tibia.

AFIP Case No. 1154417: **A,** anteroposterior view; **B,** oblique arteriogram.

DIAGNOSIS AND GRADE.—Ewing's sarcoma, tibia; growth rate III.

LIFE INFORMATION.—Male, 18 years; survived 32 months.

LOCATION.—A diffuse tumor eccentrically located in the proximal tibial metaphysis, extending into the epiphysis.

SIZE.—7 × 6 × 6 cm.

MINERALIZATION OF TUMOR.—None.

DESTRUCTION.—Permeative pattern.

PROLIFERATION.—Limited to a single lamina of periosteal new bone, with small Codman's triangle (**A, arrow**).

DIFFERENTIAL DIAGNOSIS	PROBABILITY
Osteosarcoma	.91
Ewing's sarcoma	.07
Fibrosarcoma	< .01
Reticulum cell sarcoma	< .01

COMMENT: In the arteriogram, the extraosseous tumor is outlined by an increased number of vessels which contribute to an over-all increased density. Some of these vessels have a bizarre course and may be regarded as pathologic tumor vasculature, strongly suggestive of malignancy. Another significant sign, the arteriovenous shunt, is not present here. On the whole, arteriography is a rather disappointing resource for determining whether a tumor is benign or malignant.

The generally round tumor in an eccentric location without involvement of the shaft and the coarse periosteal response are damaging to the diagnosis of Ewing's sarcoma.

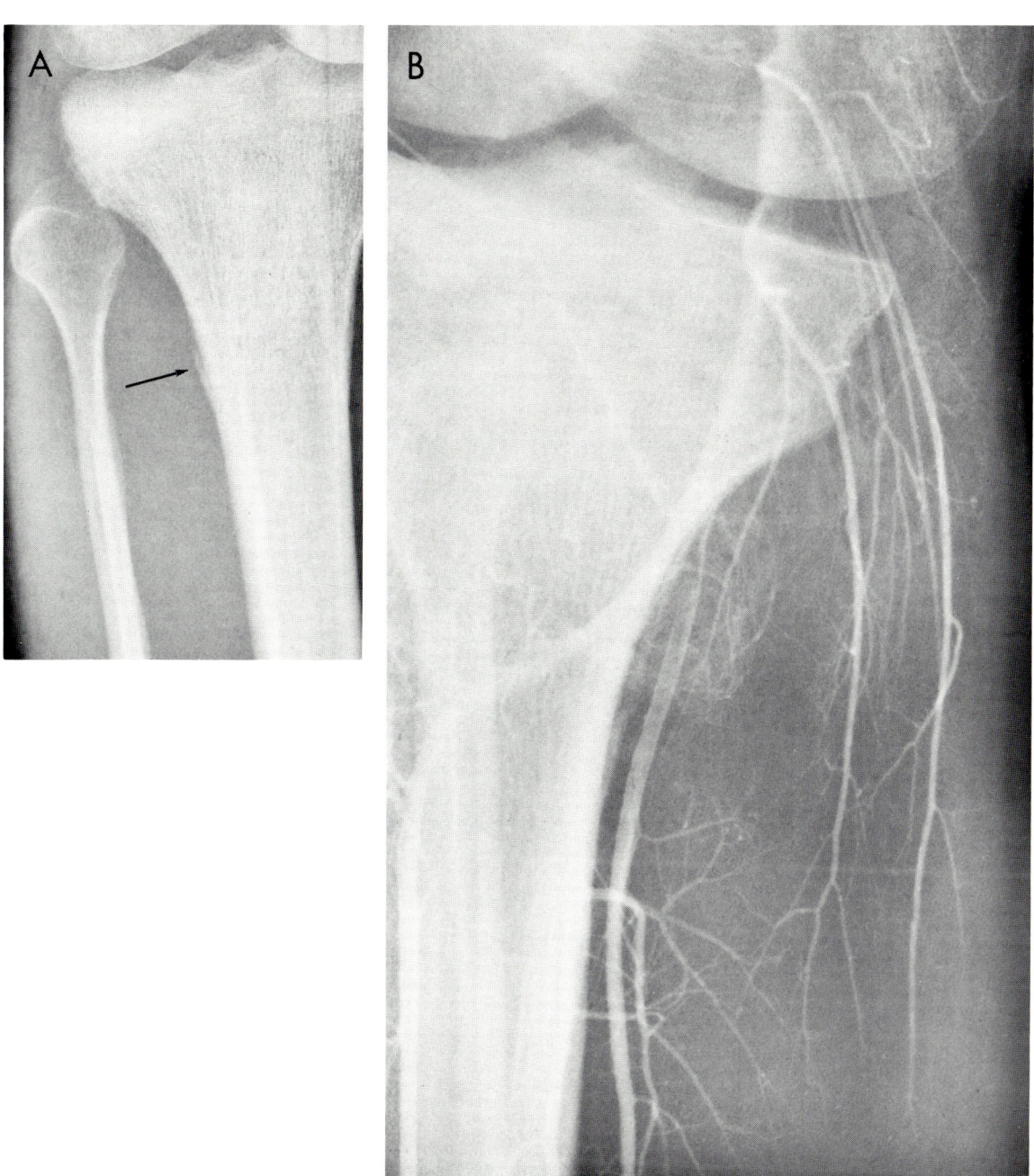

Figure 151 · Ewing's Sarcoma of Tibia

Figure 152.—Ewing's sarcoma of the pubis.

AFIP Case No. 1163562: Anteroposterior projection.

DIAGNOSIS AND GRADE.—Ewing's sarcoma, pubis; growth rate III.
LIFE INFORMATION.—Male, 30 years; survival unknown.
LOCATION.—Diffuse involvement of the entire ischium.
SIZE.—8 × 4 cm.
MINERALIZATION OF TUMOR.—None.
DESTRUCTION.—Permeative pattern with a few foci of moth-eaten bone destruction.
PROLIFERATION.—A few foci of mottled increased density medially. On the whole there is surprisingly little evidence of proliferative change.

DIFFERENTIAL DIAGNOSIS	PROBABILITY
Reticulum cell sarcoma	.90
Fibrosarcoma	.06
Ewing's sarcoma	.02
Osteosarcoma	< .01
Chondrosarcoma	< .01

COMMENT: In contrast to the tumor in Figure 149, *A,* there is little proliferative response. The histologic diagnosis submitted by the contributor was reticulum cell sarcoma. The radiologic differential diagnosis between these two tumors in spongy bone is very difficult.

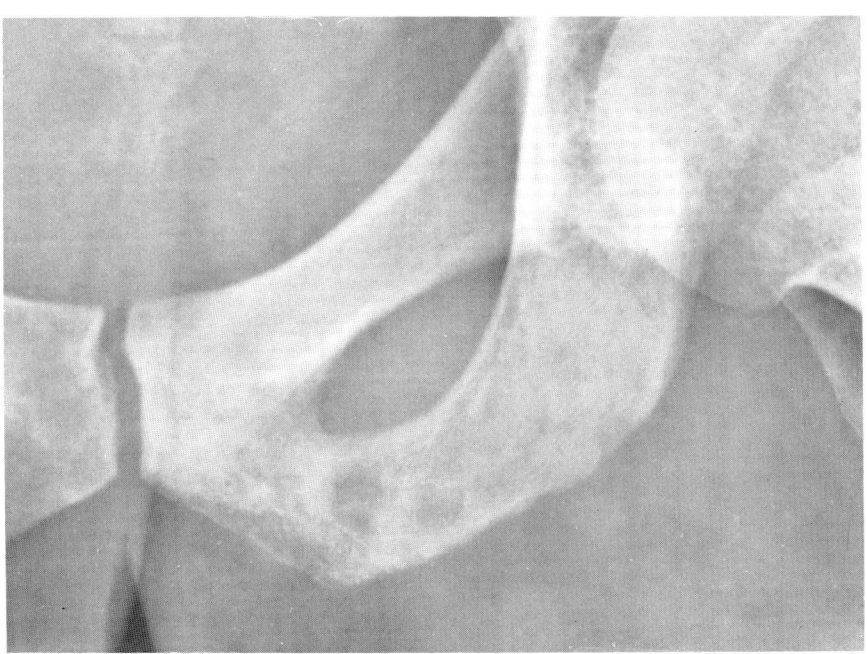

Figure 153.—Reticulum cell sarcoma of the femur.

AFIP Case No. 871328: Anteroposterior projection.

DIAGNOSIS AND GRADE.—Reticulum cell sarcoma, femur; growth rate III.
LIFE INFORMATION.—Female, 79 years; survived one week after diagnosis.
LOCATION.—A lesion in the proximal shaft of the femur.

SIZE.—15 × 7 cm.
MINERALIZATION OF TUMOR.—None.
DESTRUCTION.—Permeated pattern.
PROLIFERATION.—Slight mottling in spongy bone of the intertrochanteric area.

DIFFERENTIAL DIAGNOSIS	PROBABILITY
Reticulum cell sarcoma	.98
Osteosarcoma	.01
Fibrosarcoma	< .01

COMMENT: A basic problem to be answered in a case of reticulum cell sarcoma is "Is this a primary or a secondary tumor?" In this instance, the location of the lesion and the rapid demise strongly suggest metastatic tumor.

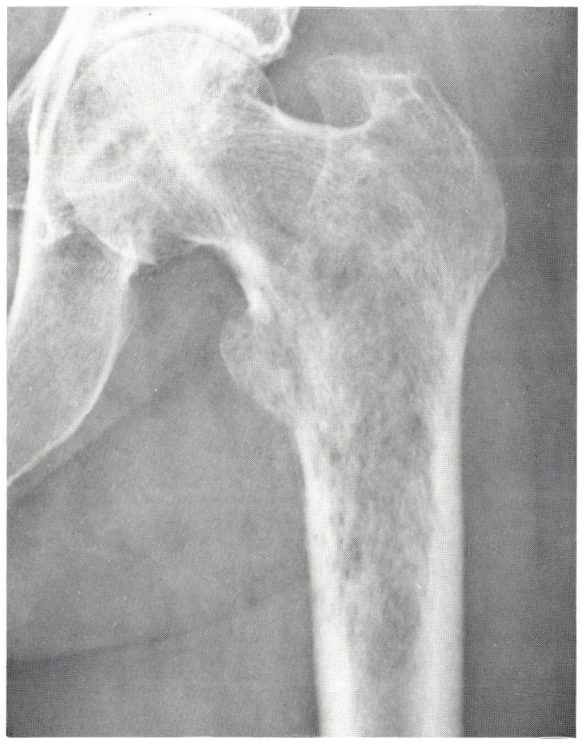

Figure 153 · Reticulum Cell Sarcoma

Figure 154.—Reticulum cell sarcoma of the femur.

AFIP Case No. 1114607: Anteroposterior projection.

DIAGNOSIS AND GRADE.—Reticulum cell sarcoma, femur; growth rate III.

LIFE INFORMATION.—Male, 27 years; alive more than three years after onset.

LOCATION.—A diffuse lesion centered in the distal femoral metaphysis, extending proximally into the shaft and distally into the epiphysis and subarticular cortex.

SIZE.—15 × 9 cm.

MINERALIZATION OF TUMOR.—None.

DESTRUCTION.—Permeative; with a long pathologic fracture which shows evidence of healing.

PROLIFERATION.—A diffuse mottled increased density in spongy bone, with a rather hard, irregular appearing lamina of subperiosteal new bone.

DIFFERENTIAL DIAGNOSIS	PROBABILITY
Reticulum cell sarcoma	.97
Fibrosarcoma	.01
Ewing's sarcoma	< .01
Osteosarcoma	< .01

COMMENT: The lack of distinctness of the permeative pattern and the regularity of the periosteal new bone suggest healing following treatment. In the expanded computer program, reticulum cell sarcoma appears to be a stronger diagnosis than we have previously experienced with this type.

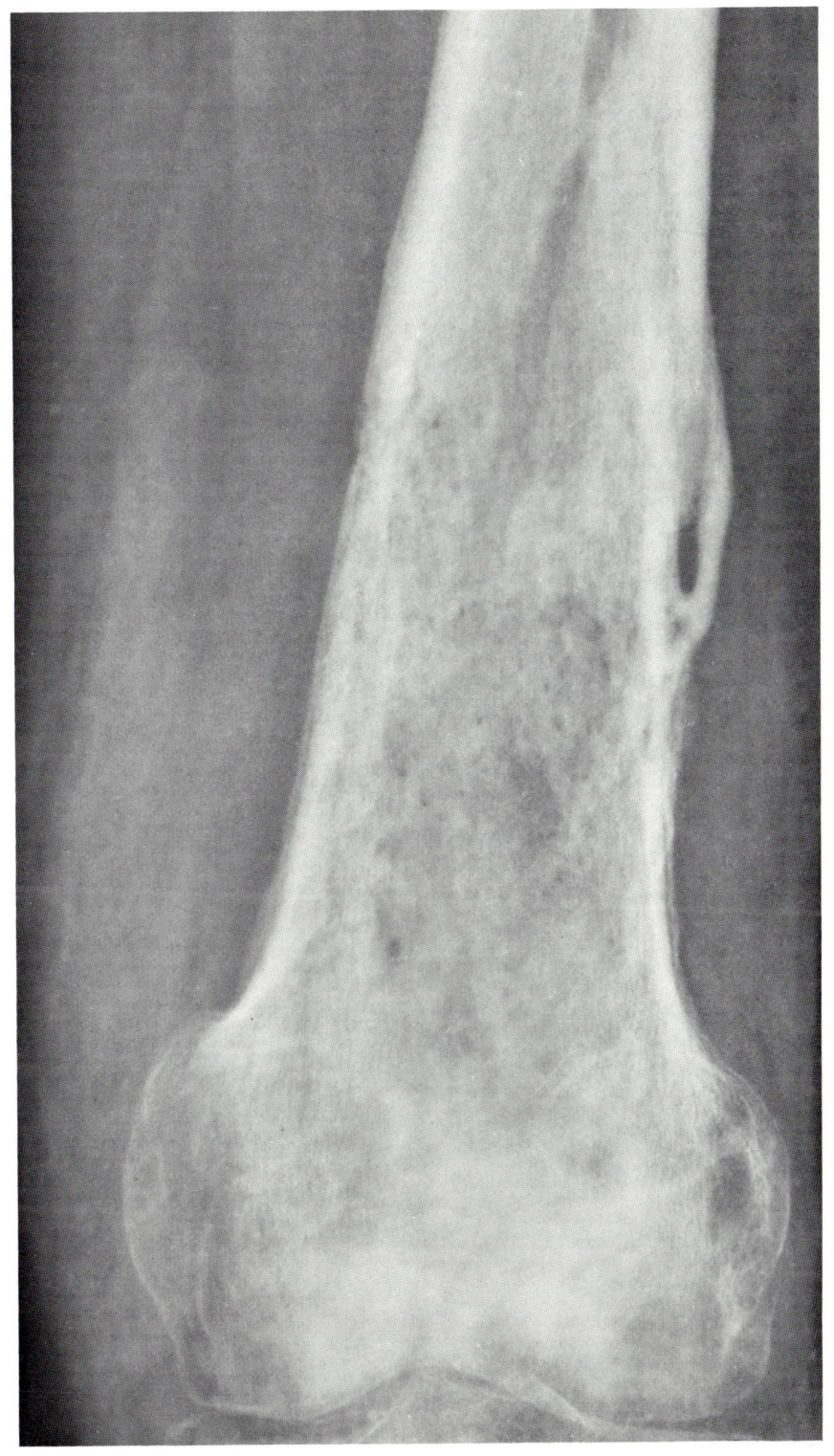

Figure 154 · Reticulum Cell Sarcoma

Figure 155.—Reticulum cell sarcoma of the clavicle.

AFIP Case No. 1119586: Anteroposterior views—**A,** initial study; **B,** 11 weeks later; **C,** 42 months later, after radiotherapy.

DIAGNOSIS AND GRADE.—Reticulum cell sarcoma, clavicle; growth rate III.
LIFE INFORMATION.—Male, 53 years; alive 3½ years after onset.
LOCATION.—A diffuse lesion centered in the distal half of the clavicle.
SIZE.—7 × 3 cm.
MINERALIZATION OF TUMOR.—None.
DESTRUCTION.—Permeative, with moth-eaten components appearing at 11 weeks (**B**) to nearly total loss of structure.
PROLIFERATION.—Irregular, imperfect laminae of periosteal new bone which appear to expand into the soft tissue mass (**B**).

DIFFERENTIAL DIAGNOSIS	PROBABILITY
Reticulum cell sarcoma	.94
Fibrosarcoma	.04
Osteosarcoma	< .01
Chondrosarcoma	< .01

COMMENT: There is a definite suggestion that a very irregular, patchy periosteal response is being displaced into the soft tissues by the expanding tumor (**B, arrows**). Following radiation therapy, with complete healing, the restored outer third of the clavicle is of much greater caliber than the original bone.

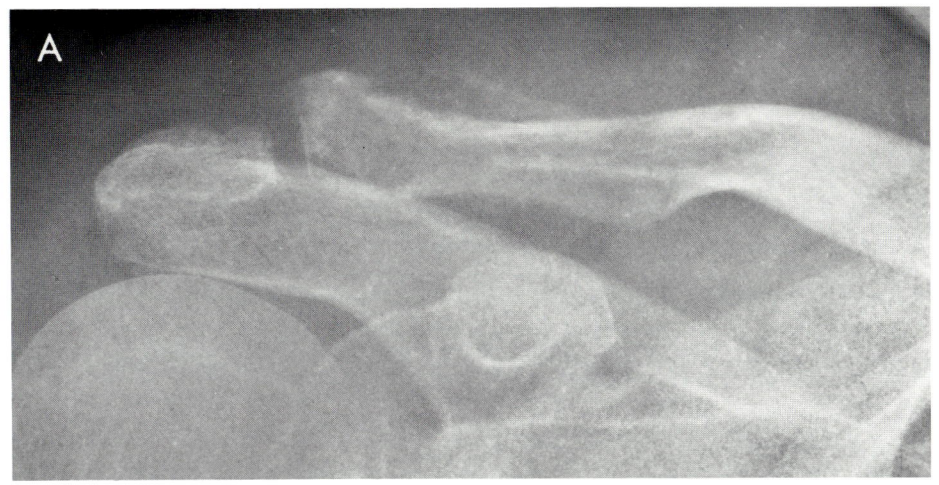

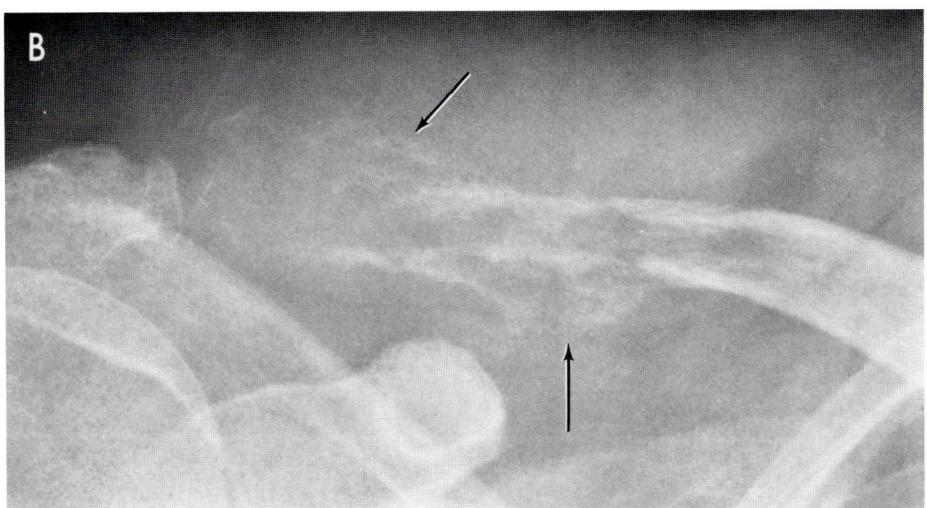

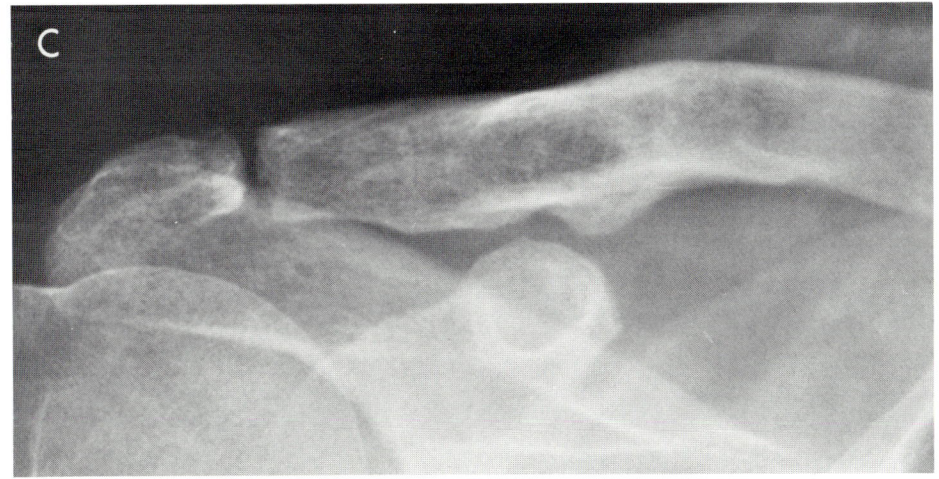

Figure 155 · Reticulum Cell Sarcoma / 365

Figure 156.—Reticulum cell sarcoma of the tibia.

AFIP Case No. 1101897: Oblique projection.

DIAGNOSIS AND GRADE.—Reticulum cell sarcoma, tibia; growth rate III.

LIFE INFORMATION.—Male, 51 years; alive four years after onset.

LOCATION.—A diffuse tumor involving the midshaft of the tibia; soft tissue extension.

SIZE.—13 × 6 cm.

MINERALIZATION OF TUMOR.—None.

DESTRUCTION.—Permeative pattern, with confluent holes (see Comment).

PROLIFERATION.—None.

DIFFERENTIAL DIAGNOSIS	PROBABILITY
Reticulum cell sarcoma	.91
Fibrosarcoma	.04
Osteosarcoma	.03
Chondrosarcoma	.01

COMMENT: A typical case of reticulum cell sarcoma. The principal difficulty is distinguishing between moth-eaten and permeative bone destruction. Because the pattern consists basically of elongated tunnels in dense cortex, without segmental loss of bone, the pattern is more consistent with permeative than with moth-eaten bone destruction, in which the individual holes tend to be round.

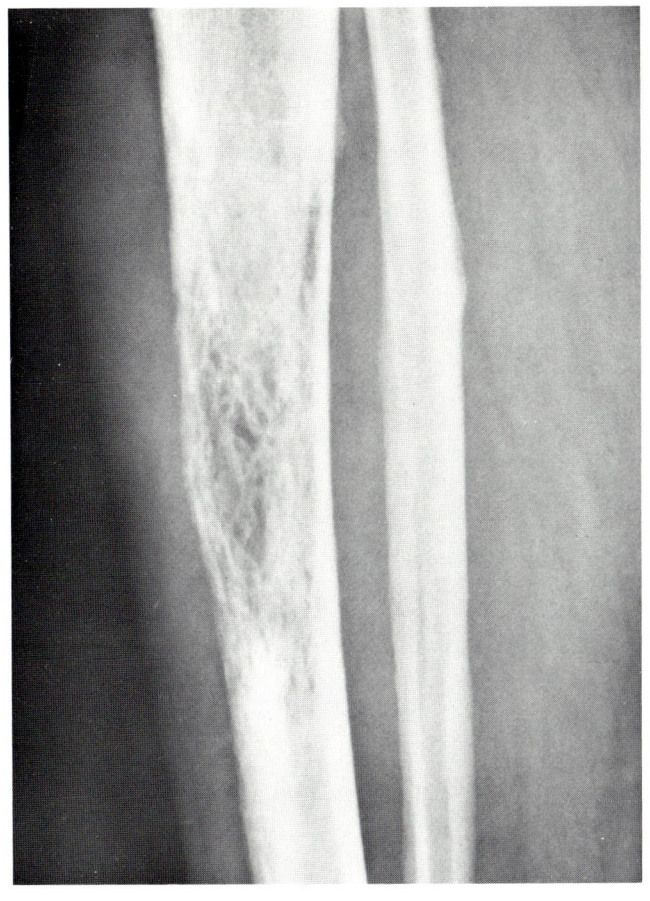

Figure 156 · Reticulum Cell Sarcoma / 367

Figure 157.—Reticulum cell sarcoma of the pelvis.

AFIP Case No. 1218013: Anteroposterior projection.

DIAGNOSIS AND GRADE.—Reticulum cell sarcoma, pelvis; growth rate III.
LIFE INFORMATION.—Male, 22 years; survival unknown.
LOCATION.—A diffuse tumor involving the medial half of the ilium and the sacroiliac joint.
SIZE.—10 × 9 cm.
MINERALIZATION OF TUMOR.—None.
DESTRUCTION.—Moth-eaten pattern.
PROLIFERATION.—Diffuse mottling throughout spongy bone.

DIFFERENTIAL DIAGNOSIS	PROBABILITY
Reticulum cell sarcoma	.81
Ewing's sarcoma	.08
Fibrosarcoma	.05
Osteosarcoma	.03
Chondrosarcoma	< .01

COMMENT: As in Ewing's sarcoma of the pelvis, identification of histologic type is based on recognition of the cause of increased density. Careful study of mottled areas near the tumor edge reveals individual trabeculae to be progressively thickened, due to deposition of reactive bone on the spongy network. This case resembles Ewing's sarcomas in Figures 146 and 149 in problems of differentiation between round cell tumor and osteosarcoma or chondrosarcoma. In any case the pattern is that of a malignant aggressive tumor.

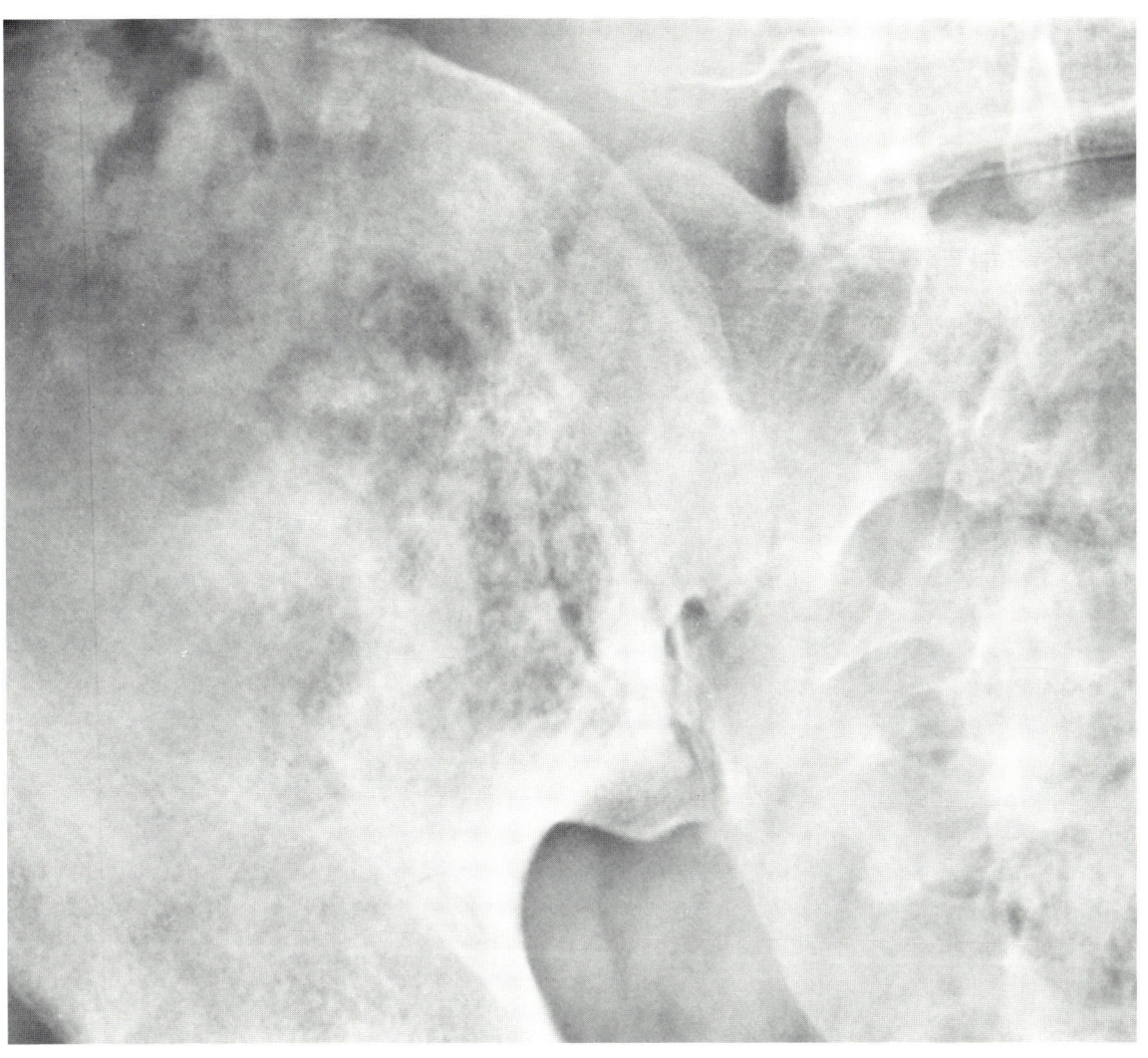

Figure 157 · Reticulum Cell Sarcoma / 369

Figure 158.—Reticulum cell sarcoma of the hip, pelvis and femur.

AFIP Case No. 692946: **A,** anteroposterior projection.

DIAGNOSIS AND GRADE.—Reticulum cell sarcoma, hip and pelvis; growth rate III.

LIFE INFORMATION.—Female, 17 years; survived 14 months.

LOCATION.—A diffuse tumor involving the proximal end of the femur, acetabulum and ilium.

SIZE.—Total area of involvement about 20 × 15 cm.

MINERALIZATION OF TUMOR.—None.

DESTRUCTION.—Combination of moth-eaten and permeative pattern throughout; pathologic fracture of femoral neck.

PROLIFERATION.—Residual spongy structural elements in the proximal femur and pelvis increased in thickness and density; scant irregular periosteal response.

DIFFERENTIAL DIAGNOSIS	PROBABILITY
Reticulum cell sarcoma	.78
Fibrosarcoma	.18
Osteosarcoma	.02
Ewing's sarcoma	< .01

COMMENT: An advanced tumor with surprisingly long survival. The question of a metastatic tumor would need to be raised here.

AFIP Case No. 584949: **B,** anteroposterior projection.

DIAGNOSIS AND GRADE.—Reticulum cell sarcoma, femur; growth rate III.

LIFE INFORMATION.—Female, 43 years; survived three months.

LOCATION.—A diffuse tumor centrally located in proximal shaft and metaphysis.

SIZE.—8 × 3 cm.

MINERALIZATION OF TUMOR.—None.

DESTRUCTION.—Permeative pattern en face (**x**).

PROLIFERATION.—A single short lamina of subperiosteal new bone at lower margin of tumor, reflecting Codman's triangle (**arrow**).

DIFFERENTIAL DIAGNOSIS	PROBABILITY
Reticulum cell sarcoma	.74
Osteosarcoma	.16
Fibrosarcoma	.08
Chondrosarcoma	< .01

COMMENT: The nonspecific appearance and location might well represent a metastatic tumor. The very short survival time supports this possibility.

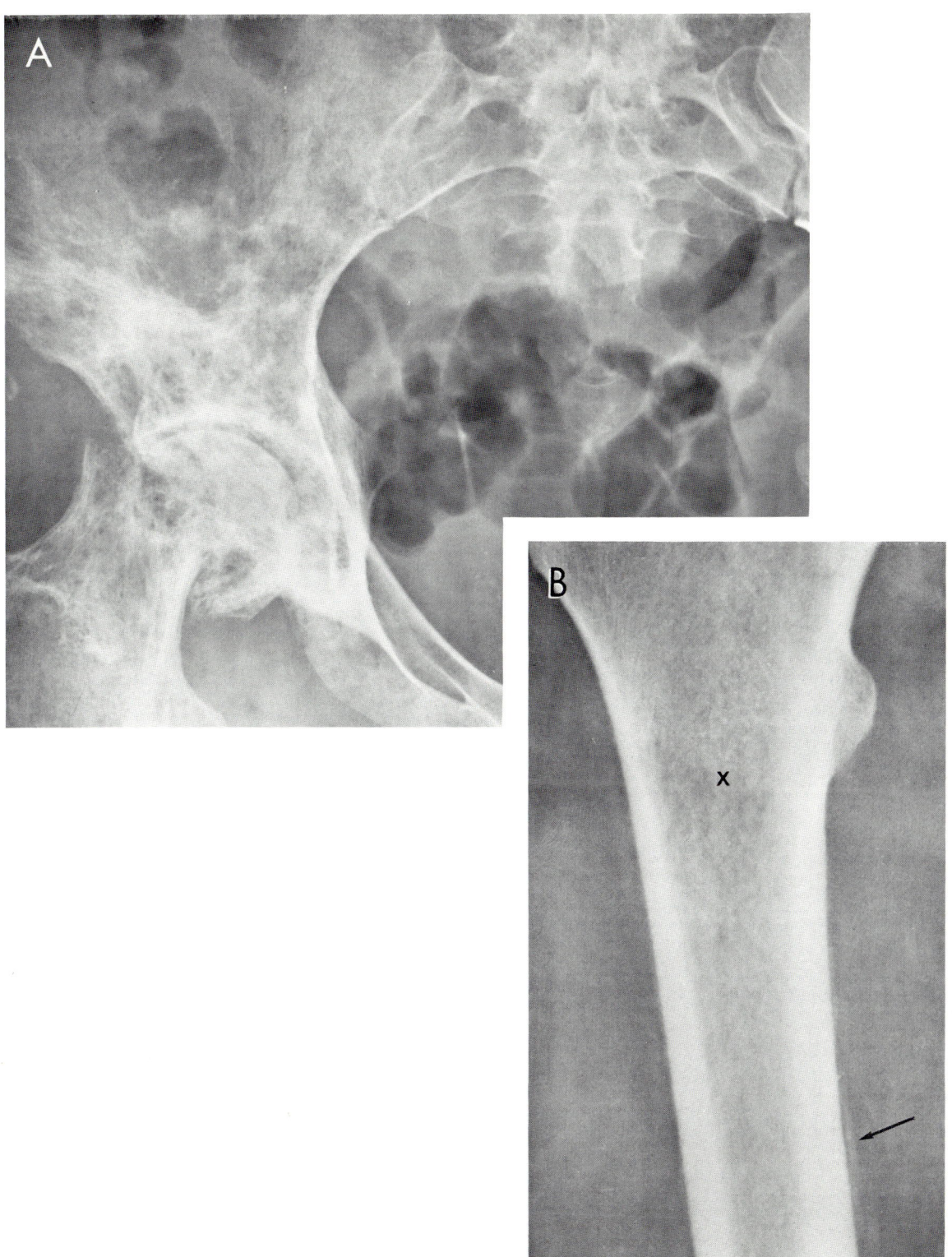

Figure 158 · Reticulum Cell Sarcomas

Figure 159.—Reticulum cell sarcoma of the femur.

AFIP Case No. 517287: **A,** initial lateral examination. *On next text page:* **B,** three weeks later, after radiation therapy; **C,** fracture, years later; **D,** subsequent pseudarthrosis; **E,** residual changes.

DIAGNOSIS AND GRADE.—Reticulum cell sarcoma, femur; growth rate III.

LIFE INFORMATION.—Female, 23 years; well 19 years after onset.

LOCATION.—A diffuse lesion centered in the distal shaft, extending into the metaphysis and epiphysis; huge extraosseous extension.

SIZE.—25 × 15 cm.

MINERALIZATION OF TUMOR.—Ill-defined reticulate pattern of calcific density scattered throughout the extraosseous component (**A, arrows**), persisting during radiation therapy and becoming more concentrated (**B**).

DESTRUCTION.—Initially (**A, a**) permeative pattern; ultimately (**E, e**) extreme osteoporosis and multiple small foci of geographic bone destruction (see Comment).

PROLIFERATION.—Initially a diffuse mottled increase of density in spongy bone (**A, b**); ultimately a dense contiguous reticulation of reactive bone (see Comment); a few indistinct spicules of reactive bone extending posteriorly into the tumor.

DIFFERENTIAL DIAGNOSIS	PROBABILITY
Reticulum cell sarcoma	.71
Ewing's sarcoma	.21
Osteosarcoma	.05
Fibrosarcoma	.01

(*Continued.*)

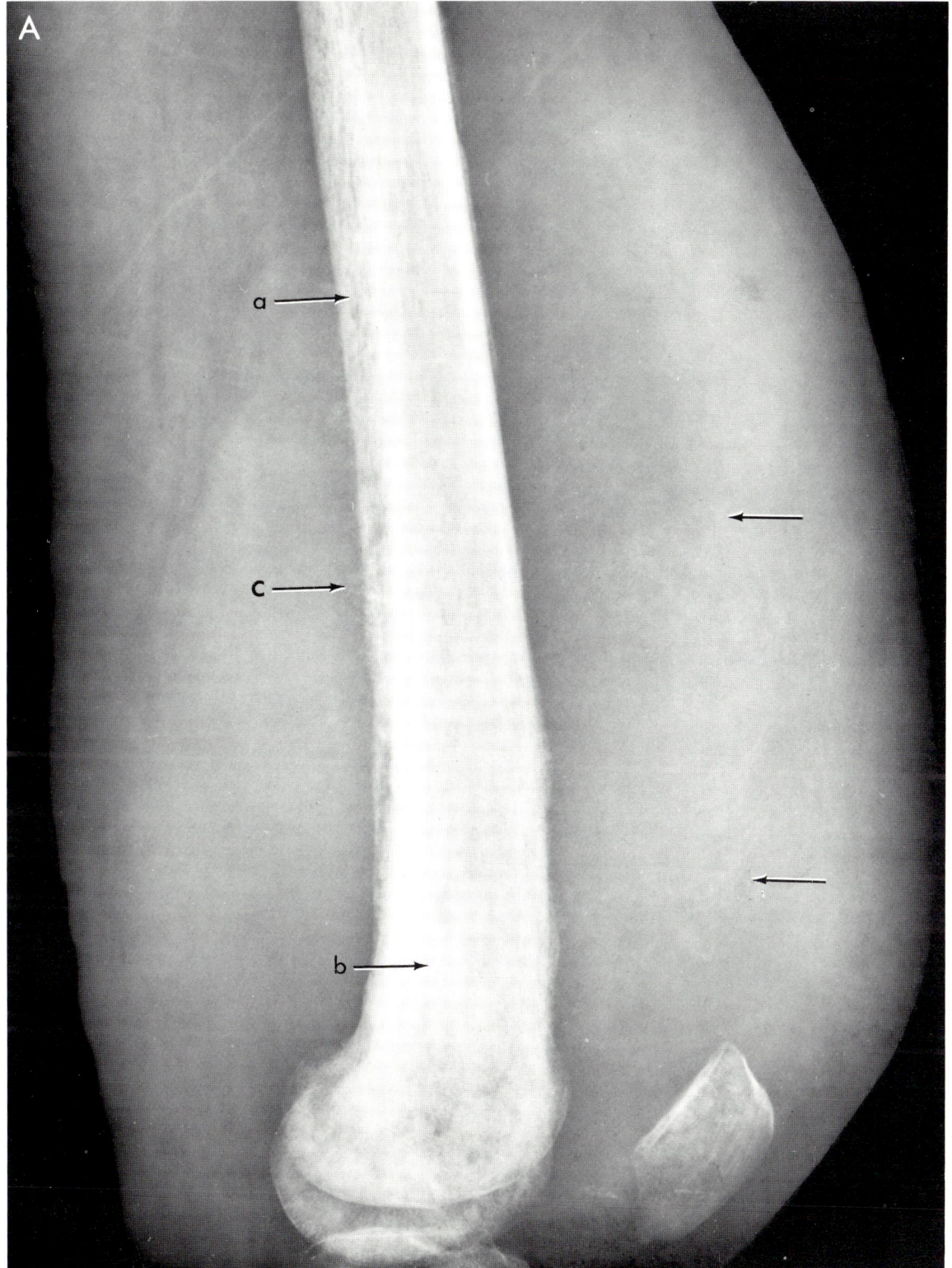

Figure 159 · Reticulum Cell Sarcoma / 373

Figure 159 (cont.).—Reticulum cell sarcoma of the femur.

B, three weeks after initial examination, following radiation therapy; **C,** fracture, years later; **D,** subsequent pseudarthrosis; **E,** residual changes.

COMMENT: This extraordinary case shows a number of interesting changes. The initial picture (**A**) of permeative bone destruction, mottled proliferative response and a vague lumpy periosteal reaction is quite typical. However, there are a few spicules (**A, c**), a very rare finding in reticulum cell sarcoma. Furthermore, there is the problem of reticulated increased density in the soft tissues (**A, arrows**), which is most conveniently interpreted as calcification in overgrown necrotic tumor. The early healing following radiation therapy (**B**) requires no special comment. Owing to the extent of the primary lesion, the entire femoral shaft was irradiated. A number of years later the femur has fractured through the subtrochanteric shaft (**C**). The fracture is essentially transverse, a kind that ordinarily is the result of abnormality in the bony structure, in this instance presumably an increased brittleness due to the radiation therapy. With the passage of time the fracture does not heal but forms a pseudarthrosis (**D, d**). The bone formerly occupied by the tumor assumes a bizarre appearance of a reticulate pattern of medullary and endosteal increased density, with normal cortex eroded by multiple foci of geographic bone destruction, causing a pockmarked appearance (**E, e**). This resembles changes often seen in bone many years after radium poisoning, in which case the radiolucent areas in the cortex probably represent fibrous replacement of bone. The dense areas are probably a combination of necrotic bone and calcified scar tissue.

The patient gets around well despite her handicap.

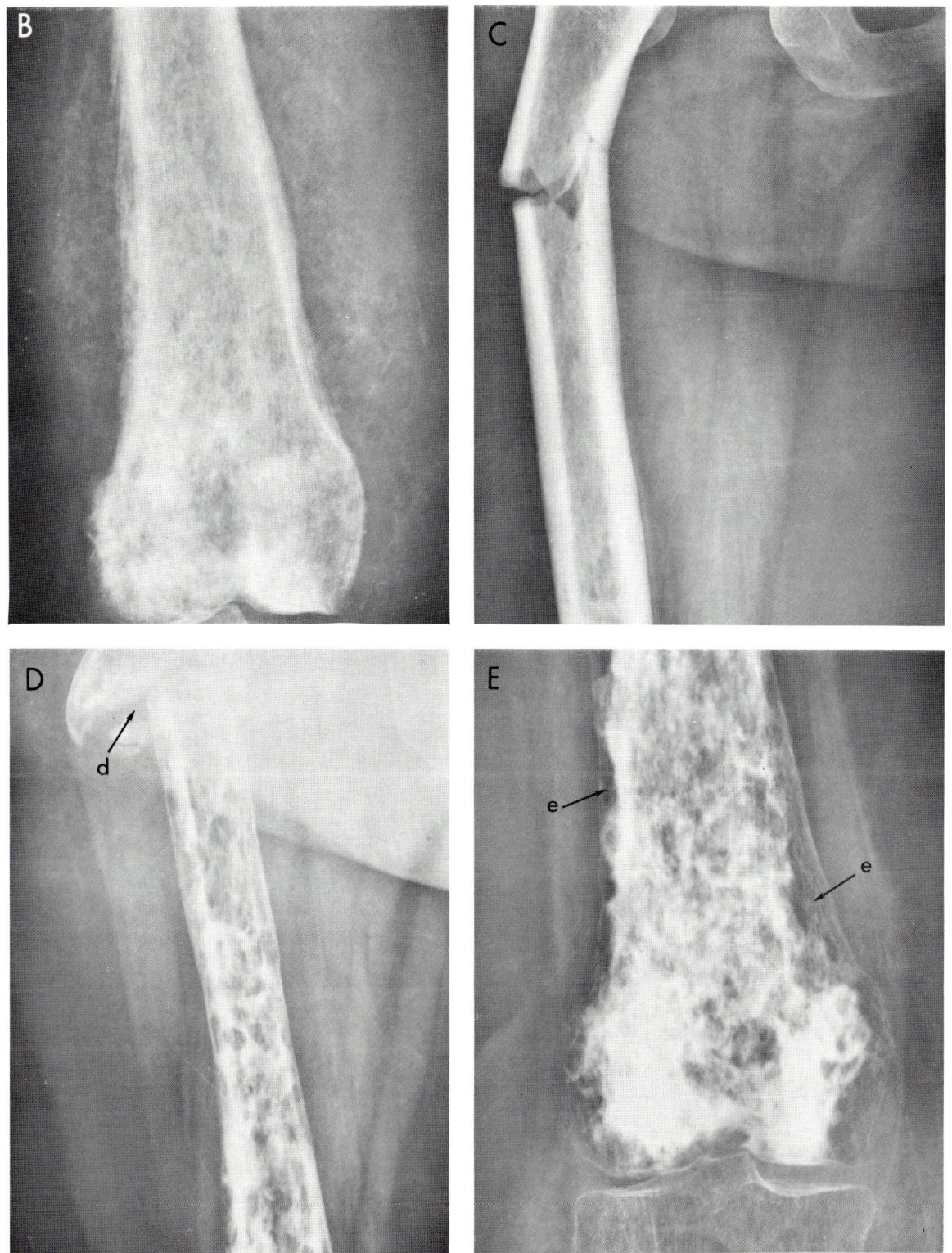

Figure 159 · Reticulum Cell Sarcoma

Figure 160.—Reticulum cell sarcoma of the humerus.

AFIP Case No. 1145778: Anteroposterior views—**A**, initial examination; **B**, 19 months later, after radiation therapy.

DIAGNOSIS AND GRADE.—Reticulum cell sarcoma, humerus; growth rate III.
LIFE INFORMATION.—Male, 27 years; radiation therapy four years after onset.
LOCATION.—A lesion in the proximal metaphysis of the shaft; extraosseous soft tissue extension.
SIZE.—Estimated 8 × 7 cm.
MINERALIZATION OF TUMOR.—None.
DESTRUCTION.—Permeative; total cortical penetration (**A**).
PROLIFERATION.—Mottled reactive areas in spongy bone of metaphysis. After irradiation (**B**) metaphysial cortex is sharper and trabecular pattern of spongy bone is reestablished.

DIFFERENTIAL DIAGNOSIS	PROBABILITY
Reticulum cell sarcoma	.66
Ewing's sarcoma	.23
Osteosarcoma	.10
Fibrosarcoma	< .01

COMMENT: Another example of response to irradiation.

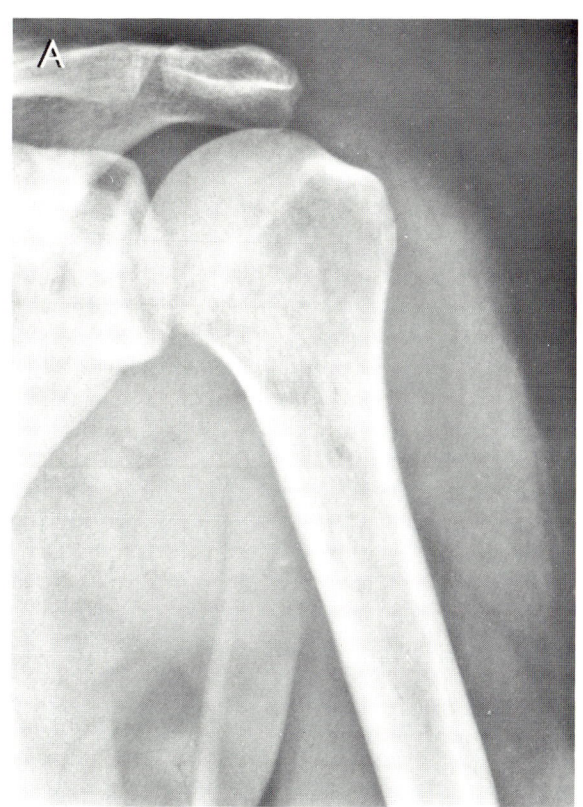

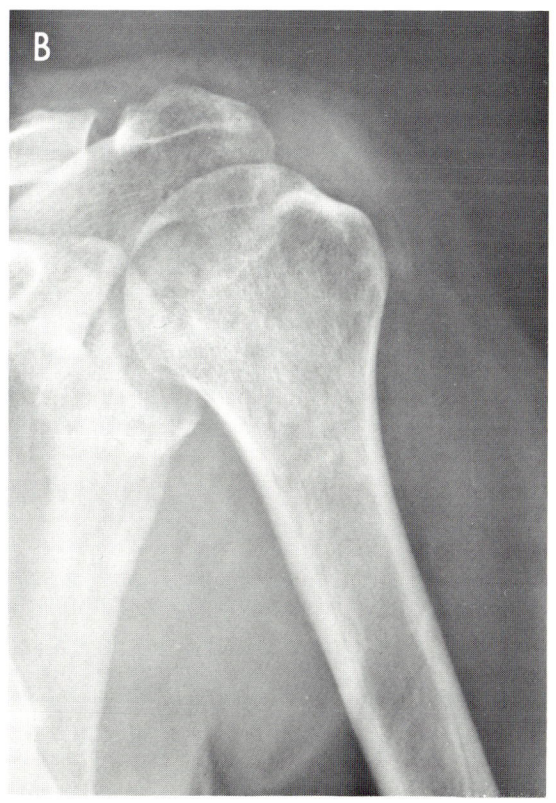

Figure 160 · Reticulum Cell Sarcoma / 377

Figure 161.—Reticulum cell sarcoma of the tibia.

AFIP Case No. 1115234: Anteroposterior projection.

DIAGNOSIS AND GRADE.—Reticulum cell sarcoma, tibia; growth rate III.

LIFE INFORMATION.—Female, 14 years; survival unknown.

LOCATION.—A diffuse tumor eccentrically centered on the growth plate of the proximal tibia, involving epiphysis and proximal metaphysis.

SIZE.—4 × 3 cm.

MINERALIZATION OF TUMOR.—None.

DESTRUCTION.—Permeative; slight cancellous reduction (**arrow**).

PROLIFERATION.—Faint mottling throughout medullary spongy bone; no periosteal response.

DIFFERENTIAL DIAGNOSIS	PROBABILITY
Fibrosarcoma	.49
Osteosarcoma	.38
Reticulum cell sarcoma	.08
Ewing's sarcoma	.03

COMMENT: Radiologically this could be either Ewing's sarcoma or reticulum cell sarcoma.

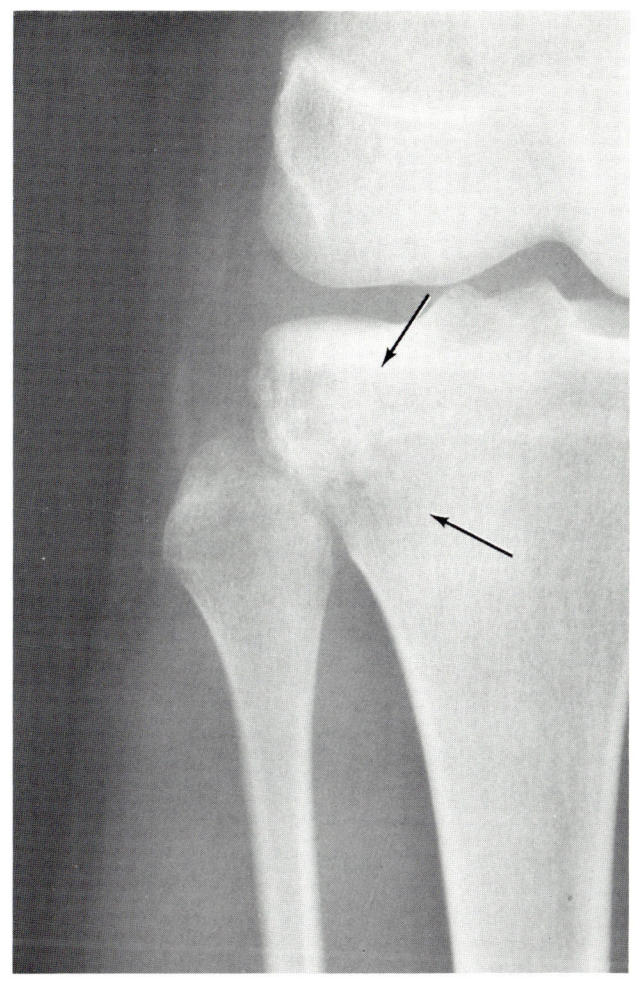

Figure 161 · Reticulum Cell Sarcoma / 379

Figure 162.—Reticulum cell sarcoma of the ilium.

AFIP Case No. 1178414: Anteroposterior views—**A,** initial examination; **B,** three months later.

DIAGNOSIS AND GRADE.—Reticulum cell sarcoma, ilium; growth rate II.

LIFE INFORMATION.—Male, 21 years; survived a year after onset.

LOCATION.—A diffuse lesion involving the lower half of the ilium.

SIZE.—Initially about 7 × 5 cm; at three months 18 × 11 cm.

MINERALIZATION OF TUMOR.—None.

DESTRUCTION.—Basically, moth-eaten throughout, with confluence of holes.

PROLIFERATION.—Extensive mottled increased density throughout with exceptionally heavy patch near the sacroiliac joint.

DIFFERENTIAL DIAGNOSIS	PROBABILITY
Reticulum cell sarcoma	.41
Ewing's sarcoma	.26
Osteosarcoma	.19
Fibrosarcoma	.12
Chondrosarcoma	< .01

COMMENT: Again a problem of distinguishing between reactive bone and tumor bone.

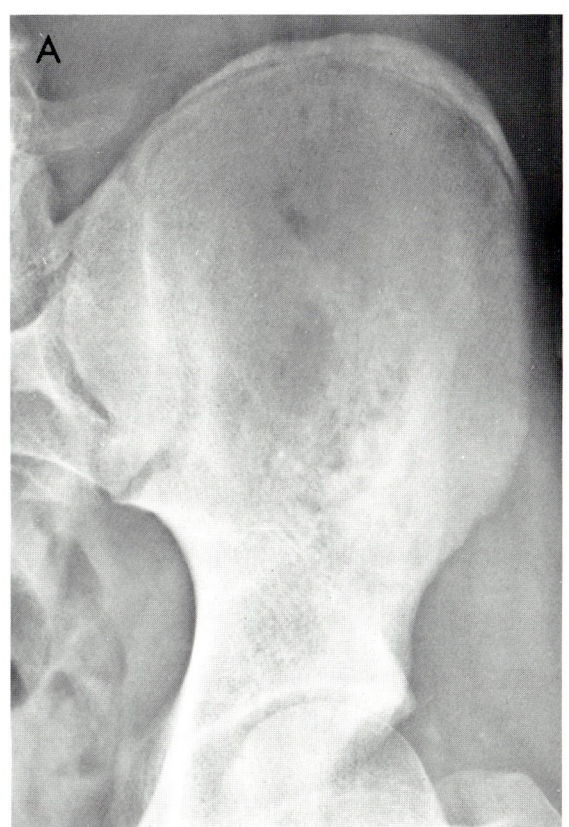
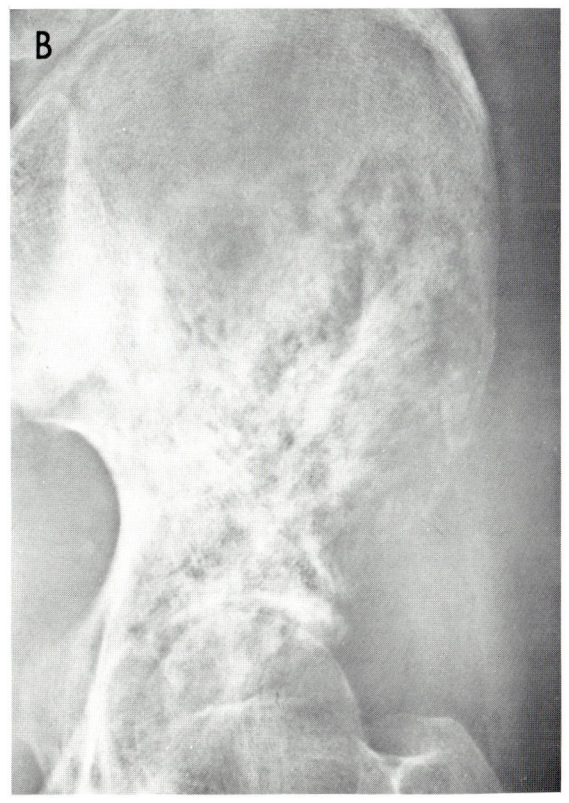

Figure 162 · Reticulum Cell Sarcoma / 381

Figure 163.—Reticulum cell sarcoma of the tibia.

AFIP Case No. 964210: **A,** anteroposterior, and **B,** lateral views.

DIAGNOSIS AND GRADE.—Reticulum cell sarcoma, tibia; growth rate IC.

LIFE INFORMATION.—Female, 74 years; survival unknown.

LOCATION.—A circumscribed tumor arising eccentrically in the upper third of the proximal metaphysis, extending into the epiphysis and subarticular cortex.

SIZE.—8 × 6 cm.

MINERALIZATION OF TUMOR.—None.

DESTRUCTION.—Geographic; total penetration of the cortex posteriorly (**B, b**), involving subarticular cortex; contour lobulated.

PROLIFERATION.—Faint mottling in intramedullary spongy bone (**A, a**); slight septation; no periosteal response.

DIFFERENTIAL DIAGNOSIS	PROBABILITY
Fibrosarcoma	.99
Osteosarcoma	.01

COMMENT: Radiologically this could pass for primary fibrosarcoma. The computer agrees.

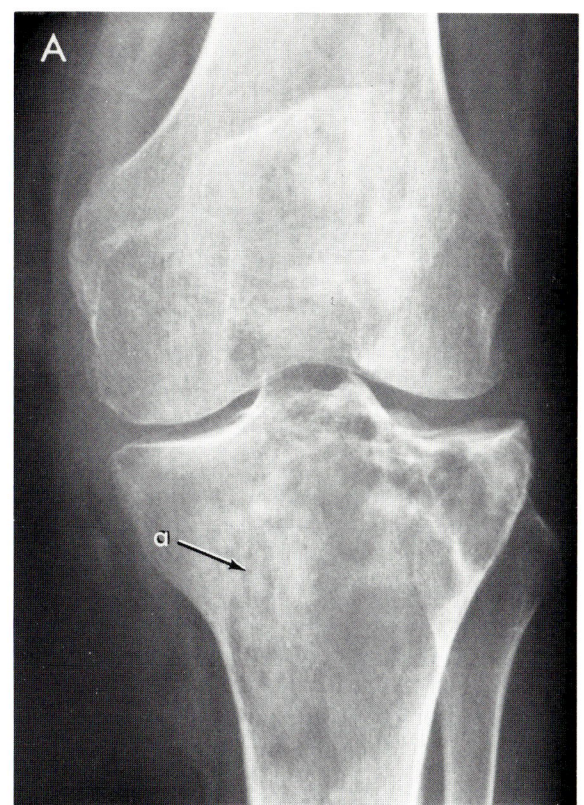
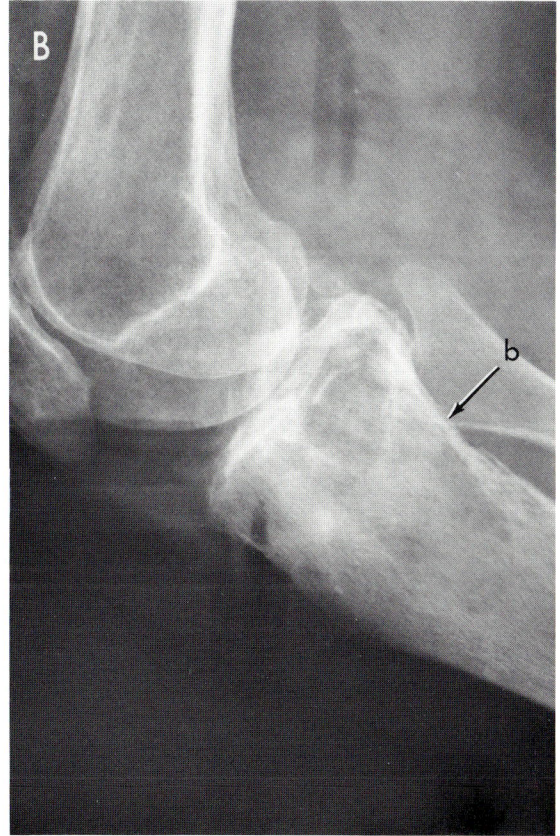

Figure 163 · Reticulum Cell Sarcoma / 383

Figure 164.—Reticulum cell sarcoma of the tibia.

AFIP Case No. 1149932: **A,** anteroposterior, and **B,** lateral views.

DIAGNOSIS AND GRADE.—Reticulum cell sarcoma, tibia; growth rate IC.
LIFE INFORMATION.—Male, 26 years; well three years after therapy.
LOCATION.—A circumscribed lesion centered eccentrically in the proximal metaphysis, extending down to the shaft.
SIZE.—5 × 3 × 2.5 cm.
MINERALIZATION OF TUMOR.—None.
DESTRUCTION.—Geographic; regular contour.
PROLIFERATION.—Faint marginal sclerosis; amorphous periosteal response laterally, except over center of lesion (**A, a**).

DIFFERENTIAL DIAGNOSIS	PROBABILITY
Nonossifying fibroma	.80
Fibrosarcoma	.13
Chondromyxoid fibroma	.04
Cyst	< .01
Villonodular synovitis	< .01
Chondrosarcoma	< .01
Cartilaginous tumor	< .01

COMMENT: Nothing here suggests reticulum cell sarcoma since most such tumors show rapid growth. Radiologically it suggests a fibrous or cystic lesion, the computer agreeing.

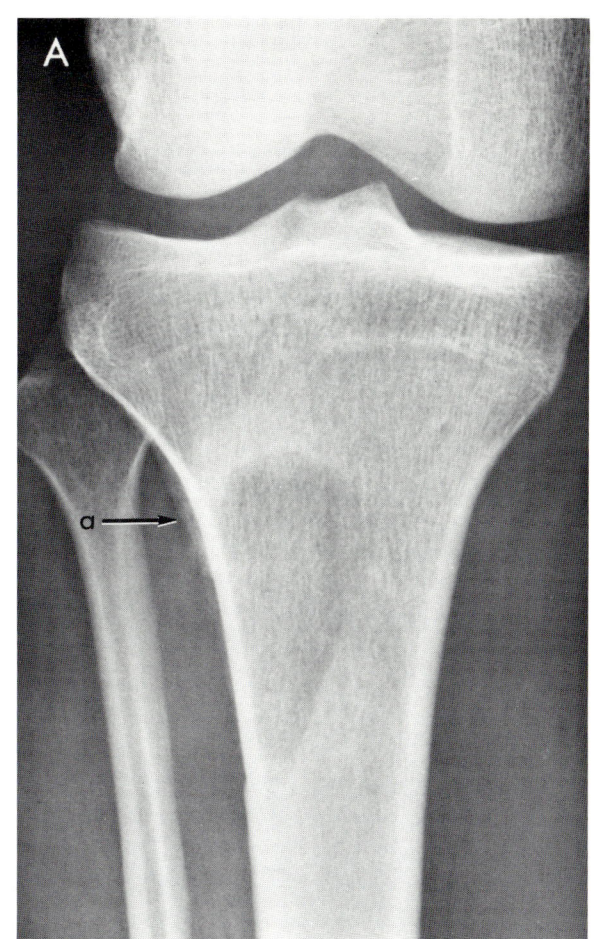
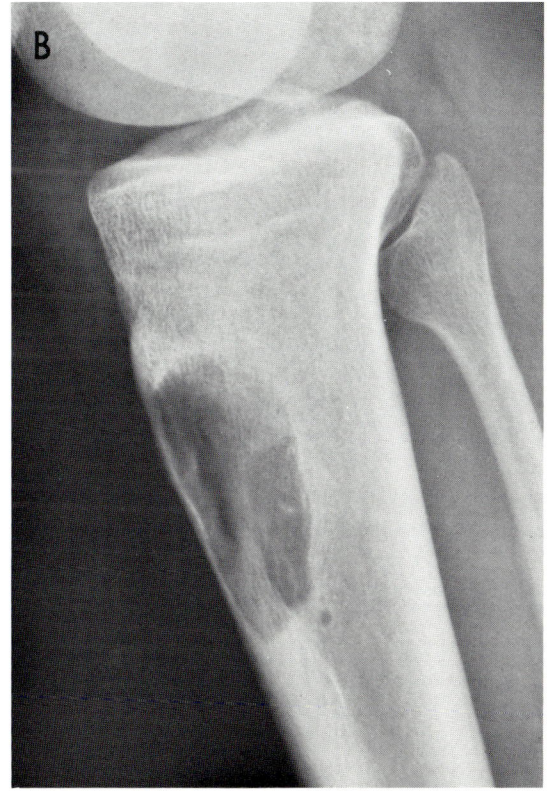

Figure 164 · Reticulum Cell Sarcoma / 385

Figure 165.—Myeloma of the skull.

AFIP Case No. 1121118: Lateral tangential projection.

DIAGNOSIS AND GRADE.—Myeloma, skull; growth rate IC.
LIFE INFORMATION.—Female, 53 years; survived 21 months.
LOCATION.—A large circumscribed lesion in the apex of the calvarium.

SIZE.—8 × 6 cm.
MINERALIZATION OF TUMOR.—None.
DESTRUCTION.—Geographic; regular margin.
PROLIFERATION.—None.

DIFFERENTIAL DIAGNOSIS	PROBABILITY
Myeloma	.94
Fibrosarcoma	.04
Chondrosarcoma	.01

COMMENT: A nonspecific pattern of bone destruction reflecting moderate growth rate.

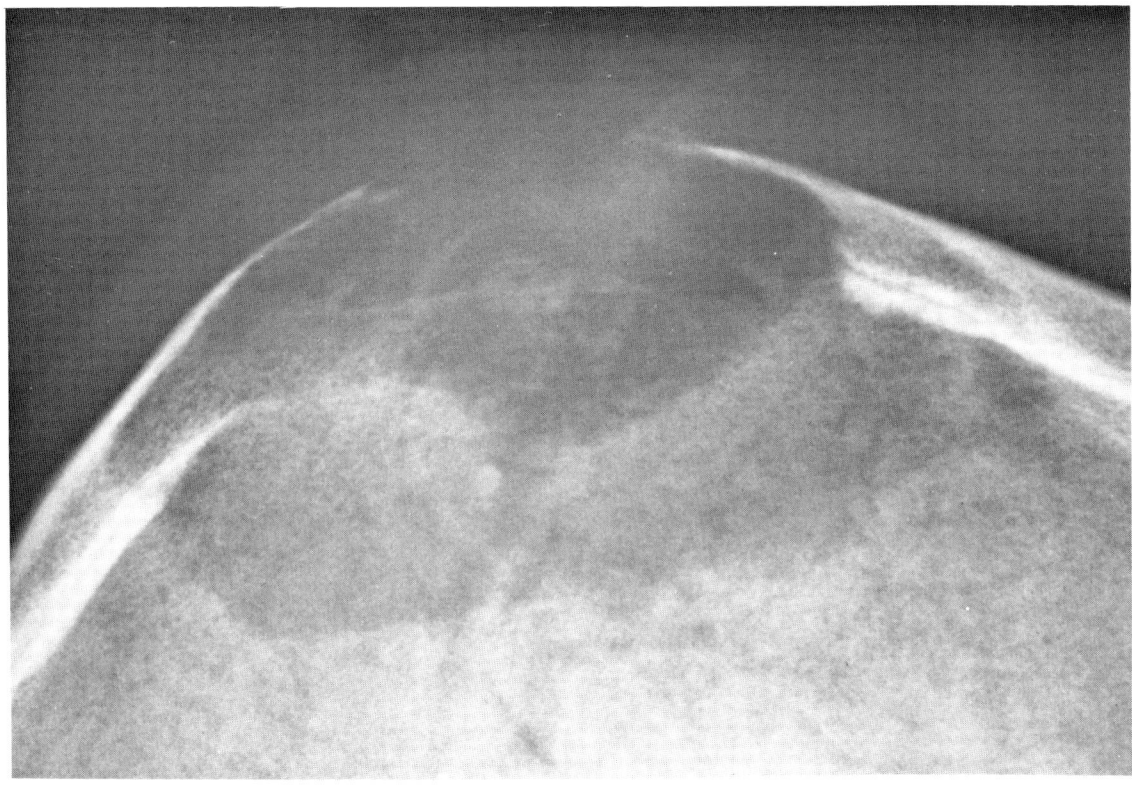

Figure 165 · Myeloma of Skull

Figure 166.—Solitary myeloma of the pelvis.

AFIP Case No. 866032: Anteroposterior projection.

DIAGNOSIS AND GRADE.—Solitary myeloma, pelvis; growth rate IC.

LIFE INFORMATION.—Male, 62 years; survival unknown.

LOCATION.—A large circumscribed lesion involving the medial three-fourths of the ilium.

SIZE.—16 × 8 cm.

MINERALIZATION OF TUMOR.—None.

DESTRUCTION.—Geographic; ragged contour.

PROLIFERATION.—Suggestion of slight sclerosis around edge of destroyed area; unusual petallike configuration of lateral margin.

DIFFERENTIAL DIAGNOSIS	PROBABILITY
Myeloma	.90
Chondrosarcoma	.07
Chondromyxoid fibroma	< .01
Cyst	< .01
Fibrosarcoma	< .01

COMMENT: A fairly typical solitary myeloma. The radiographic pattern rarely suggests a growth rate more rapid than this.

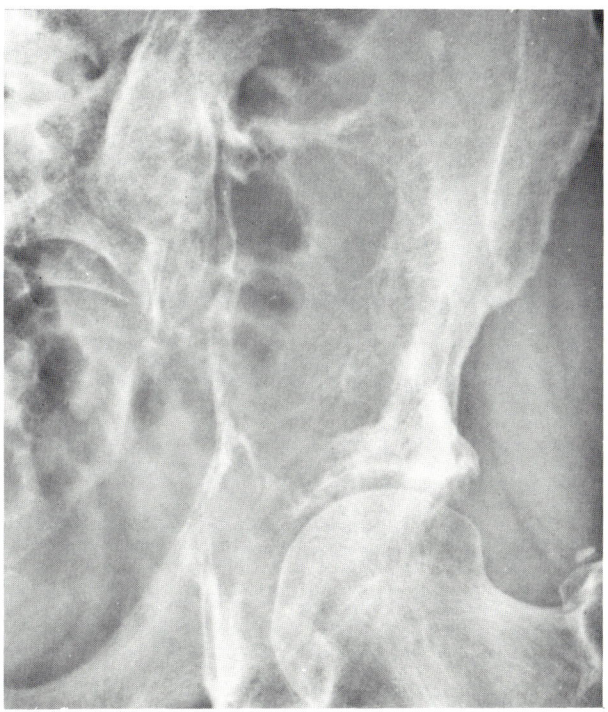

Figure 167.—Solitary myeloma of the femur.

AFIP Case No. 1067267: Anteroposterior projection.

DIAGNOSIS AND GRADE.—Solitary myeloma, femur; growth rate IB.

LIFE INFORMATION.—Male, 60 years; well five years later.

LOCATION.—A circumscribed lesion at junction of proximal shaft and metaphysis.

SIZE.—7 × 3.5 cm.

MINERALIZATION OF TUMOR.—None.

DESTRUCTION.—Geographic; lobulated contour.

PROLIFERATION.—None.

Differential Diagnosis	Probability
Myeloma	.54
Fibrosarcoma	.38
Chondrosarcoma	.04
Cartilaginous tumor	.02
Nonossifying fibroma	< .01
Chondromyxoid fibroma	< .01
Hemangio-, angiosarcoma	< .01
Cyst	< .01

COMMENT: A typical myeloma that has not penetrated the cortex. It does not have the sclerotic rim of growth rate IA.

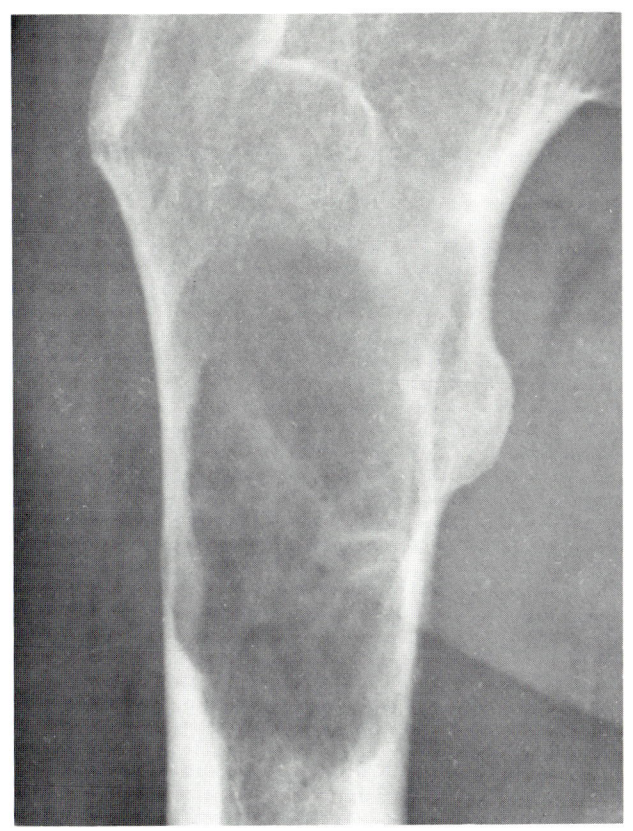

Figure 167 · Myeloma of Femur / 389

Figure 168.—Angioendothelial tumor of the humerus.

AFIP Case No. 1161437: Anteroposterior projection.

DIAGNOSIS AND GRADE.—Angioendothelial tumor, humerus; growth rate II.

LIFE INFORMATION.—Male, 41 years; survival unknown.

LOCATION.—A circumscribed lesion located centrally at the junction of the shaft and proximal metaphysis, extending to involve the entire metaphysis to the middle third of the shaft.

SIZE.—11 × 5 cm.

MINERALIZATION OF TUMOR.—None.

DESTRUCTION.—Upper half of the tumor, clearly geographic pattern; lower half basically moth-eaten, with total penetration of cortex medially and laterally.

PROLIFERATION.—Smooth expansion of the cortex around the proximal half of the tumor, with coarse septate pattern; sunburst pattern of spiculation medially, where the tumor breaks through the cortex.

DIFFERENTIAL DIAGNOSIS	PROBABILITY
Hemangio-, angiosarcoma	.90
Chondrosarcoma	.04
Osteosarcoma	.02
Fibrosarcoma	.02

COMMENT: This case seems to reflect an aggressive change of character in the lower half of a tumor which is quite encapsulated in its upper half.

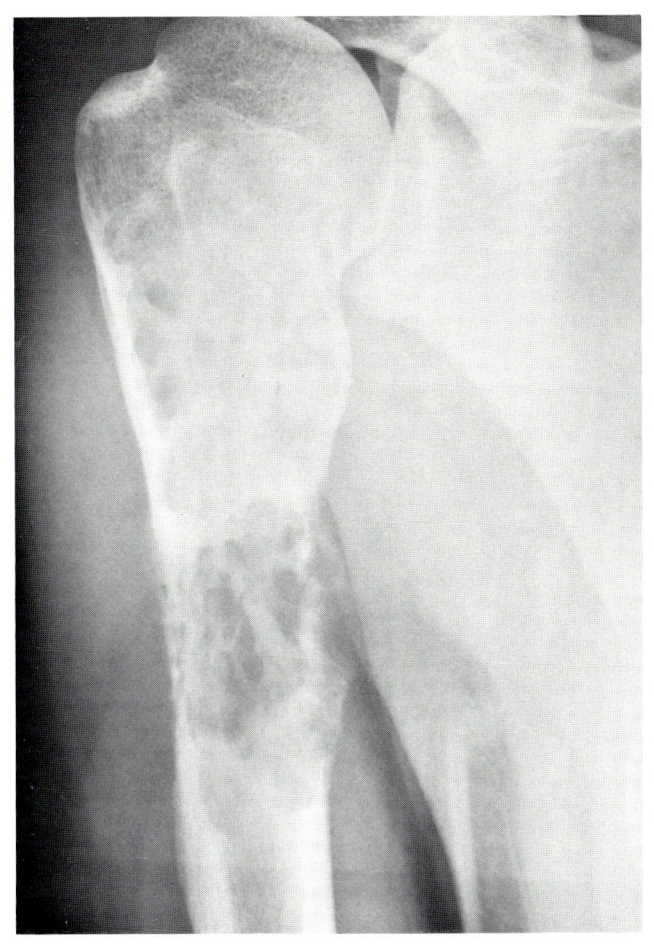

Figure 168 · Angioendothelial Tumor / 391

Figure 169.—Angiosarcoma of the humerus.

AFIP Case No. 993910: Anteroposterior views—**A,** initial study; **B,** six months later.

DIAGNOSIS AND GRADE.—Angiosarcoma, humerus; growth rate III.

LIFE INFORMATION.—Male, 17 years; survived 34 months after onset.

LOCATION.—A diffuse lesion centered on the junction of the shaft and proximal metaphysis, extending into the epiphysis and down into the shaft; large extraosseous component.

SIZE.—15 × 10 cm.

MINERALIZATION OF TUMOR.—Multiple small lumps of what appear to be cloudy tumor matrix mineralization scattered throughout the intramedullary portion; extraosseous component is radiolucent.

DESTRUCTION.—Permeative; pathologic fracture.

PROLIFERATION.—Multilaminated periosteal response.

	DIFFERENTIAL DIAGNOSIS	PROBABILITY
Exam. 1	Reticulum cell sarcoma	.69
	Ewing's sarcoma	.28
	Osteosarcoma	.01
	Fibrosarcoma	< .01
Exam. 2	Hemangio-, angiosarcoma	.90
	Fibrosarcoma	.04
	Chondrosarcoma	.04
	Cyst	.01
	Giant cell tumor	< .01
	Chondromyxoid fibroma	< .01

COMMENT: In **A,** made about two months after onset, there is already a degree of periosteal consolidation and blunting of destructive pattern which suggests a radiation effect. At six months (**B**) complete encapsulation and healing of the pathologic fracture have occurred.

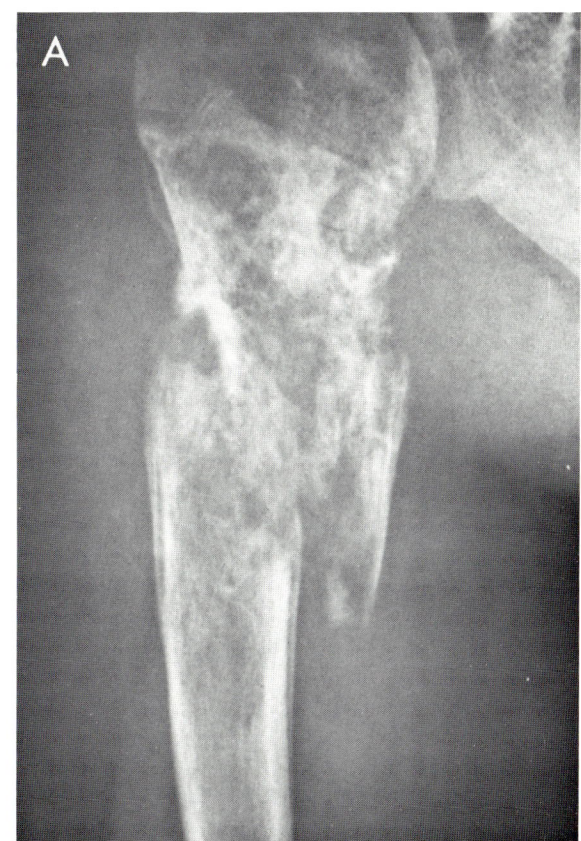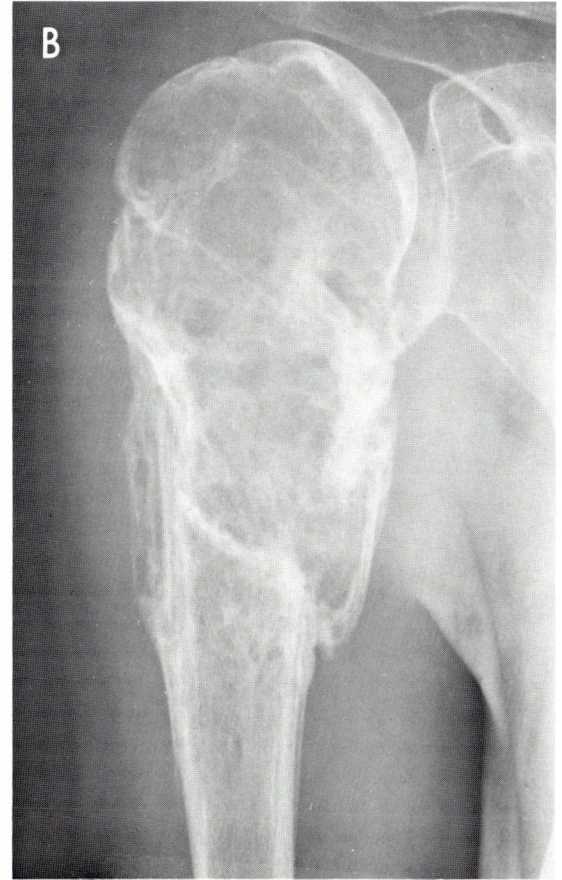

Figure 169 · Angiosarcoma of Humerus / 393

Figure 170.—Angiosarcoma of the fibula.

AFIP Case No. 1059558: **A,** anteroposterior, and **B,** lateral views.

DIAGNOSIS AND GRADE.—Angiosarcoma, fibula; growth rate IC.

LIFE INFORMATION.—Male, 27 years; well five years after onset.

LOCATION.—A circumscribed lesion centered on the cortex of the proximal metaphysis, with a soft tissue component (**B, x**) about the size of the intraosseous portion.

SIZE.—4 × 3 × 2 cm.

MINERALIZATION OF TUMOR.—None.

DESTRUCTION.—Geographic; regular contour; total penetration of cortex.

PROLIFERATION.—Dense marginal sclerosis; two buttresses at lower edge of the tumor; suggestion of a component of expanded cortex which does not encapsulate the tumor.

DIFFERENTIAL DIAGNOSIS	PROBABILITY
Cyst	.43
Fibrosarcoma	.27
Cartilaginous tumor	.11
Chondromyxoid fibroma	.06
Myeloma	.06

COMMENT: In this tumor of slow rate of growth I see nothing which points to angiosarcoma as the best diagnosis.

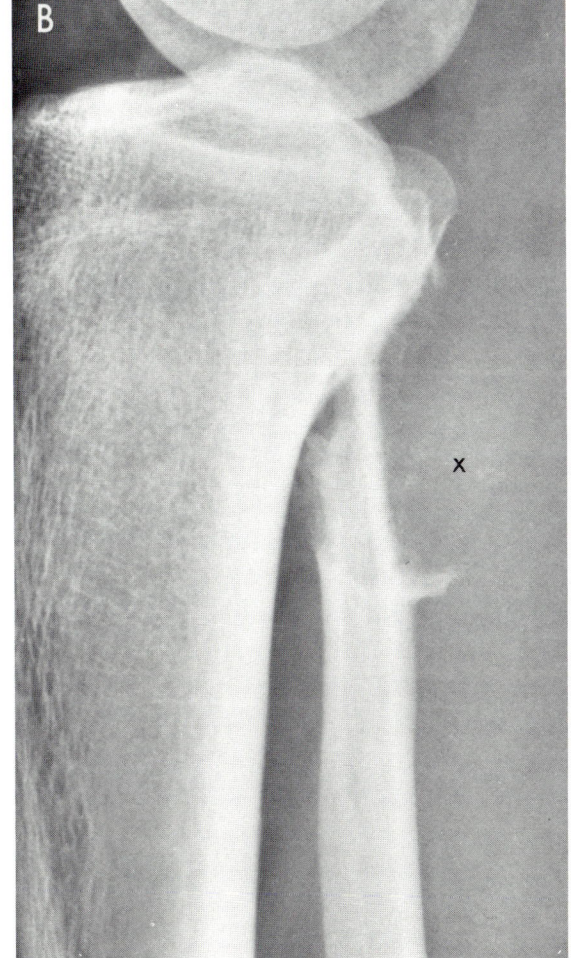

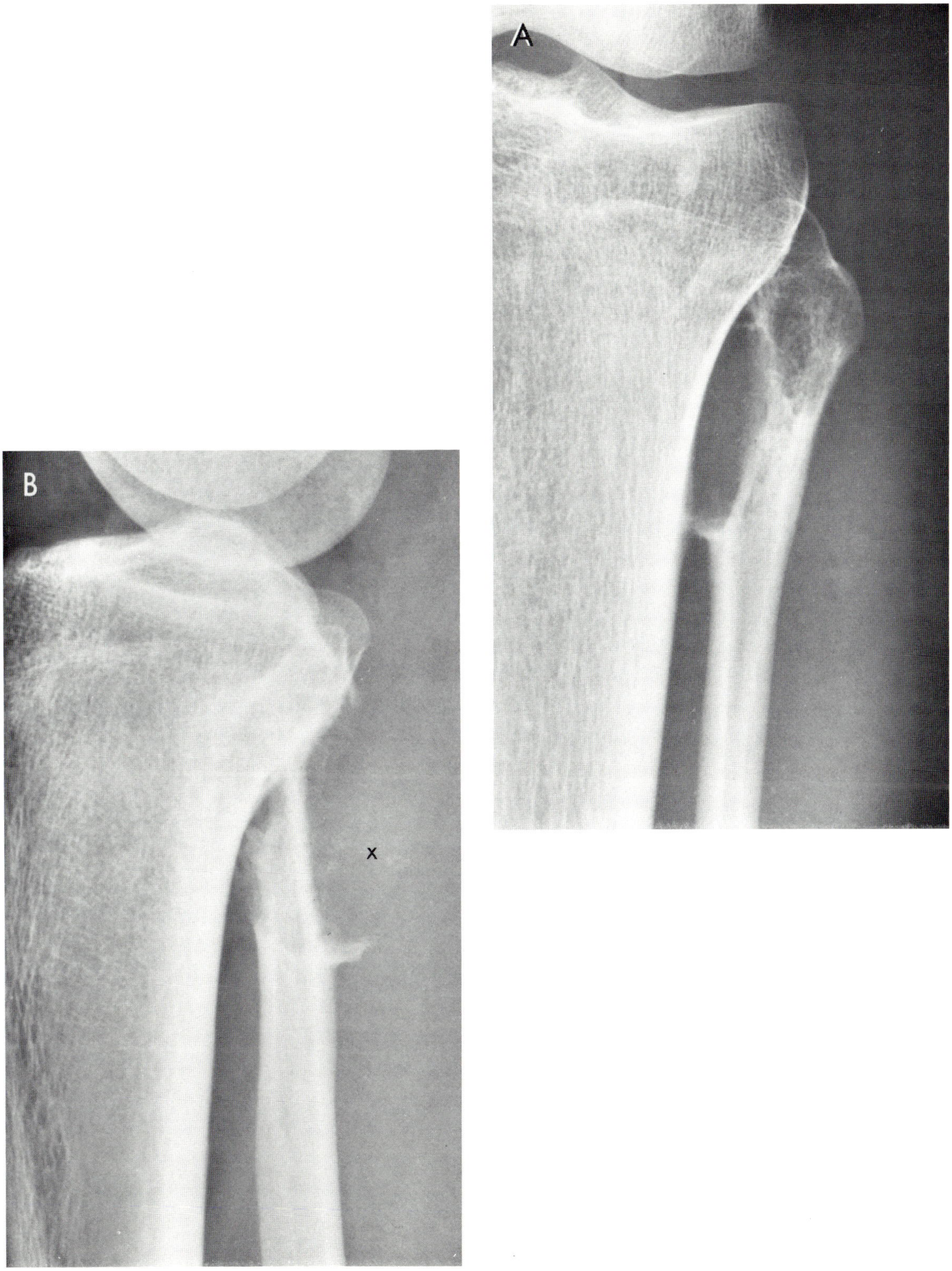

Figure 170 · Angiosarcoma of Fibula / 395

Figure 171.—Ossifying hemangiomas of the fibula and finger.

AFIP Case No. 1154127: **A,** anteroposterior, and **B,** lateral views.

DIAGNOSIS AND GRADE.—Ossifying hemangioma, fibula; growth rate IC.
LIFE INFORMATION.—Male, 5 years; survival unknown.
LOCATION.—A circumscribed lesion centered in the distal metaphysis; loss of density in the adjacent epiphysis, perhaps due to reflex hyperemia.

SIZE.—2 × 1 cm × 8 mm.
MINERALIZATION OF TUMOR.—None.
DESTRUCTION.—Geographic; regular margin (**arrows**).
PROLIFERATION.—Faint marginal sclerosis.

DIFFERENTIAL DIAGNOSIS	PROBABILITY
Chondromyxoid fibroma	.89
Osteoblastoma	.05
Cartilaginous tumor	.04
Giant cell tumor	< .01

COMMENT: A very difficult lesion to evaluate.

AFIP Case No. 1221607: **C,** posteroanterior projection.

DIAGNOSIS AND GRADE.—Ossifying hemangioma, finger; growth rate IC.
LIFE INFORMATION.—Male, 47 years; last known to be well.
LOCATION.—A parosteal soft tissue lesion medial to the proximal phalanx.

SIZE.—1.8 × 1 cm.
MINERALIZATION OF TUMOR.—None.
DESTRUCTION.—Smooth geographic saucerization of underlying cortex (**arrow**).
PROLIFERATION.—None.

DIFFERENTIAL DIAGNOSIS	PROBABILITY
Myositis ossificans	.99
Chondrosarcoma	< .01

COMMENT: This tumor is reminiscent of myositis ossificans in the hand, particularly that in Figure 125, *A* and *B*.

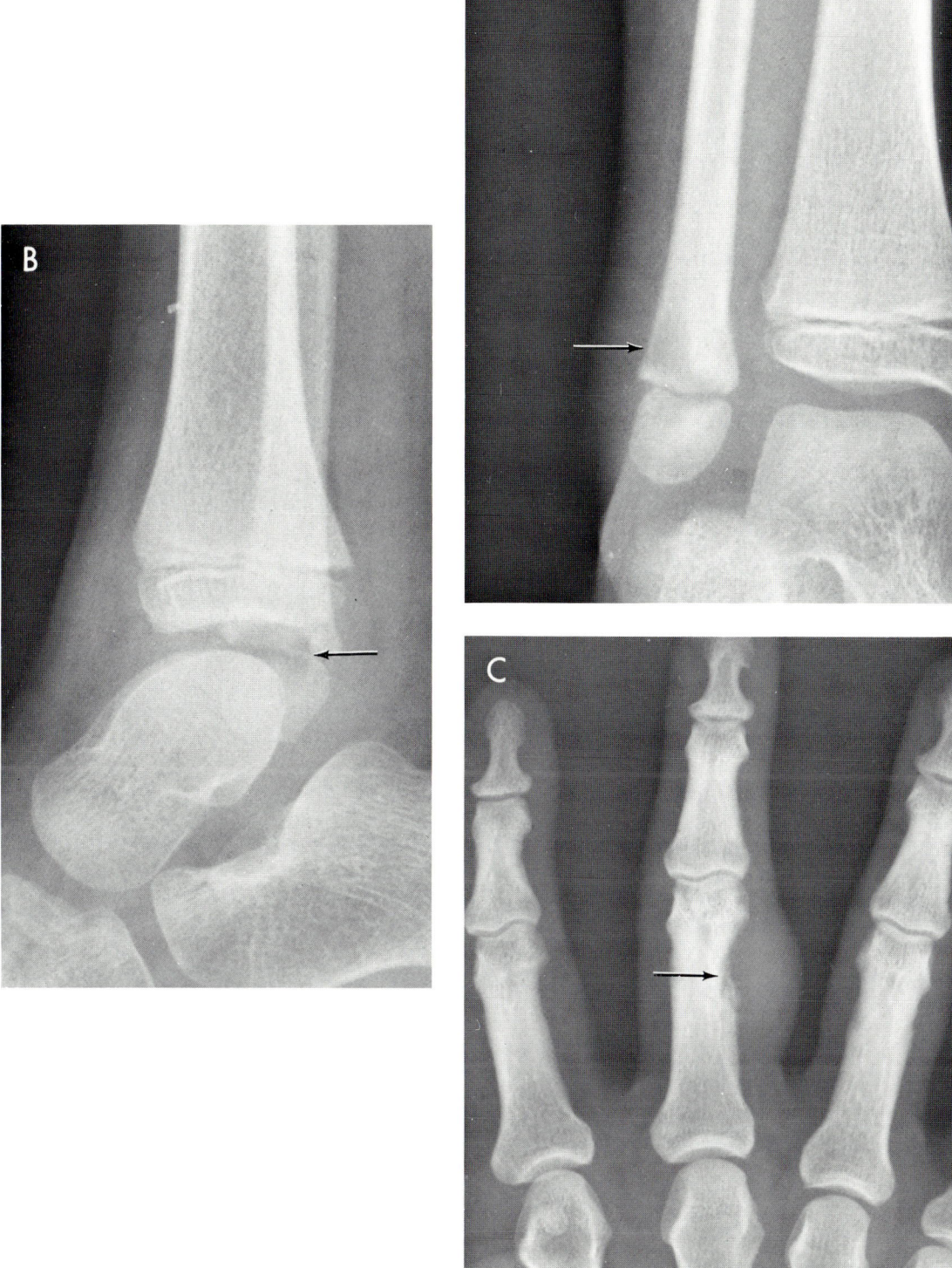

Figure 171 · Ossifying Hemangiomas / 397

Figure 172.—Angioendothelial tumor of the ilium.

AFIP Case No. 1195234: Anteroposterior projection.

DIAGNOSIS AND GRADE.—Angioendothelial tumor, ilium; growth rate IA.

LIFE INFORMATION.—Female, 55 years; symptoms for seven years before diagnosis; last known to be well.

LOCATION.—A circumscribed lesion in the upper lateral iliac crest.

SIZE.—4 × 3 cm.

MINERALIZATION OF TUMOR.—None definite.

DESTRUCTION.—Geographic; lobulated contour.

PROLIFERATION.—Dense sclerotic rim (**arrow**); honeycomb septal pattern.

DIFFERENTIAL DIAGNOSIS	PROBABILITY
Chondromyxoid fibroma	.67
Chondrosarcoma	.11
Myeloma	.07
Fibrosarcoma	.05
Cyst	.04
Cartilaginous tumor	.03

COMMENT: The lesion seems encapsulated and is quite small despite the long history. The unusual honeycomb pattern may reflect a vascular tumor. A bit more sophistication is needed for computer diagnosis.

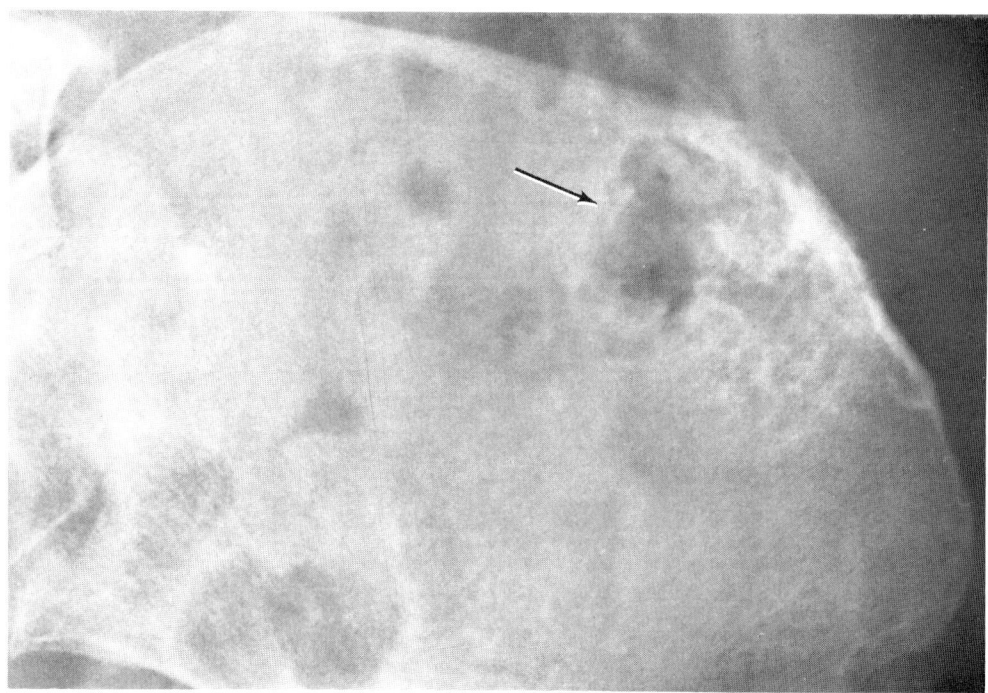

Figure 173.—Angioma of the lumbar spine.

AFIP Case No. 1117951: Lateral projection.

DIAGNOSIS AND GRADE.—Angioma, lumbar spine; not graded.
LIFE INFORMATION.—Female, 9 years; last known to be well.
LOCATION.—A circumscribed lesion in the dorsal process of L2.
SIZE.—4 × 4 cm.
MINERALIZATION OF TUMOR.—Ossified edge (**arrows**); cloudy areas of increased density.
DESTRUCTION.—The dorsal process is destroyed, perhaps moth-eaten, although the appearance may result from a combination of geographic distribution and honeycomb proliferation.
PROLIFERATION.—Ossified edge at the tumor margin, believed to represent a residual expanded shell of proliferative bone. Honeycomb pattern?

DIFFERENTIAL DIAGNOSIS	PROBABILITY
Osteoblastoma	.61
Fibrosarcoma	.38
Chondrosarcoma	< .01

COMMENT: An unusual lesion in a site where it is almost impossible to tell what is happening. The original structure may be replaced by reactive bone. I cannot account for the cloudy areas.

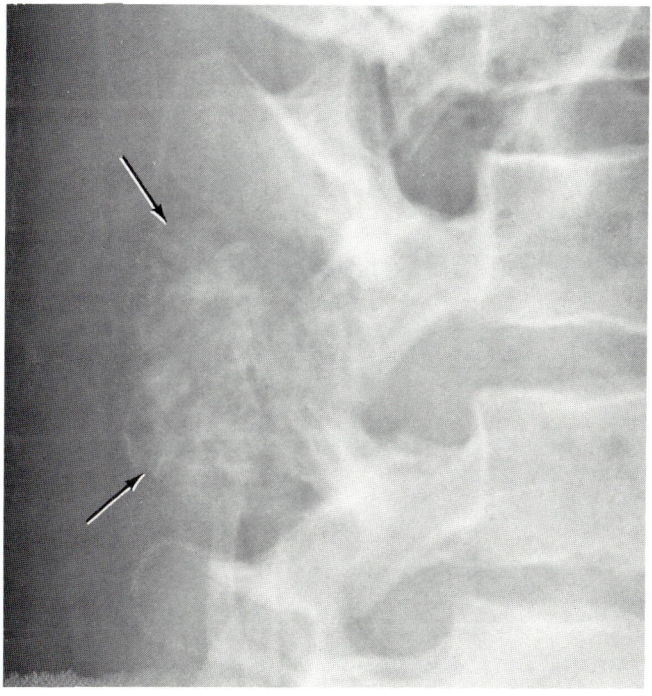

Figure 173 · Angioma of Spine

PART 7

Tumors of the Joints and Soft Tissues

Figure 174.—Villonodular synovitis of the knee and toe.

AFIP Case No. 1048447: **A,** anteroposterior projection.

DIAGNOSIS AND GRADE.—Villonodular synovitis, knee; growth rate IC.
LIFE INFORMATION.—Male, 47 years; well seven years later.
LOCATION.—Circumscribed involvement of distal femur, proximal tibia and fibula; massive involvement of knee joint and periarticular soft tissues.

SIZE.—4 × 4 cm medial tibia; 4 × 4 cm lateral tibia; 3 × 3 cm fibula.
MINERALIZATION OF TUMOR.—None.
DESTRUCTION.—Multiple areas of geographic destruction; lobulated contours.
PROLIFERATION.—Dense marginal sclerosis around areas of destruction; slight expansion of cortex in the head of the fibula.

DIFFERENTIAL DIAGNOSIS	PROBABILITY
Villonodular synovitis	100

COMMENT: Typical villonodular synovitis in bone, with multiple involvement of bones on both sides of a joint and the large nodular soft tissue mass (**x**) strongly supporting the diagnosis. There should be a break in the cortex in some projection for each lesion.

AFIP Case No. 1003495: **B,** anteroposterior projection.

DIAGNOSIS AND GRADE.—Villonodular synovitis, toe; growth rate IC.
LIFE INFORMATION.—Male, 56 years; last known to be well.
LOCATION.—Involvement of the distal two segments of the great toe immediately adjacent to the distal interphalangeal joint; soft tissue mass (**x**) medial to the bone lesion.

SIZE.—Combined size 3 × 1.5 cm.
MINERALIZATION OF TUMOR.—None.
DESTRUCTION.—One geographic area in each bone; lobulated contour.
PROLIFERATION.—Marginal sclerosis; slight expansion; septation.

DIFFERENTIAL DIAGNOSIS	PROBABILITY
Villonodular synovitis	100

COMMENT: A typical case.

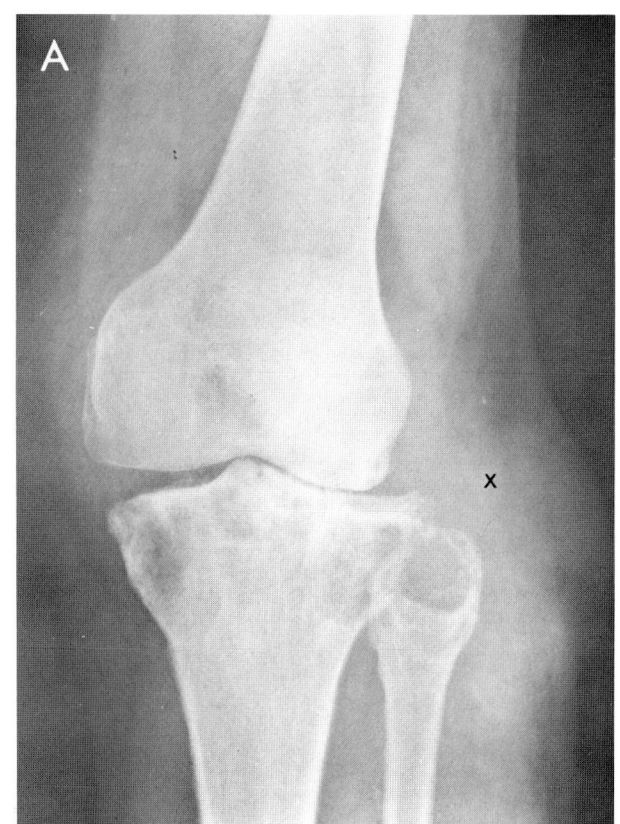
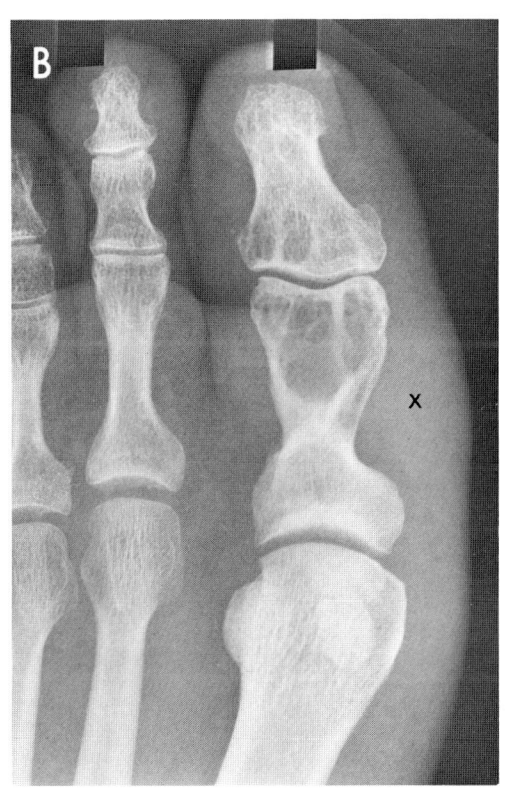

Figure 174 · Villonodular Synovitis / 403

Figure 175.—Villonodular synovitis of the femur.

AFIP Case No. 986518: Anteroposterior projection.

DIAGNOSIS AND GRADE.—Villonodular synovitis, femur; growth rate IC.
LIFE INFORMATION.—Female, 42 years; well five years later.
LOCATION.—A sharply circumscribed lesion in the superior neck.

SIZE.—3 × 3 cm.
MINERALIZATION OF TUMOR.—None.
DESTRUCTION.—Geographic: lobular outline.
PROLIFERATION.—Narrow marginal sclerosis.

DIFFERENTIAL DIAGNOSIS	PROBABILITY
Benign cartilaginous tumor	.49
Myeloma	.32
Chondromyxoid fibroma	.07
Villonodular synovitis	.05
Fibrosarcoma	.04
Chondrosarcoma	< .01
Cyst	< .01
Osteosarcoma	< .01

COMMENT: The location around the base of the neck is fairly typical of villonodular synovitis in the hip.

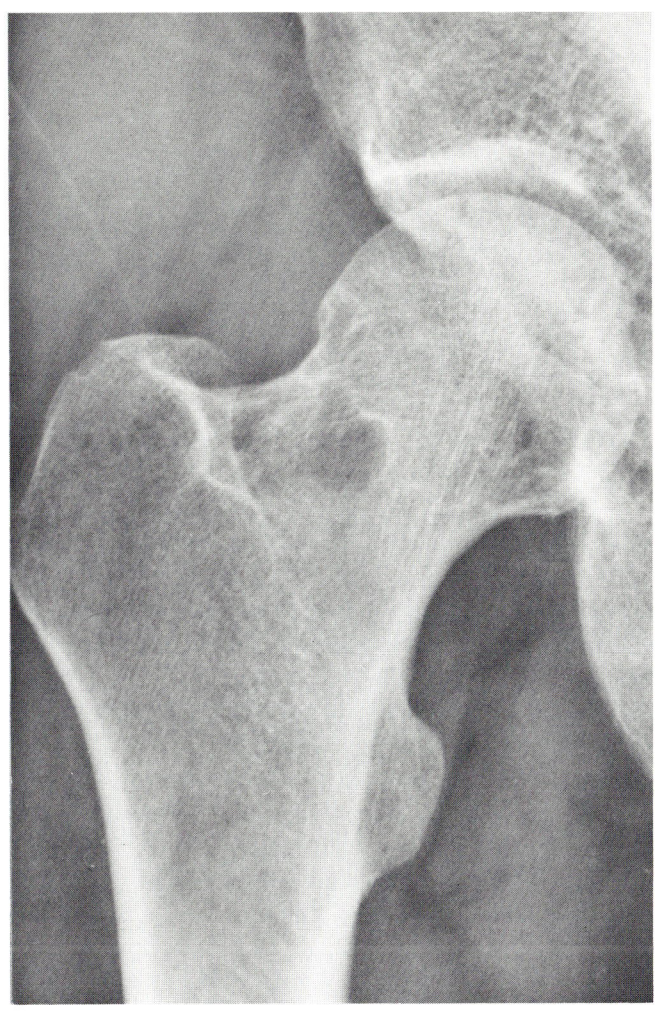

Figure 175 · Villonodular Synovitis / 405

Figure 176.—Synovial osteochondromatosis and synovial osteosarcoma of the knee.

AFIP Case No. 1173903: **A,** lateral projection.

DIAGNOSIS AND GRADE.—Synovial osteochondromatosis, knee; ungraded.
LIFE INFORMATION.—Male, 28 years; well 13 years after onset.
LOCATION.—Oval and round calcific opacities in distended knee joint.

SIZE.—The largest body 4 cm long.
MINERALIZATION OF TUMOR.—Opacities have a structured appearance, with cortex, concentric rings of mineral and more radiolucent central area.
DESTRUCTION.—None.
PROLIFERATION.—None.

DIFFERENTIAL DIAGNOSIS	PROBABILITY
Osteochondroma	.99
Osteosarcoma	< .01

COMMENT: Typical synovial osteochondromatosis.

AFIP Case No. 1094632: **B,** lateral projection.

DIAGNOSIS AND GRADE.—Synovial osteosarcoma, knee; ungraded.
LIFE INFORMATION.—Female, 39 years; last known to be well.
LOCATION.—A large ill-defined lesion in the anterior joint between the patella and the anterior tibial tubercle.

SIZE.—6 × 3 cm.
MINERALIZATION OF TUMOR.—In the center, an irregular contiguous area of matrix mineralization surrounded by a soft tissue halo.
DESTRUCTION.—None.
PROLIFERATION.—None.

DIFFERENTIAL DIAGNOSIS	PROBABILITY
Osteochondroma	.98
Osteosarcoma	.01

COMMENT: This rare lesion is characterized by bone formation centrally. It is much less well organized than the usual synovial osteochondroma, a clue to its malignant status.

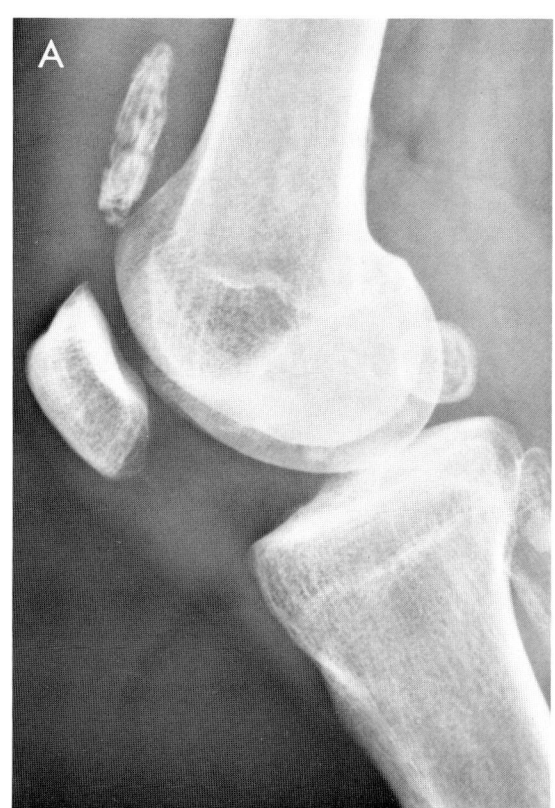
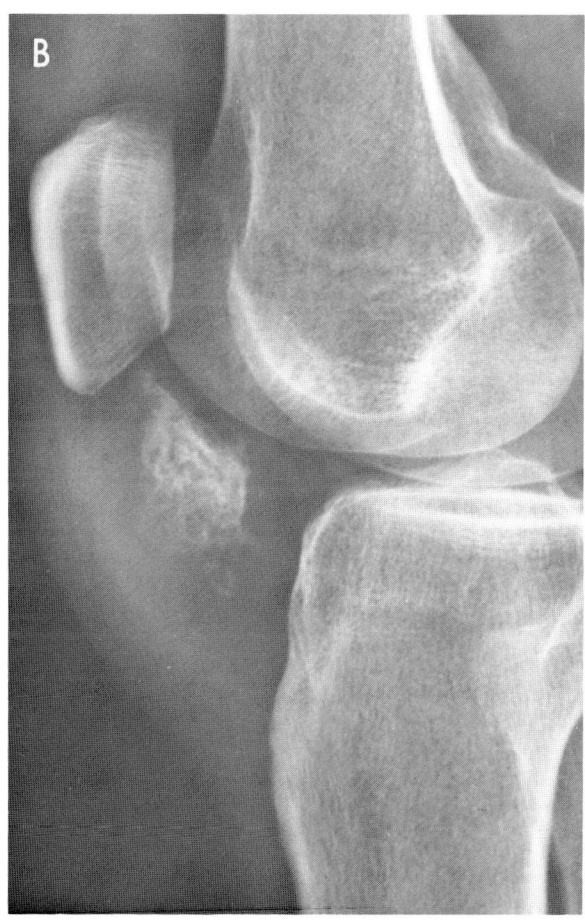

Figure 176 · Osteochondromatosis & Osteosarcoma

Figure 177.—Synovial chondrosarcomas of fingers.

AFIP Case No. 1139304: **A,** posteroanterior projection.

DIAGNOSIS AND GRADE.—Synovial chondrosarcoma, finger; ungraded.
LIFE INFORMATION.—Male, 22 years; last known to be well.
LOCATION.—An ill-defined soft tissue mass surrounding the metacarpophalangeal articulation of the middle finger.
SIZE.—3 × 3 cm.
MINERALIZATION OF TUMOR.—Floccules throughout the mass.
DESTRUCTION.—Irregular geographic erosion of lateral articular cortex of the middle metacarpal (**arrow**).
PROLIFERATION.—None.

DIFFERENTIAL DIAGNOSIS	PROBABILITY
Chondrosarcoma	.88
Benign cartilaginous tumor	.11

COMMENT: A typical synovial chondrosarcoma of a joint.

AFIP Case No. 1159465: **B,** oblique projection.

DIAGNOSIS AND GRADE.—Synovial chondrosarcoma, finger; ungraded.
LIFE INFORMATION.—Male, 44 years; well four years later.
LOCATION.—An ill-defined mass involving the distal two segments of the little finger.
SIZE.—3.5 × 2.5 × 2.5 cm.
MINERALIZATION OF TUMOR.—Multiple floccules of calcified tumor matrix throughout the soft tissue lesion.
DESTRUCTION.—None.
PROLIFERATION.—An amorphous periosteal response in bone adjacent to the tumor.

DIFFERENTIAL DIAGNOSIS	PROBABILITY
Chondrosarcoma of mesenchymal or synovial origin	.99
Osteosarcoma	< .01

COMMENT: The tumor centers on the distal interphalangeal articulation, a strong clue to its origin.

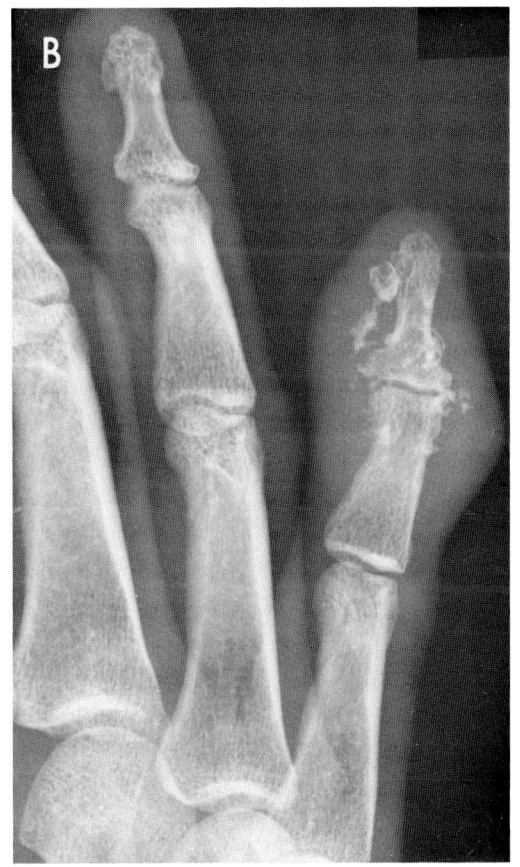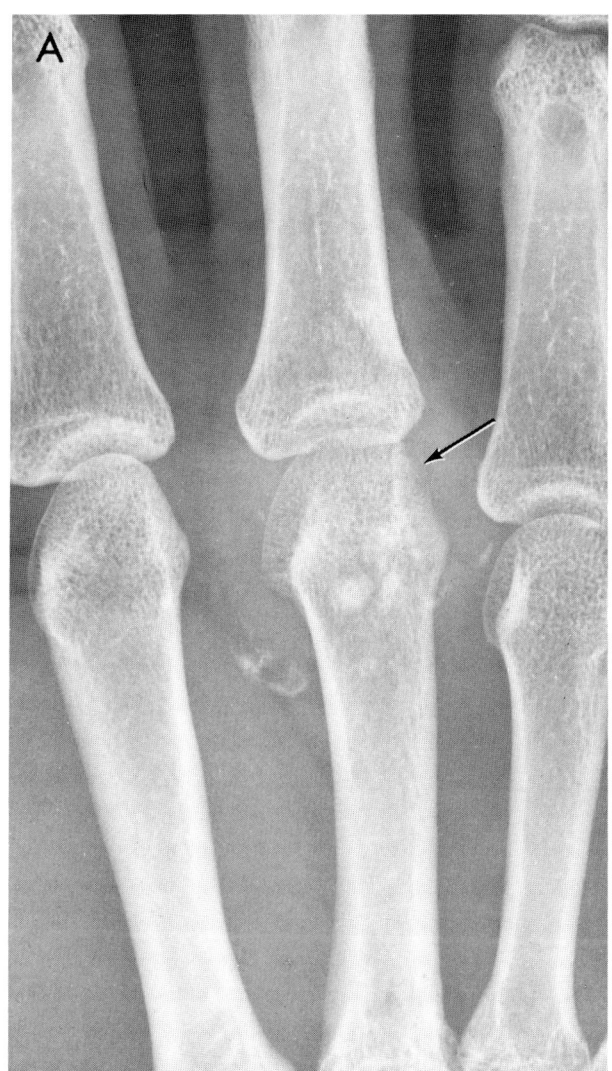

Figure 177 · Synovial Chondrosarcomas / 409

Figure 178.—Synovial sarcoma of the foot; vertebral synovioma.

AFIP Case No. 1220441: **A,** oblique projection.

DIAGNOSIS AND GRADE.—Synovial sarcoma, foot; ungraded.
LIFE INFORMATION.—Female, 15 years; lived 26 months after onset.
LOCATION.—An ill-defined soft tissue tumor between the first and second metatarsals.

SIZE.—7 × 4 cm.
MINERALIZATION OF TUMOR.—None.
DESTRUCTION.—Localized smooth erosion of opposing surfaces of the first and second metatarsals (**arrows**), apparently due to external pressure from the tumor.
PROLIFERATION.—None.

DIFFERENTIAL DIAGNOSIS	PROBABILITY
Synovial sarcoma	.79
Sarcoma	.19
Myositis ossificans	.01
Fibrosarcoma	.01

COMMENT: The tumor must have grown very slowly to have produced the smooth erosion accompanied by reconstruction of underlying cortex.

AFIP Case No. 910828: **B,** anteroposterior projection.

DIAGNOSIS AND GRADE.—Synovioma, T12 and rib; growth rate III.
LIFE INFORMATION.—Female, 54 years; lived 15 months.
LOCATION.—Lesion of the body and pedicles of T12 and adjacent rib.

SIZE.—7 × 2.5 cm.
MINERALIZATION OF TUMOR.—None.
DESTRUCTION.—Ill-defined permeative pattern; penetration of cortex.
PROLIFERATION.—Mottled focal areas of increased density.

DIFFERENTIAL DIAGNOSIS	PROBABILITY
Reticulum cell sarcoma	.98
Fibrosarcoma	.01
Hemangio-, angiosarcoma	< .01

COMMENT: Bone destruction is believed to be permeative because, despite extensive bone loss, the vertebral cortex is fairly visible. Clearly the pedicles are gone.

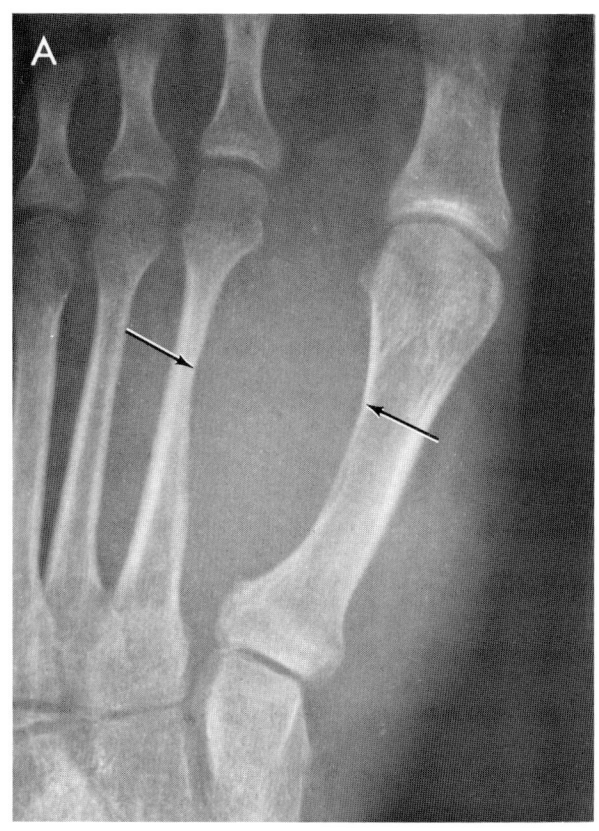
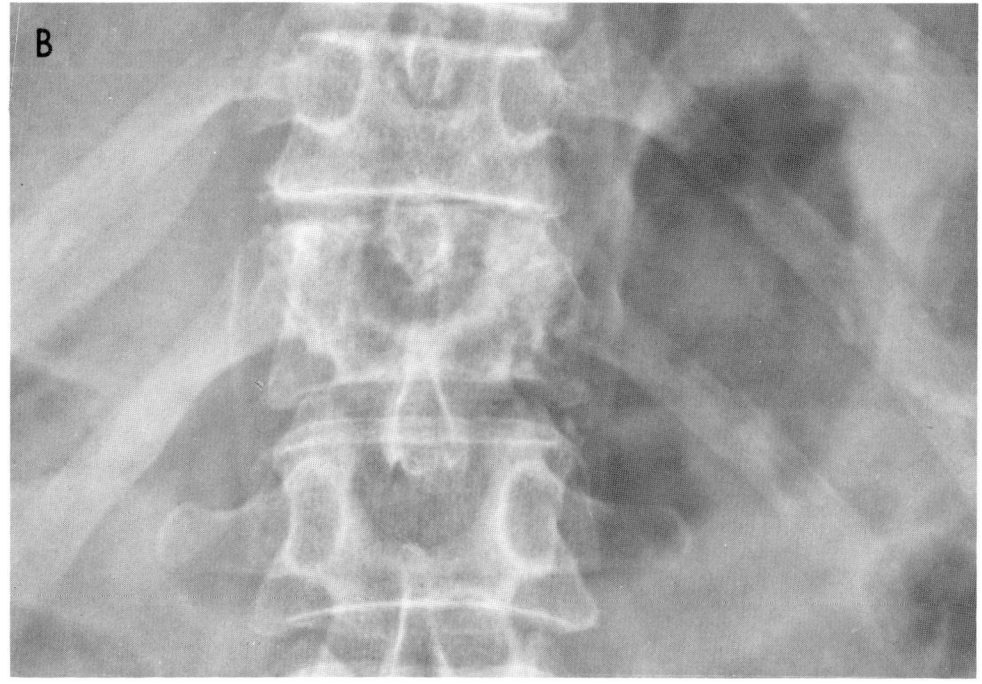

Figure 178 · Synovial Sarcoma; Synovioma / 411

PART 8

Miscellaneous Tumors

Figure 179.—Adamantinoma of the fibula.

AFIP Case No. 1050813: **A,** anteroposterior, and **B,** lateral views.

DIAGNOSIS AND GRADE.—Adamantinoma, fibula; growth rate IC.

LIFE INFORMATION.—Male, 28 years; survival unknown.

LOCATION.—A large circumscribed lesion which has completely overgrown its location in the distal shaft and metaphysis.

SIZE.—$11 \times 6 \times 6$ cm.

MINERALIZATION OF TUMOR.—None.

DESTRUCTION.—Geographic; lobulated contour; total destruction of cortex laterally, anteriorly and medially.

PROLIFERATION.—A 3 cm expansion of cortex posteriorly, with moderate residual septation; no encapsulation of the tumor by the periosteal response; large buttresses at the upper margin of the lesion.

DIFFERENTIAL DIAGNOSIS	PROBABILITY
Adamantinoma	.71
Hemangio-, angiosarcoma	.19
Fibrosarcoma	.05
Myeloma	.01
Chondrosarcoma	.01
Chondromyxoid fibroma	< .01
Cyst	< .01

COMMENT: The principal information offered by the radiograph is that the lesion is growing moderately slowly. Having seen an adamantinoma in this unusual location, we have the basis for diagnosing another.

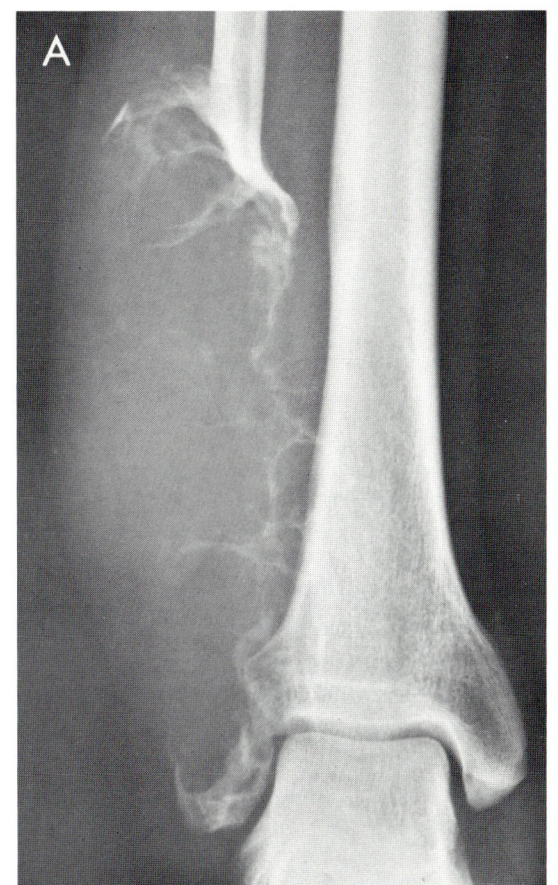
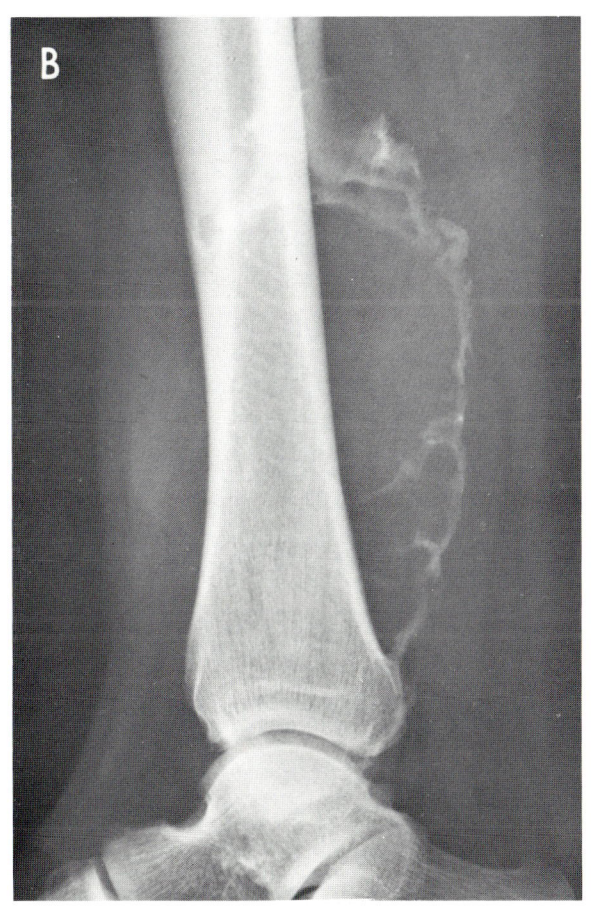

Figure 179 · Adamantinoma of Fibula / 415

Figure 180.—Adamantinoma of the tibia.

AFIP Case No. 1122932: **A,** anteroposterior view, initial examination; **B,** anteroposterior, and **C,** tangential views seven months later.

DIAGNOSIS AND GRADE.—Adamantinoma, tibia; growth rate IA.

LIFE INFORMATION.—Male, 82 years; survival unknown.

LOCATION.—A circumscribed lesion located centrally in the junction of the middle and lower thirds of the shaft, extending into the soft tissues.

SIZE.—Initially $7 \times 3 \times 2.5$ cm; seven months later, $8 \times 3.5 \times 3$ cm.

MINERALIZATION OF TUMOR.—None.

DESTRUCTION.—Geographic; lobulated contour. Initially the cortex is incompletely penetrated; later there is a large defect in the anterior cortex (**c**).

PROLIFERATION.—Faint marginal sclerosis; slight septation; expanded shell medially, laterally and anteriorly.

DIFFERENTIAL DIAGNOSIS	PROBABILITY
Adamantinoma	.49
Myeloma	.37
Fibroma	.07
Chondromyxoid fibroma	.03
Fibrosarcoma	.01
Chondrosarcoma	< .01
Benign cartilaginous tumor	< .01
Cyst	< .01

COMMENT: This adamantinoma is typical in terms of its location and rate of growth. Nothing in the radiographic pattern specifically identifies it as an adamantinoma, however.

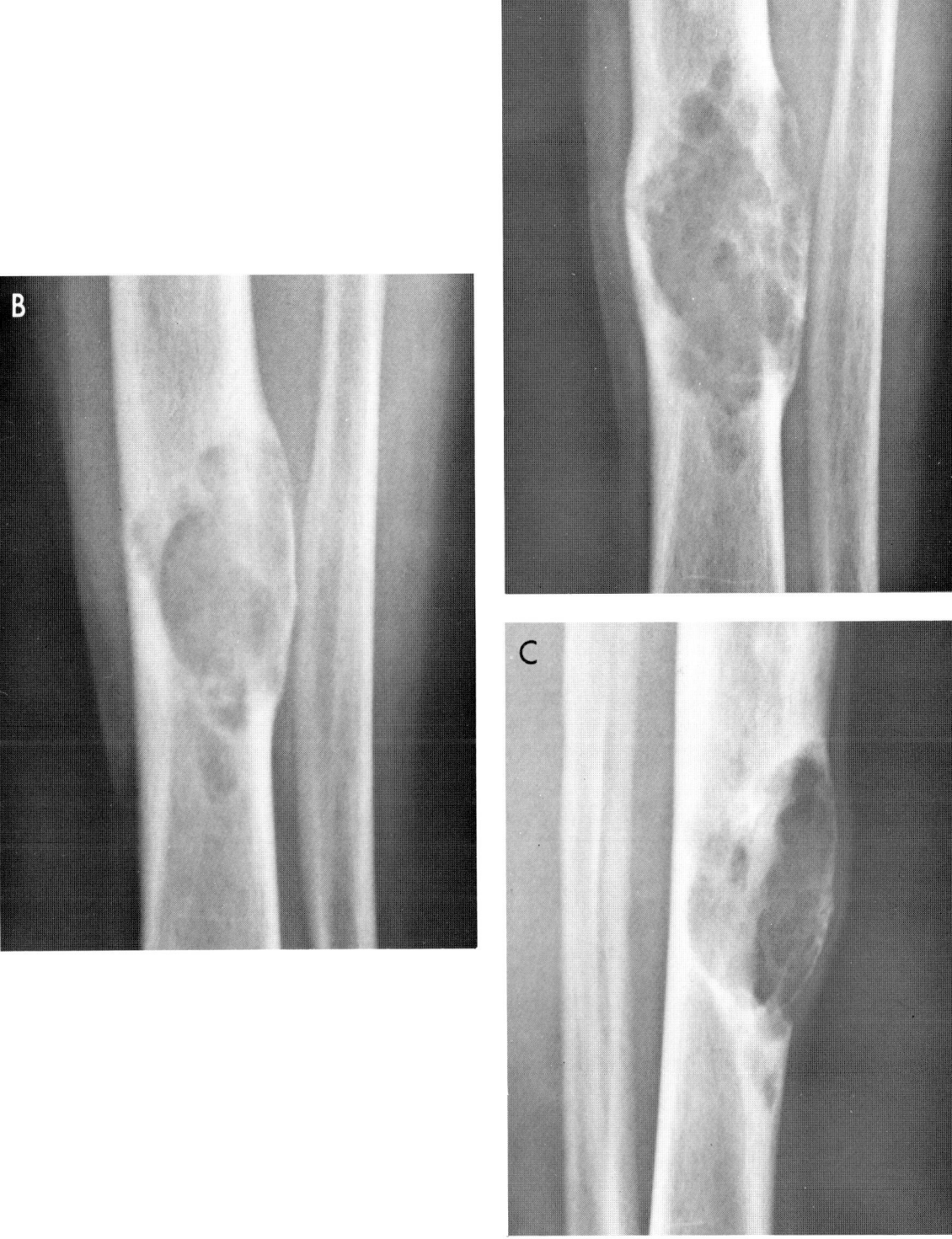

Figure 180 · Adamantinoma of Tibia

Figure 181.—Adamantinoma of the femur.

AFIP Case No. 1144688: Oblique projection.

DIAGNOSIS AND GRADE.—Adamantinoma, femur; growth rate IC.

LIFE INFORMATION.—Female, 37 years; survival unknown.

LOCATION.—A circumscribed lesion centrally located in the distal shaft near its junction with the metaphysis; no extraosseous tumor.

SIZE.—3 × 3 cm.

MINERALIZATION OF TUMOR.—None.

DESTRUCTION.—Geographic; ragged contour.

PROLIFERATION.—No marginal sclerosis; moderate amorphous reaction over site of maximal penetration.

DIFFERENTIAL DIAGNOSIS	PROBABILITY
Fibrosarcoma	.86
Chondrosarcoma	.07
Adamantinoma	.06

COMMENT: Radiologically this is a moderately slowly growing lesion which has little or nothing to identify it as an adamantinoma.

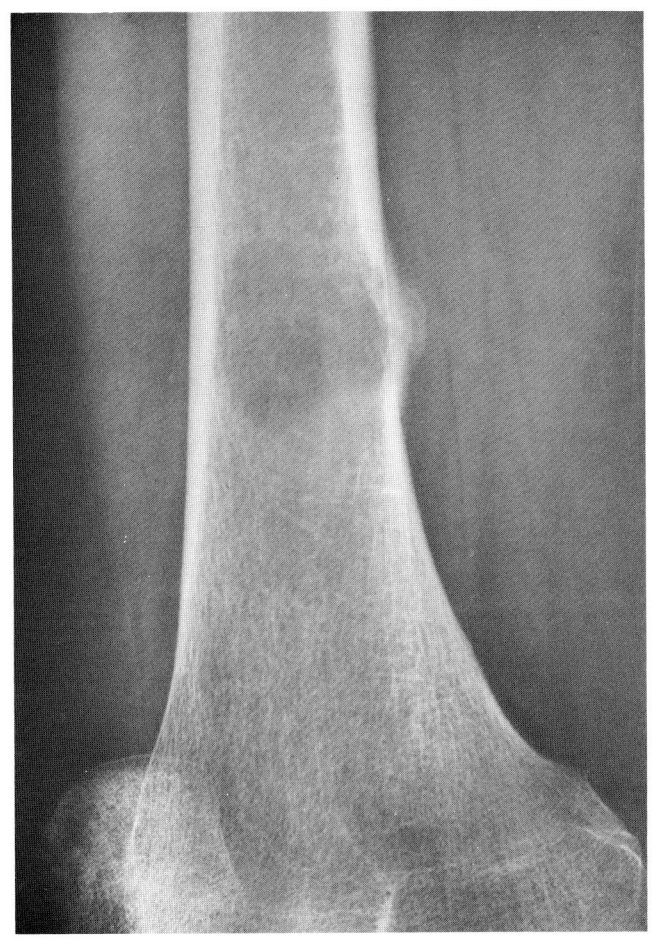

Figure 181 · Adamantinoma of Femur / 419

Figure 182.—Chordomas of the spine.

AFIP Case No. 1209110: **A,** anteroposterior, and **B,** lateral views.

DIAGNOSIS AND GRADE.—Chordoma, lumbar spine; growth rate IC.
LIFE INFORMATION.—Male, 73 years; survival unknown.
LOCATION.—A large soft tissue mass (**A, x**) in the right paraspinal region, with apparent involvement of lower three lumbar segments.

SIZE.—15 × 12 cm.
MINERALIZATION OF TUMOR.—None.
DESTRUCTION.—Smooth, geographic erosion of the lateral and posterior aspects of L3–5; regular contour.
PROLIFERATION.—Smooth anterior displacement of posterior cortex of L3–5.

DIFFERENTIAL DIAGNOSIS	PROBABILITY
Chordoma	100

COMMENT: A large chordoma presenting as an abdominal tumor. In a similar case the sacrum was involved.

AFIP Case No. 950076: **C,** lateral projection.

DIAGNOSIS AND GRADE.—Chordoma, cervical spine; growth rate II.
LIFE INFORMATION.—Male, 75 years; survived 54 months.
LOCATION.—A large soft tissue mass (**x**) on the anterior surface of the upper cervical spine, involving C2.

SIZE.—7 × 4 cm.
MINERALIZATION OF TUMOR.—None.
DESTRUCTION.—Moth-eaten destruction of the upper anterior surface of the body of C2.
PROLIFERATION.—None.

DIFFERENTIAL DIAGNOSIS	PROBABILITY
Chordoma	.98
Synovial sarcoma	< .01
Soft tissue sarcoma	< .01
Fibrosarcoma	< .01

COMMENT: A typical chordoma of the upper cervical spine.

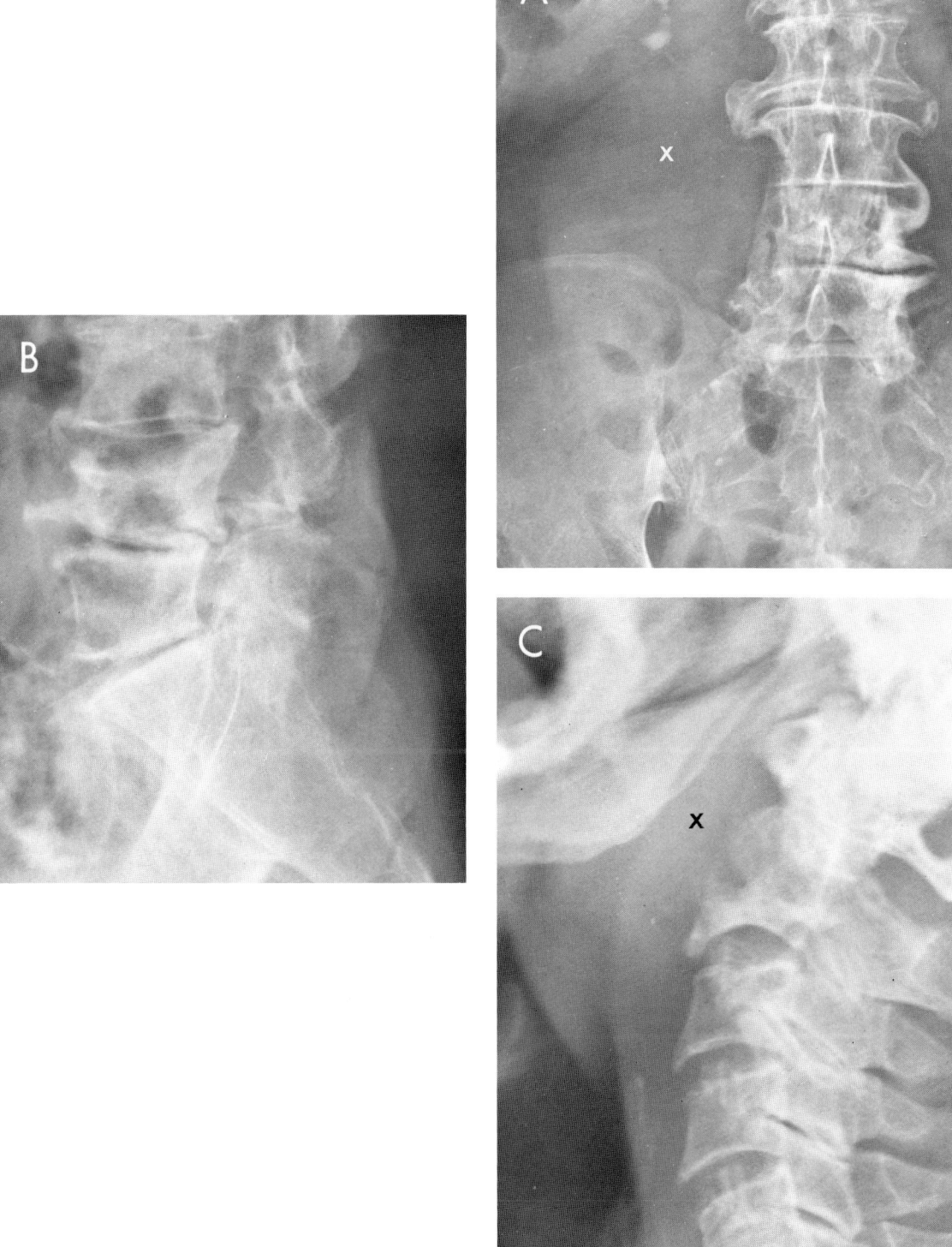

Figure 182 · Chordomas of Spine

Figure 183.—Chordomas of the cervical spine and sacrum.

AFIP Case No. 807795: **A,** lateral projection.

DIAGNOSIS AND GRADE.—Chordoma, cervical spine; not graded.
LIFE INFORMATION.—Male, 65 years; survived nearly two years.
LOCATION.—Large soft tissue mass (**x**) on the anterior surface of the mid-cervical spine, with extensive involvement of C4.

SIZE.—8 × 3 cm.
MINERALIZATION OF TUMOR.—None.
DESTRUCTION.—Severe compression fracture of C4, with displacement of some fragments anteriorly.
PROLIFERATION.—None.

DIFFERENTIAL DIAGNOSIS	PROBABILITY
Chordoma	.68
Myeloma	.30
Giant cell tumor	.01
Fibrosarcoma	< .01

COMMENT: A typical picture.

AFIP Case No. 1165358: **B,** anteroposterior projection.

DIAGNOSIS AND GRADE.—Chordoma, sacrum; growth rate IB.
LIFE INFORMATION.—Male, 71 years; low back pain for several years; survived nine months after diagnosis; radiation therapy not effective.
LOCATION.—Large circumscribed lesion in the midline.

SIZE.—9 × 9 cm.
MINERALIZATION OF TUMOR.—None.
DESTRUCTION.—Geographic; regular contour.
PROLIFERATION.—Dense marginal sclerosis (**arrows**); slight septation; expanded shell over 1 cm encapsulating the lesion.

DIFFERENTIAL DIAGNOSIS	PROBABILITY
Myeloma	.73
Chordoma	.15
Giant cell tumor	.10
Cyst	< .01
Fibrosarcoma	< .01

COMMENT: A typical chordoma of the sacrum. Myeloma is much commoner, as reflected in the order of probabilities.

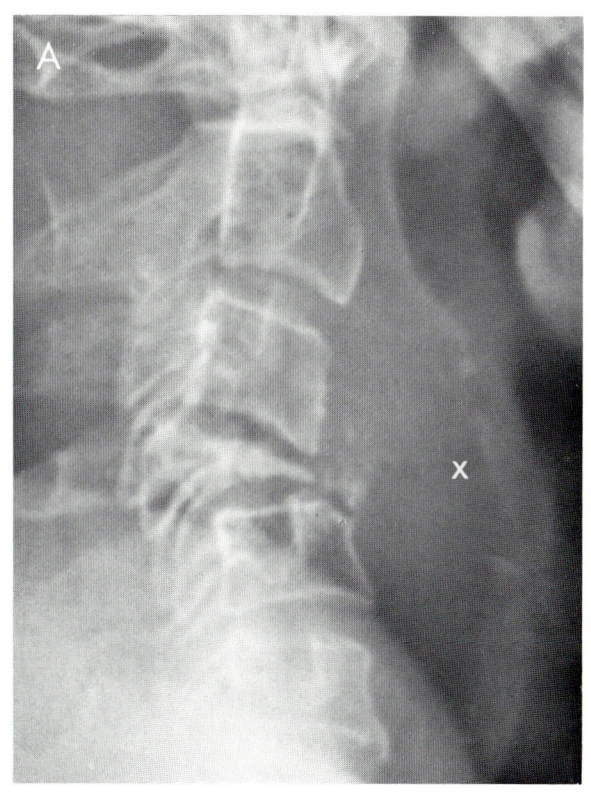

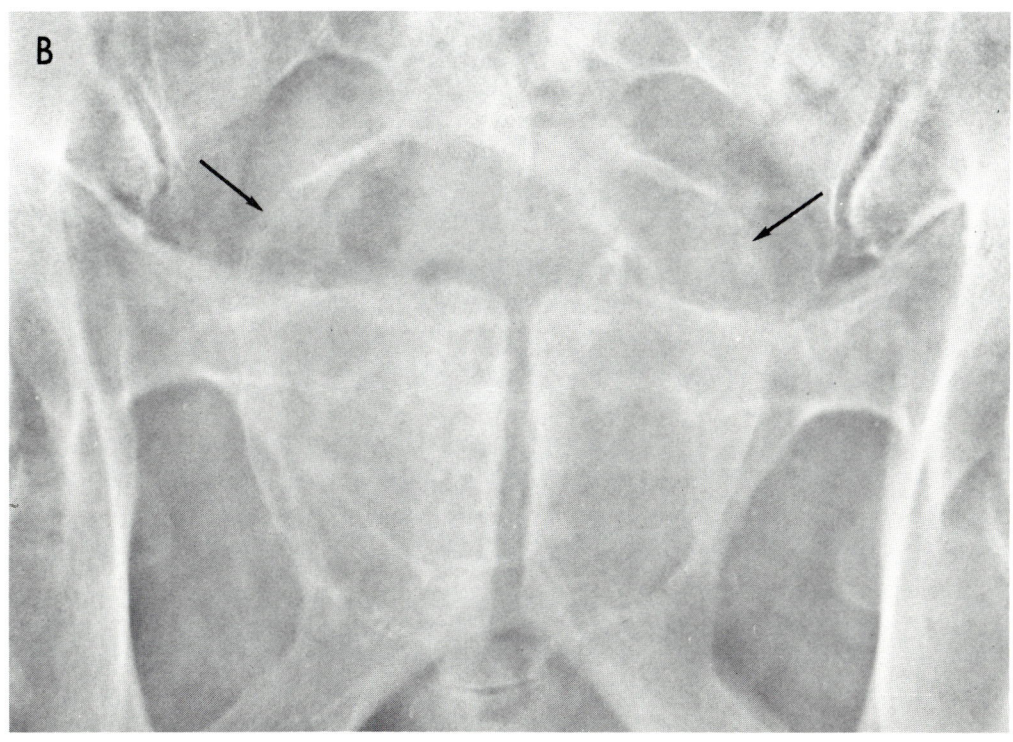

Figure 183 · Chordomas of Spine / 423

Figure 184.—Lipomas of the humerus.

AFIP Case No. 1033960: **A,** anteroposterior projection.

DIAGNOSIS AND GRADE.—Lipoma, humerus; growth rate IA.
LIFE INFORMATION.—Female, 34 years; survival unknown.
LOCATION.—A small circumscribed lesion centered eccentrically in the region of the greater tuberosity, extending into the proximal metaphysis.
SIZE.—2 × 2 cm.
MINERALIZATION OF TUMOR.—A dense ring of calcific density in the center of the tumor which does not conform to the usual pattern in cartilaginous and bone-forming lesions, has no trabecular structure and may represent deposition of calcium in tissue rather than bone.
DESTRUCTION.—Geographic; regular contour; no penetration of cortex.
PROLIFERATION.—A faint zone of marginal sclerosis.

DIFFERENTIAL DIAGNOSIS	PROBABILITY
Lipoma	.99
Chondrosarcoma	< .01
Osteosarcoma	< .01

COMMENT: A picture somewhat like that of chondroblastoma.

AFIP Case No. 1058001: **B,** anteroposterior, and **C,** body section.

DIAGNOSIS AND GRADE.—Lipoma, humerus; growth rate IA.
LIFE INFORMATION.—Male, 26 years; survival unknown.
LOCATION.—A circumscribed lesion centered eccentrically in the proximal epiphysis, involving the subarticular cortex.
SIZE.—2 × 2 × 2 cm.
MINERALIZATION OF TUMOR.—None.
DESTRUCTION.—Geographic; lobulated contour.
PROLIFERATION.—Dense sclerotic rim.

DIFFERENTIAL DIAGNOSIS	PROBABILITY
Chondroblastoma	.72
Villonodular synovitis	.26
Lipoma	.01
Benign cartilaginous tumor	< .01

COMMENT: In no way distinguishable radiologically from chondroblastoma.

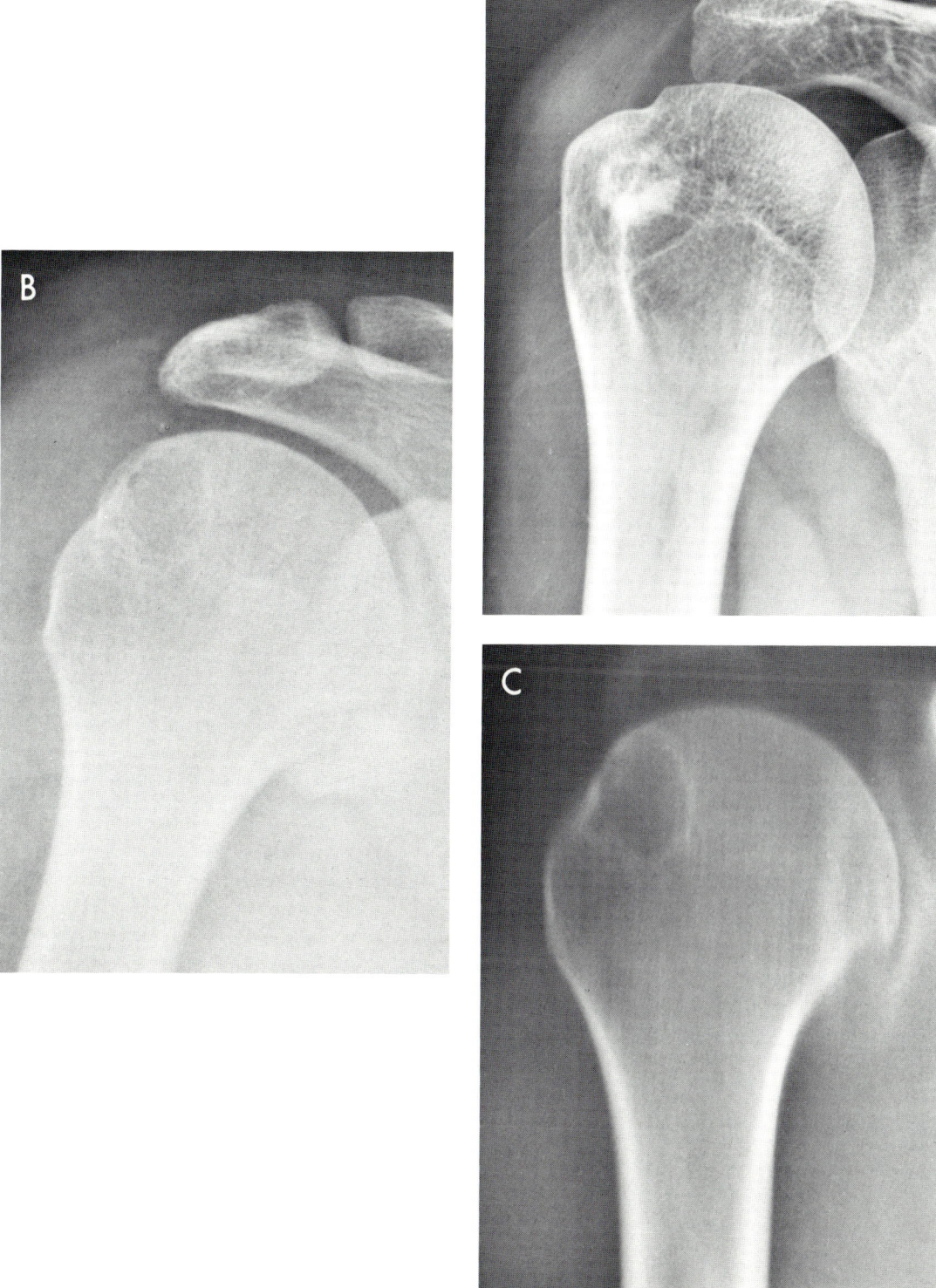

Figure 184 · Lipomas of Humerus / 425

Figure 185.—Lipoma of the femur.

AFIP Case No. 982228: **A,** anteroposterior, and **B,** lateral views.

DIAGNOSIS AND GRADE.—Lipoma, femur; growth rate IA.
LIFE INFORMATION.—Female, 63 years; survival unknown.
LOCATION.—A circumscribed lesion centered in the proximal shaft, extending into the intertrochanteric area; no extraosseous extension.
SIZE.—7 × 2.5 × 2.5 cm.
MINERALIZATION OF TUMOR.—A few floccules of calcific density near the margin of the cystic area.
DESTRUCTION.—Geographic; lobulated contour.
PROLIFERATION.—A dense sclerotic rim completely surrounding the lesion; no significant expansion of the cortex; a few incomplete septa.

DIFFERENTIAL DIAGNOSIS	PROBABILITY
Myeloma	.61
Fibrosarcoma	.24
Benign cartilaginous tumor	.05
Nonossifying fibroma	.05
Chondrosarcoma	.01
Chondromyxoid fibroma	.01
Cyst	< .01

COMMENT: Radiologically this lipoma appears to be quite inactive. This is a favorite site for other types of bone tumors, but the computer is confused, never having heard of lipoma in this location except as a remote possibility.

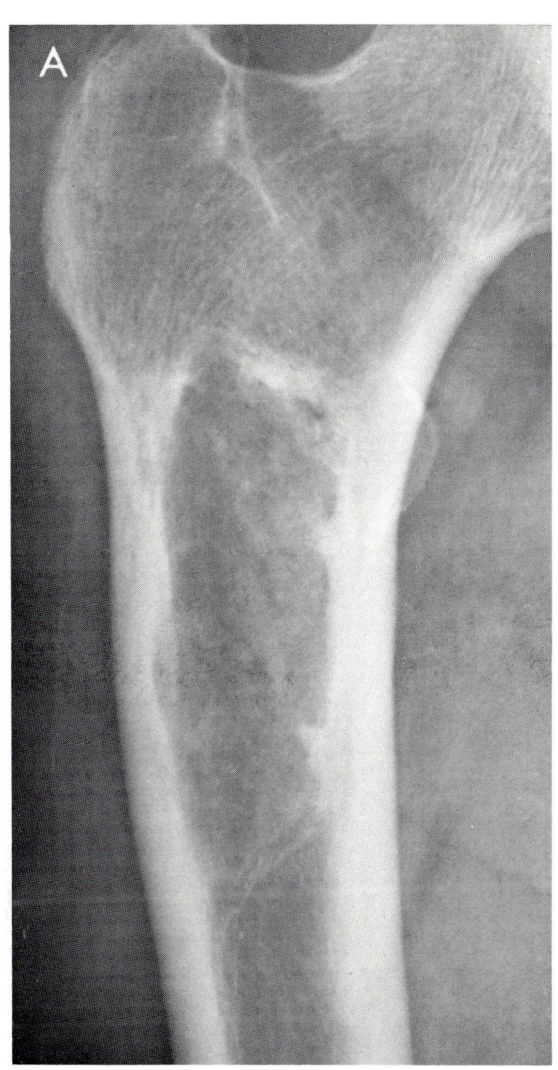
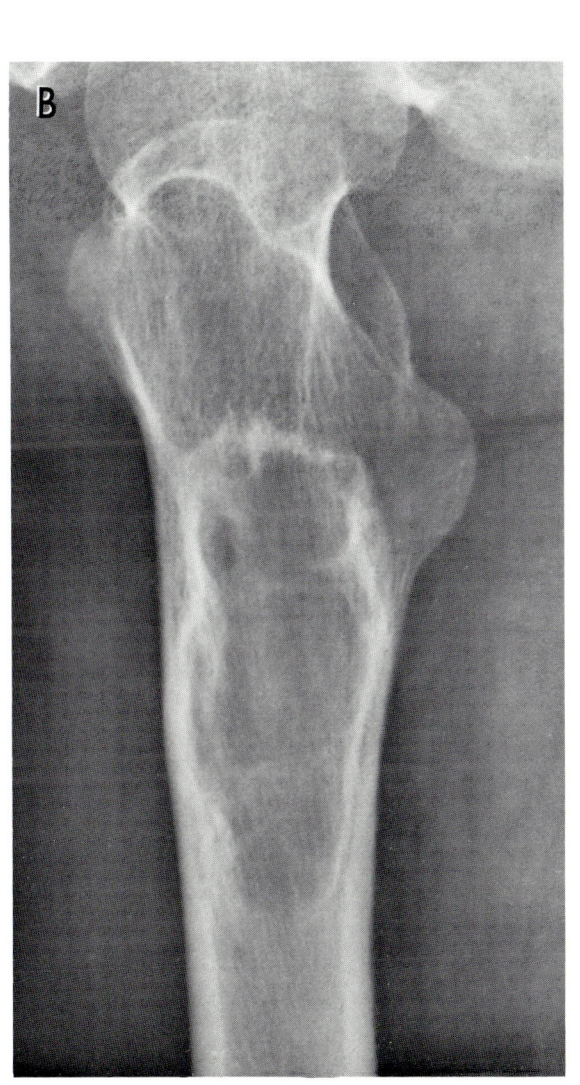

Figure 185 · Lipoma of Femur

Figure 186.—Myxolipoma of the femur.

AFIP Case No. 1068166: Anteroposterior projection.

DIAGNOSIS AND GRADE.—Myxolipoma, femur; growth rate IA.
LIFE INFORMATION.—Male, 2 years; well five years after onset.
LOCATION.—A circumscribed lesion centered in the intertrochanteric area of the proximal femur, spreading down to involve the shaft.
SIZE.—3 × 1.5 cm.
MINERALIZATION OF TUMOR.—None.
DESTRUCTION.—Geographic; lobulated contour; incomplete penetration of the cortex.
PROLIFERATION.—Broad sclerosis around the upper margin of the lesion.

DIFFERENTIAL DIAGNOSIS	PROBABILITY
Nonossifying fibroma	.80
Benign cartilaginous tumor	.14
Chondromyxoid fibroma	.02
Cyst	.01
Fibrosarcoma	< .01
Osteosarcoma	< .01

COMMENT: Radiologically this seems to be an impossible lesion to diagnose. Differential diagnosis should include xanthoma and histiocytosis X. The correct diagnosis is included as a rare possibility by the computer.

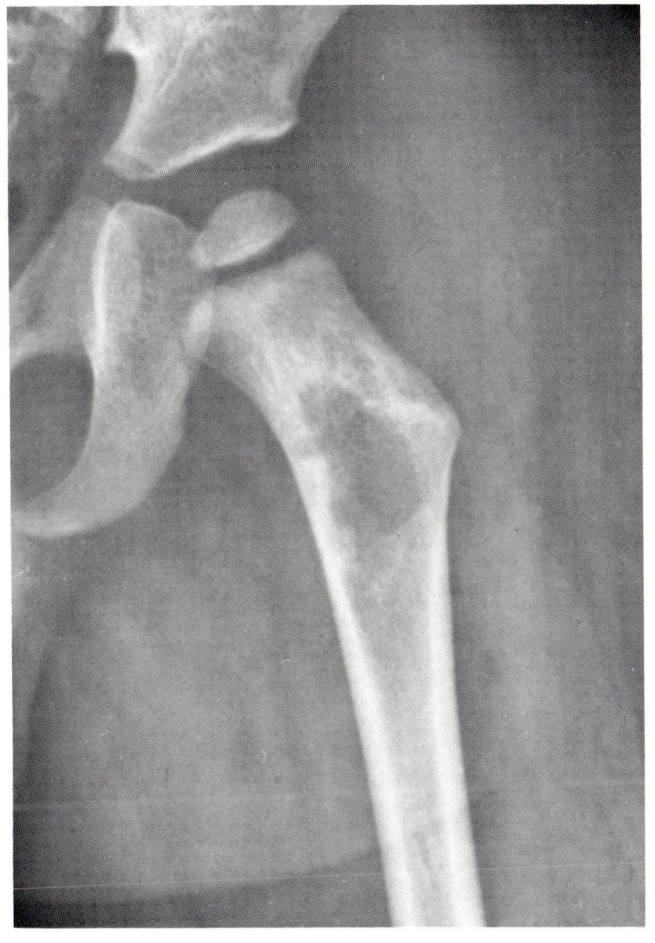

Figure 186 · Myxolipoma of Femur / 429

Figure 187.—Osteosarcoma in Paget's disease.

AFIP Case No. 1128364: Anteroposterior projection.

DIAGNOSIS AND GRADE.—Osteosarcoma in Paget's disease, humerus; growth rate II.

LIFE INFORMATION.—Female, 63 years; died seven months after onset.

LOCATION.—An ill-defined lesion centered at the junction of the metaphysis and epiphysis of the proximal humerus; medial soft tissue extension.

SIZE.—6 × 5 cm.

MINERALIZATION OF TUMOR.—Several flocculent areas of tumor matrix mineralization.

DESTRUCTION.—Moth-eaten in the humeral head; total penetration of the cortex; permeative pattern in the shaft, a part of Paget's disease.

PROLIFERATION.—None beyond that observed in Paget's disease.

DIFFERENTIAL DIAGNOSIS	PROBABILITY
Reticulum cell sarcoma	.79
Fibrosarcoma	.15
Osteosarcoma	.05

COMMENT: A typical osteosarcoma in Paget's disease in terms of its high degree of malignancy and scant tumor bone formation. The computer does not know about Paget's disease.

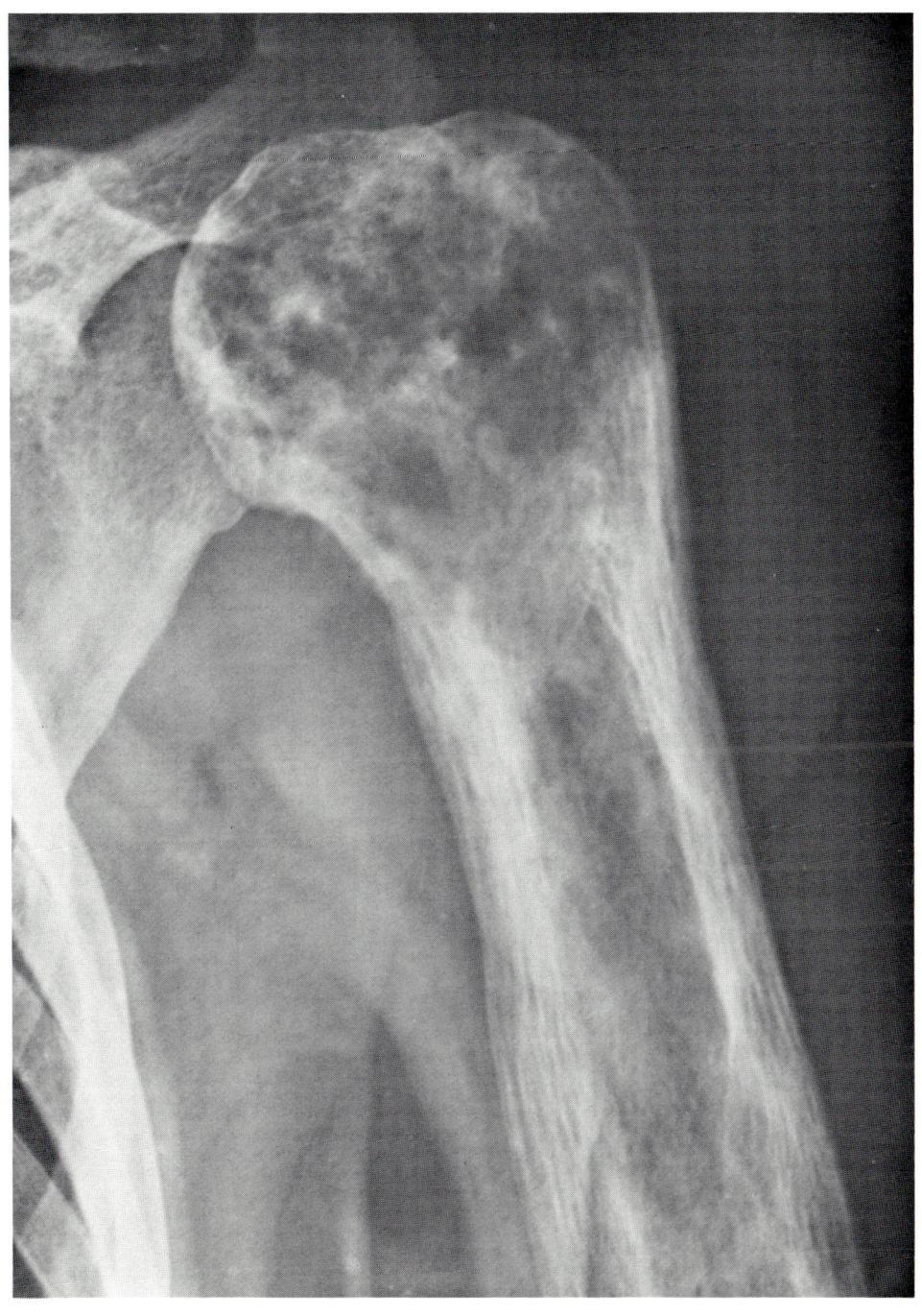

Figure 187 · Osteosarcoma in Paget's Disease / 431

Figure 188.—Metastasis in the tibia from a primary tumor in the lung.

AFIP Case No. 1180666: Anteroposterior projection.

DIAGNOSIS AND GRADE.—Metastasis to tibia, from primary in lung; growth rate III.

LIFE INFORMATION.—Female, 37 years; survived eight months.

LOCATION.—A poorly circumscribed lesion centered eccentrically in the proximal shaft; large extraosseous extension.

SIZE.—5 × 5 cm.

MINERALIZATION OF TUMOR.—None.

DESTRUCTION.—Permeative; total penetration of cortex.

PROLIFERATION.—Small Codman's triangle (**arrow**).

DIFFERENTIAL DIAGNOSIS	PROBABILITY
Osteosarcoma	.60
Fibrosarcoma	.32
Reticulum cell sarcoma	.06
Ewing's sarcoma	< .01
Chondrosarcoma	< .01

COMMENT: Because of its location at the level of the nutrient foramen, metastatic tumor should be suspected. However, the extraosseous extension is much larger than ordinarily seen in a secondary neoplasm. No probability matrix for metastatic tumors has been included in the computer.

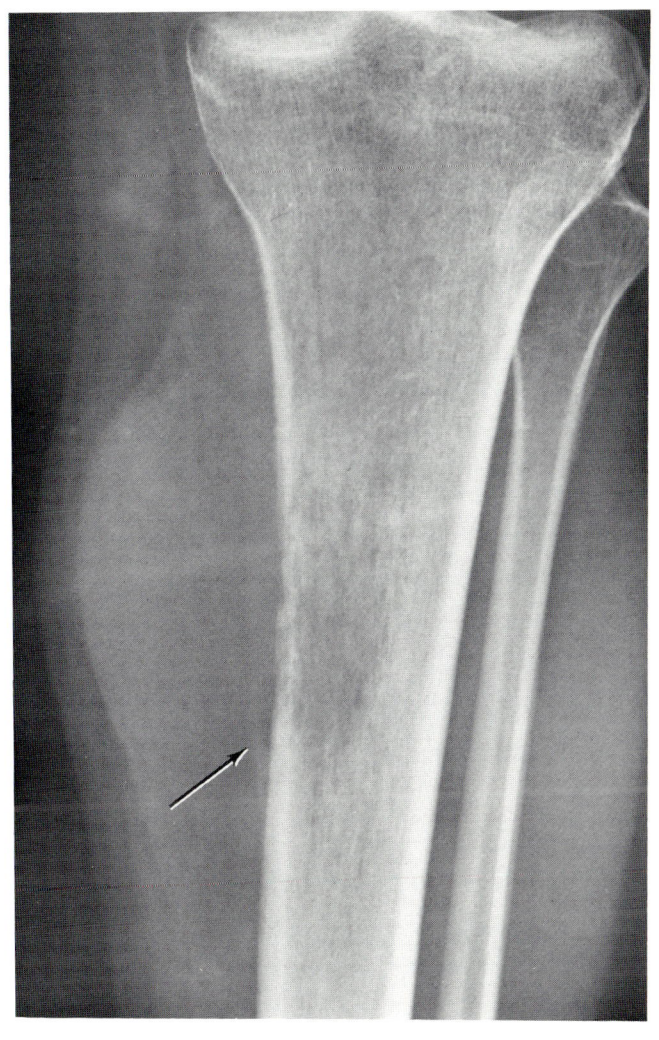

Figure 188 · Tibial Metastasis from Lung / 433

Figure 189.—Metastasis in the humerus from a carcinoma of the prostate.

AFIP Case No. 1199710: Anteroposterior projection.

DIAGNOSIS AND GRADE.—Metastasis to humerus, from prostate; ungraded.
LIFE INFORMATION.—Male, 70 years; last known to be alive.
LOCATION.—Diffuse involvement of the entire humerus.

SIZE.—About 30 × 5 cm.
MINERALIZATION OF TUMOR.—None.
DESTRUCTION.—Permeative pattern throughout.
PROLIFERATION.—Diffuse mottling in the spongy ends of the humerus; coarse hair-on-end spiculation from the cortical surface perpendicularly into the extraosseous tumor surrounding the shaft.

DIFFERENTIAL DIAGNOSIS	PROBABILITY
Reticulum cell sarcoma	.98
Osteosarcoma	< .01
Fibrosarcoma	< .01

COMMENT: An especially florid case of proliferative spiculation excited by metastatic carcinoma of the prostate. None of the computer diagnoses seem appropriate. Metastatic tumor is the only diagnosis.

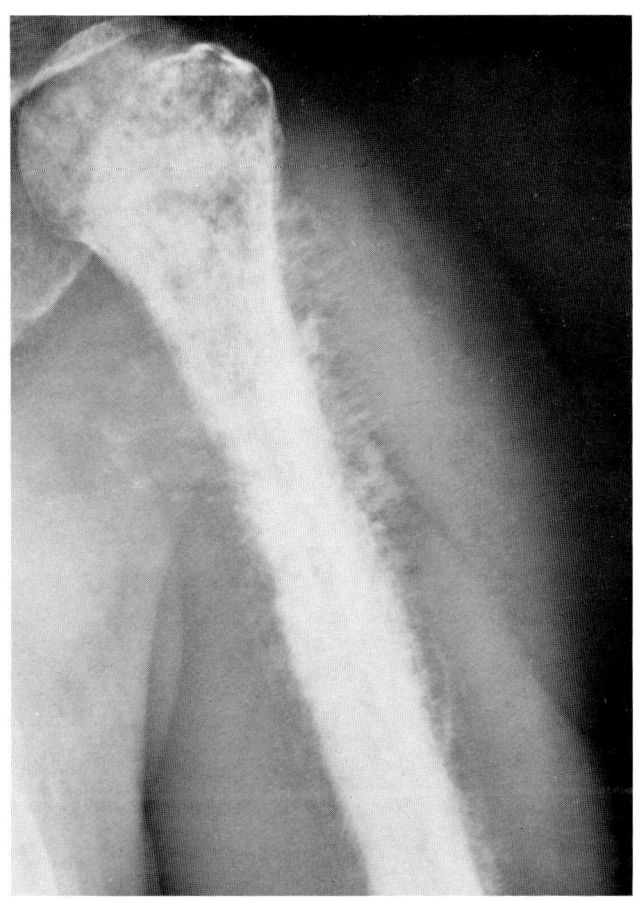

Figure 189 · Humeral Metastasis from Prostate / 435

CONTRIBUTORS OF AFIP RADIOGRAPHS

Figure		Figure	
18	1190412: Giant cell tumor. R. M. Canidy, M.D., St. Anne's Hospital, Chicago.	33	1148441: Giant cell tumor. R. V. Hussey, U.S.A.F. M.C., 807th Medical Group, March Air Force Base, Calif.
19	1080027: Giant cell tumor. S. Mamlick, M.D., Stevens Clinic Hospital, Welch, W.Va.	34	1151077: Giant Cell tumor. P. E. Siebert, M.D., Fitzsimons General Hospital, Denver, Colo.
20	1135211: Giant cell tumor. K. Flachs, M.D., Veterans Administration Hospital, Buffalo, N.Y.	35	1195256: Cystic giant cell tumor. A. S. Carlson, M.D., Community Hospital, Glen Cove, N.Y.
21	1147238: Giant cell tumor. E. R. Jacobs, M.D., National Orthopaedic and Rehabilitation Hospital, Arlington, Va.	36	1022639: Bone cyst. J. R. John, M.D., Medical Center Clinic, Pensacola, Fla.
22	1016356: Giant cell tumor. W. L. Bonnet, M.D., Helen Fuld Hospital, Trenton, N.J.	37, A	1027619: Bone cyst. H. M. Simon, Jr., M.D., Hialeah Hospital, Hialeah, Fla.
23, A	996237: Giant cell tumor. K. M. Keane, M.D., Badgerow Building, Sioux City, Iowa.	37, B	1087809: Bone cyst. J. W. Linden, M.D., Santa Clara, Calif.
23, B	1163342: Giant cell tumor. S. H. Macht, M.D., Washington County Hospital Association, Hagerstown, Md.	38	1194303: Bone cyst. H. S. Weens, M.D., Grady Memorial Hospital, Atlanta, Ga.
24	1171403: Giant cell tumor. W. F. Scott, M.D., Medical Laboratory Associates, Birmingham, Ala.	39, 40	1193759: Bone cyst. Chief of Radiology, Orange Memorial Hospital, Orlando, Fla.
25	1160108: Giant cell tumor. C. D. Rosenthal, M.D., St. Margaret Hospital, Hammond, Ind.	41	1111366: Cystic giant cell tumor. Chief of Radiology, Public Health Service, Alaska Native Medical Center, Anchorage.
26	1175158: Giant cell tumor. G. F. Dobel, U.S.N. M.C., United States Naval Hospital, Great Lakes, Ill.	42	1165684: Bone cyst. L. S. Smith, M.D., Floyd Hospital, Rome, Ga.
27, A	910821: Giant cell tumor. E. H. White, M.D., Cincinnati, Ohio.	43	1213808: Bone cyst. E. W. Ylitah, U.S.A. M.C., Fourth United States Army Laboratory, Fort Sam Houston, Tex.
27, B	1157309: Giant cell tumor. E. M. Auringer, M.D., Hornell, N.Y.	44, A	1120445: Bone cyst. H. C. Alfred, M.D., U.S. Air Force Hospital, Kessler Air Force Base, Miss.
28	1188553: Giant cell tumor. R. F. Scalf, M.D., Saints Mary and Elizabeth Hospital, Louisville, Ky.	44, B	1065938: Bone cyst. H. L. Twigg, M.D., Georgetown University Hospital, Washington, D.C.
29	1109956: Giant cell tumor: D. L. McRae, M.D., Montreal Neurological Institute, Montreal, Canada.	45, A	1126687: Bone cyst. Chief of Radiology Service, Madigan General Hospital, Tacoma, Wash.
30	819218: Giant cell tumor: E. C. Kley, M.D., St. Clare Hospital, Denville, N.J.	45, B	1035921: Bone cyst. R. L. Bosman, U.S.A. M.C., Landstuhl Army Medical Center, New York, N.Y.
31	1129479: Giant cell tumor. S. H. Huff, Jr., M.D., Anderson Memorial Hospital, Anderson, S.C.	46	978219: Bone cyst. Chief of Radiology, Langley Air Force Hospital, Langley Field, Va.
32	1155465: Giant cell tumor. R. J. Atkinson, M.D., U.S. Air Force Hospital, Elmendorf, Alaska.		

Figure	
47	1129433: Bone cyst. H. C. Alfred, U.S. Air Force Hospital, Kessler Air Force Base, Miss.
48	1152297: Fibrosarcoma. R. G. Reinbold, U.S.A. M.C., U.S. Army Hospital, Munich, Germany.
49	1081826: Fibrosarcoma. A. Hedegaard, M.D., Visalia, Calif.
50, A, B	1061467: Fibrosarcoma. L. Ehrlich, M.D., Chief of Radiology, San Patricio Veterans Administration Hospital, San Juan, Puerto Rico.
50, C	907257: Fibrosarcoma. W. R. Howard, M.D., Children's Hospital, Columbus, Ohio.
51, A	1035222: Fibrosarcoma. Chief of Radiology, U.S. Naval Hospital, San Diego, Calif.
51, B	1128996: Fibrosarcoma. L. M. Warshaw, M.D., St. Patrick's Hospital, Lake Charles, La.
52	1106260: Fibrosarcoma. P. J. Trier, M.D., Veterans Administration Hospital, Des Moines, Iowa.
53	949448: Fibrosarcoma. J. G. Wood, M.D., Wood, Vkosskuhldr & Associates, Flagstaff, Ariz.
54	1096840: Fibrosarcoma. Chief of Radiology, D.H.S.A.N. Hospital, Anchorage, Alaska.
55	1081268: Fibrosarcoma. Chief of Radiology, Veterans Administration Hospital, Temple, Tex.
56	1063737: Fibrosarcoma. M. Green, M.D., MacNeal Memorial Hospital, Berwyn, Ill.
57	1065289: Fibrosarcoma. C. H. Burge, M.D., Methodist Hospital, Houston, Tex.
58, A, B	1028513: Fibrosarcoma. Chief of Radiology, Westover Air Force Base, Mass.
58, C, D	1165869: Fibrosarcoma. Chief of Radiology, Tripler General Hospital, Honolulu, Hawaii.
59, A	1002914: Chondromyxoid fibroma. T. D. Moberg, M.D., Luther Hospital, Eau Claire, Wis.
59, B	1009537: Chondromyxoid fibroma. Chief of Radiology, Mercy Hospital, Charlotte, N.C.
60	933894: Chondromyxoid fibroma. F. Stuttle, M.D., Peoria, Ill.
61	932830: Chondromyxoid fibroma. L. C. Hamilton, U.S.A. M.C., Walter Reed General Hospital, Washington, D.C.
62	1189541: Chondromyxoid fibroma. P. T. Webster, M.D., Purdue University Hospital, Lafayette, Ind.
63, A	1080586: Chondromyxoid fibroma. J. F. Weigen, M.D., Palo Alto Medical Clinic, Palo Alto, Calif.
63, B, C	1004844: Chondromyxoid fibroma. A. C. Wyman, M.D., Alexandria, Va.
64	1207088: Chondromyxoid fibroma: Chief of Radiology, Southside Hospital, Bay Shore, N.Y.
65	795574: Chondromyxoid fibroma: G. C. Walter, M.D., St. Joseph's Hospital, Lewiston, Idaho.
66, A	972983: Chondromyxoid fibroma. Chief of Radiology, Veterans Administration Hospital, White River Junction, Vt.
66, B	1035794: Chondromyxoid fibroma. T. B. Drotning, U.S.A. M.C., Reynolds Army Hospital, Fort Sill, Okla.
67, A, B	1167299: Fibroxanthoma. L. C. Hamilton, U.S.A. M.C., Walter Reed General Hospital, Washington, D.C.
67, C, D	1207290: Fibroxanthoma. G. E. Maddock, M.D., Ehrling Bergquist U.S. Air Force Hospital, Offutt Air Force Base, Neb.
68, A	1164168: Fibroxanthoma. W. Becker, U.S.A. M.C., William Beaumont General Hospital, El Paso, Tex.
68, B	1158190: Fibroxanthoma. J. B. Tully, M.D., St. Joseph Hospital, Orange, Calif.
69, A	1155055: Fibroxanthoma. W. A. Stevens, M.D., St. Joseph's Hospital, Syracuse, N.Y.
69, B	1142240: Fibroxanthoma. W. C. Yarbrough, M.D., General Hospital, Greenville, Miss.
70, A	1004238: Periosteal fibroma. Chief of Radiology, Veterans Administration Hospital, Topeka, Kans.
70, B	1115976: Fibroxanthoma. F. M. Grossman, U.S.A.F. M.C., MacDill Air Force Base, Fla.
71	1156660: Fibroxanthoma. Chief of Radiology, Public Health Service, Alaska Native Medical Center, Anchorage.
72, A	1037533: Fibrous osteoma. R.

Contributors of AFIP Radiographs / 437

Figure	
72, B	W. Spicher, U.S.N. M.C., U.S. Naval Hospital, Chelsea, Mass. 1048662: Ossifying fibroma. Chief of Radiology, U.S. Air Force Hospital, Lackland Air Force Base, Tex.
73	1036261: Fibrous osteoma. L. C. Hamilton, U.S.A. M.C., Walter Reed General Hospital, Washington, D.C.
74, A	1188917: Cortical desmoid. M. Moskowitz, M.D., Middlesex Memorial Hospital, Middletown, Conn.
74, B	1105882: Cortical desmoid. R. Ellis., M.D., Wilford Hall U.S. Air Force Hospital, Lackland Air Force Base, Tex.
75, A	1131478: Cortical desmoid. W. R. Laughlin, U.S.A. M.C., Fort Sam Houston, Tex.
75, B	1201001: Cortical desmoid. W. D. Greenough, M.D., U.S. Army Hospital, Fort Carson, Colo.
76	1200002: Cortical desmoid. W. N. Zuck, U.S.A.F. M.C., Maxwell Air Force Base, Fla.
77	1190741: Chondrosarcoma. Chief of Radiology, Madigan General Hospital, Tacoma, Wash.
78	9082676: Chondrosarcoma. G. W. McCall, M.D., Tuberculosis Hospital (Clinic), Bristol Memorial Hospital, Bristol, Tenn.
79	1130060: Chondrosarcoma. G. F. Lull, Jr., M.D., Veterans Administration Hospital, Phoenix, Ariz.
80	1109753: Chondrosarcoma. Chief of Radiology, Trinity Lutheran Hospital, Kansas City, Mo.
81	850094: Chondrosarcoma. E. Burkhalter, M.D., Veterans Administration Center, Temple, Tex.
82	1130957: Chondrosarcoma. M. D. Sacks, M.D., Veterans Administration Hospital, Cleveland, Ohio.
83, A	1154401: D. E. Red, U.S.A.F. M.C., U.S. Air Force Hospital, Wright-Patterson Air Force Base, Ohio.
83, B	1203575: Chondrosarcoma. E. E. Fox, M.D., Veterans Administration Center, Sioux Falls, S.D.
84	1010529: Chondrosarcoma. Chief of Radiology, St. John's McNamara Hospital, Rapid City, S.D.
85	1181318: Chondrosarcoma. G. W. Sengpiel, M.D., St. Joseph's Hospital, Milwaukee, Wis.
86	1135837: Chondrosarcoma. R. L. Smith, M.D., Doctors' Hospital, Coral Gables, Fla.
87	1182899: Chondrosarcoma. S. J. Bocick, M.D., Bethlehem Steel Corporation, Sparrows Point, Md.
88, A	1194779: Chondrosarcoma. W. N. Zuck, U.S.A.F. M.C., U.S. Air Force Hospital, Maxwell Air Force Base, Ala.
88, B, C	1142139: Chondrosarcoma. L. D. Miller, M.D., Mercy Hospital, Denver, Colo.
89	1170056: Chondrosarcoma. Chief of Radiology, U.S. Naval Hospital, Bethesda, Md.
90	1100836: Chondrosarcoma. J. F. Shaw, M.D., Veterans Administration Hospital, Topeka, Kans.
91	1138139: Chondrosarcoma. J. M. Dennis, M.D., University Hospital, Baltimore, Md.
92, A	1074141: Chondroblastoma. L. S. Snell, M.D., Idaho Falls, Idaho.
92, B	1162659: Chondroblastoma. E. T. Campbell, M.D., Washington County Hospital Association, Hagerstown, Md.
93, A	909973: Cystic chondroblastoma. L. C. Hamilton, U.S.A. M.C., Walter Reed Army Hospital, Washington, D.C.
93, B	1154601: Chondroblastoma. Chief of Radiology, U.S. Air Force Hospital, Wright-Patterson Air Force Base, Ohio.
94	1053068: Chondroblastoma. D. H. Williams, M.D., Weirton General Hospital, Weirton, W.Va.
95, A	1142245: Chondroblastoma. J. Israel, M.D., Clara Maass Memorial Hospital, Belleville, N.J.
95, B	1099859: Chondroblastoma. D. Kingsley, M.D., U.S. Naval Hospital, Newport, R.I.
96	1180671: Chondroblastoma. L. T. Brown, U.S.N. M.C., National Navy Medical Center, Bethesda, Md.
97, A	909010: Chondroblastoma. A. W. Perlman, M.D., Cincinnati.
97, B	1173043: Periosteal chondroma.

Figure	
	E. K. Poole, U.S.N. M.C., U.S. Naval Hospital, Corpus Christi, Tex.
98, A	1187793: Periosteal chondroma. T. E. Whiteside, Jr., M.D., Emory University Clinic, Atlanta, Ga.
98, B	1015416: Synovial chondroma. S. Reitman, U.S.N. M.C., U.S. Naval Hospital, Newport, R.I.
99, A	1135669: Periosteal chondroma. G. W. Bylsma, M.D., Charles F. Kettering Memorial Hospital, Kettering, Ohio
99, B	1219380: Cortical chondroma. S. M. Bronson, M.D., Memorial Hospital, Johnson City, Tenn.
100	1044761: Periosteal chondroma. S. Reitman, U.S.N. M.C., U.S. Naval Hospital, Newport, R.I.
101, A, B	1154288: Enchondroma. D. C. Hill, M.D., North Miami General Hospital, North Miami, Fla.
101, C	904008: Chondroma. J. R. Amberg, M.D., Veterans Administration Hospital, San Francisco.
102, A	1115991: Osteosarcoma. L. C. Hamilton, U.S.A. M.C., Walter Reed General Hospital, Washington, D.C.
102, B	1071103: Osteosarcoma. H. L. Tseng, M.D., Provident Hospital, Inc., Baltimore, Md.
103	1072069: Osteosarcoma. L. J. Malielski, M.D., St. Mary's Hospital, Kankakee, Ill.
104	1102907: Osteosarcoma. D. B. Rulon, U.S.N. M.C., U.S. Naval Hospital, Oakland, Calif.
105	1185558: Osteosarcoma. T. A. Tristan, M.D., The Harrisburg Polyclinic Hospital, Harrisburg, Pa.
106	1051392: Osteosarcoma. Chief of Radiology, Histopathology Center, Travis Air Force Base, Calif.
107	1102182: Osteosarcoma. B. E. Greenberg, M.D., Veterans Administration Hospital, Memphis, Tenn.
108	1115305: Osteosarcoma. H. L. Pope, M.D., U.S. Naval Hospital, Camp Le Jeune, N.C.
109	1081977: Osteosarcoma. R. Barden, M.D., Philadelphia.
110	1058661: Osteosarcoma. Chief of Radiology, Children's Hospital, Baltimore, Md.

Figure	
111	1165589: Osteosarcoma. R. A. McIntyre, M.D., Medical Arts X-ray, Carlsbad, N.M.
112, A, B	1169622: Parosteal sarcoma. R. J. Kurth, U.S.A.F. M.C., Wilford Hall Air Force Hospital, Lackland Air Force Base, Tex.
112, C	962302: Parosteal sarcoma. Chief of Radiology, Group Health Hospital, Seattle, Wash.
113	1011399: Parosteal sarcoma. L. H. Hansen, M.D., Mercy Hospital, Denver, Colo.
114	1200785: Parosteal sarcoma. S. G. Parker, M.D., Decatur, Ill.
115	1166130: Parosteal sarcoma. Chief of Radiology, Veterans Administration Center, Wichita, Kan.
116	840231: Parosteal sarcoma. R. H. Baehr, M.D., A. T. & S. F. Hospital Association, Topeka, Kan.
117, A, B	1011792: Parosteal sarcoma. H. Murphy, M.D., Murphy-Jones Orthopedic Clinic, Little Rock, Ark.
117, C	1071994: Parosteal sarcoma. P. R. Dirkse, M.D., St. Francis Hospital, Peoria, Ill.
118	1138854: Parosteal sarcoma. E. W. Rice, M.D., King's Daughters Hospital, Martinsburg, W.Va.
119	1027447: Parosteal sarcoma. M. Eskridge, M.D., Mobile Infirmary, Mobile, Ala.
120	740221: Parosteal sarcoma. J. M. Morgan, M.D., Veterans Administration Hospital, Birmingham, Ala.
121	1072072: Myositis ossificans. K. R. Gross, M.D., Lakewood General Hospital, Tacoma, Wash.
122	1100080: Myositis ossificans. J. R. Matheson, M.D., Utah Valley Hospital, Provo, Utah.
123	1084305: Myositis ossificans. W. Lawrence, M.D., Veterans Administration Hospital, Shreveport, La.
124	1174968: Myositis ossificans. Drs. Adkins, Bunting, Friedlander, and Pederson, Bishop Clarkson Memorial Hospital, Omaha, Neb.
125, A, B	1024980: Myositis ossificans. R. Terry, M.D., Strong Memorial Hospital, Rochester, N.Y.
125, C-E	1209621: Myositis ossificans.

Figure	
	Chief of Radiology, St. Anne's Hospital, Chicago.
126	1172087: Myositis ossificans. W. T. Mezaros, M.D., Illinois Masonic Hospital Association, Chicago.
127	1171688: Myositis ossificans. G. R. Schultze, M.D., Baltimore.
128	1139372: Myositis ossificans. J. C. Crumley, M.D., Blount Professional Building, Knoxville, Tenn.
129	1159474: Myositis ossificans. L. Cordero, Jr., M.D., Universidad de Cuenca, Cuenca, Ecuador.
130	1087799: Myositis ossificans. E. H. Wicker, M.D., St. Michael's Hospital, Texarkana, Ark.
131, A, B	1162291: Osteoblastoma. L. C. Hamilton, U.S.A. M.C., Walter Reed General Hospital, Washington, D.C.
131, C, D	1141563: Osteoblastoma. J. S. Garrison, III, U.S.N. M.C., U.S. Naval Hospital, Portsmouth, Va.
132	1194334: Osteoblastoma. Chief of Radiology, Notre Dame Hospital, Montreal, Canada.
133	1097658: Osteoblastoma. J. S. Garrison, III, U.S.N. M.C., U.S. Naval Hospital, Portsmouth, Va.
134	1127146: Osteoblastoma. L. C. Hamilton, U.S.A. M.C., Walter Reed General Hospital, Washington, D.C.
135, A	1164270: Osteoblastoma. W. Kennedy, M.D., Anderson Memorial Hospital, Anderson, S.C.
135, B	1111241: Osteoblastoma. J. H. Payne, M.D., Ireland Army Hospital, Fort Knox, Ky.
136	1189453: Osteoblastoma. Chief of Radiology, U.S. Air Force Hospital, Travis Air Force Base, Calif.
137, A, B	708055:Osteoid osteoma. E. P. McKeown, M.D., Tripler Army Hospital, Honolulu, Hawaii.
137, C, D	1163873: Osteoid osteoma. R. Curry, M.D., Orange Memorial Hospital, Orlando, Fla.
138, A, B	111591: Osteoid osteoma. R. J. Atkinson, M.D., U.S. Air Force Hospital, Elmendorf, Alaska.
138, C, D	1143115: Osteoid osteoma. S. Rogoff, M.D., University of Rochester, Rochester, N.Y.
139, A, B	1157466: Osteoid osteoma. G.

Figure	
	F. Monzingo, U.S.A. M.C., Sandia Base Hospital, Albuquerque, New Mexico.
139, C, D	1179739: Osteoid osteoma. Chief of Radiology, Klinik Sonnehof, Bucherstrasse, Bern, Switzerland.
140, A, B	1177642: Osteoid osteoma. T. Dixon, Jr., U.S.A. M.C., Kenner Army Hospital, Fort Lee, Va.
140, C, D	1169564: Osteoid osteoma. Chief of Radiology, DeWitt Army Hospital, Fort Belvoir, Va.
141	1130688: Ewing's sarcoma. C. R. Hoffman, M.D., Medical Towers Building, Louisville, Ky.
142, A	1136657: Ewing's sarcoma. Chief of Radiology, Wheelock Memorial Hospital, Goodrich, Mich.
142, B	1154814: Ewing's sarcoma. D. E. Chandler, U.S.N. M.C., U.S. Naval Hospital, San Diego, Calif.
143	704565: Ewing's sarcoma. W. F. Hansen, U.S.N. M.C., U.S. Naval Hospital, San Albans, Long Island, N.Y.
144	1136228: Ewing's sarcoma. Chief of Radiology, Elliot Community Hospital, Keene, N.H.
145	1163189: Ewing's sarcoma. L. A. Davis, M.D., Children's Hospital, Louisville, Ky.
146	1042686: Ewing's sarcoma. R. D. Gregory, Jr., M.D., Memorial Mission Hospital, Asheville, N.C.
147	1062430: Ewing's sarcoma. J. Ziskind, M.D., Veterans Administration Hospital, New Orleans, La.
148	1154985: Ewing's sarcoma. R. E. Campbell, M.D., Colbert County Hospital, Sheffield, Ala.
149, A	933964: Ewing's sarcoma. M. W. Olson, U.S.N. M.C., U.S. Naval Hospital, Oakland, Calif.
149, B	1080037: Ewing's sarcoma. H. Plenk, M.D., St. Marks Hospital, Salt Lake City, Utah.
150, A	957122: Ewing's sarcoma. Chief of Radiology, Fort Eustis, Va.
150, B	1208176: Ewing's sarcoma. G. F. Dobel, U.S.N. M.C., U.S. Naval Hospital, Great Lakes, Ill.
151	1154417: Ewing's sarcoma. L.

Figure	
	C. Hamilton, U.S.A. M.C., Walter Reed General Hospital, Washington, D.C.
152	1163562: Ewing's sarcoma. P. E. Duvall, M.D., U.S. Naval Hospital, Memphis, Tenn.
153	871328: Reticulum cell sarcoma. E. Spiro, M.D., General Hospital, Portsmouth, Ohio.
154	1114607: Reticulum cell sarcoma. P. J. Trier, M.D., Veterans Administration Center, Des Moines, Iowa.
155	1119586: Reticulum cell sarcoma. J. H. Urich, M.D., Little Company of Mary Hospital, Evergreen Park, Ill.
156	1101897: Reticulum cell sarcoma. C. J. Romeo, M.D., Veterans Administration Center, Dublin, Ga.
157	1218013: Reticulum cell sarcoma. O. T. Stone, M.D., U.S. Air Force Hospital, Kessler Air Force Base, Miss.
158, A	692946: Reticulum cell sarcoma. S. P. Barden, M.D., Leila Hospital, Battle Creek, Mich.
158, B	584949: Reticulum cell sarcoma. H. Plenk, M.D., St. Marks Hospital, Salt Lake City, Utah.
159	517287: Reticulum cell sarcoma. J. H. Walker, M.D., The Mason Clinic, Seattle, Wash.
160	1145778: Reticulum cell sarcoma. L. C. Hamilton, U.S.A. M.C., Walter Reed General Hospital, Washington, D.C.
161	1115234: Reticulum cell sarcoma. Chief of Radiology, Columbia Hospital of Richland County, Columbia, S.C.
162	1178414: Reticulum cell sarcoma. N. R. Blemly, U.S.N. M.C., Walter Reed General Hospital, Washington, D.C.
163	964210: Reticulum cell sarcoma. Drs. Foster, Graham & Darling, O'Connor Hospital, San Jose, Calif.
164	1149932: Reticulum cell sarcoma. L. C. Hamilton, U.S.A. M.C., Walter Reed General Hospital, Washington, D.C.
165	1121118: Myeloma. G. E. Irwin, Jr., M.D., Brokaw Hospital, Normal, Ill.
166	866032: Solitary myeloma. E. Fox, M.D., Veterans Administration Hospital, Sioux Falls, S.D.
167	1067267: Solitary myeloma. Chief of Radiology, St. Mary's Hospital, Rochester, N.Y.
168	1161437: Angioendothelial tumor. J. Allen, M.D., Charleston General Hospital, Charleston, W. Va.
169	993910: Angiosarcoma. O. K. Stewart, M.D., Duke University Medical Center, Durham, N.C.
170	1059558: Angiosarcoma. S. B. Sternlieb, M.D., Wilkes-Barre, Pa.
171, A, B	1154127: Ossifying hemangioma. K. Morris, M.D., Shaw Air Force Base, S.C.
171, C	1221607: Ossifying hemangioma. R. H. Keller, M.D., Murray, Utah.
172	1195234: Angioendothelial tumor. S. M. Rogoff, M.D., Strong Memorial Hospital, Rochester, N.Y.
173	1117951: Angioma. E. R. Jacobs, M.D., National Orthopedic & Rehabilitation Hospital, Arlington, Va.
174, A	1048447: Nodular synovitis. C. J. Romeo, M.D., Veterans Administration Center, Dublin, Ga.
174, B	1003495: Nodular synovitis. Chief of Radiology, Lakeview Clinic, Suffolk, Va.
175	986518: Nodular synovitis. C. L. Dale, M.D., Hinsdale Sanitarium and Hospital, Hinsdale, Ill.
176, A	1173903: Synovial osteochondromatosis: O. E. Crews, U.S.N. M.C., U.S. Naval Hospital, San Francisco.
176, B	1094632: Synovial osteosarcoma. S. H. Macht, M.D., Washington County Hospital, Hagerstown, Md.
177, A	1139304: Synovial chondrosarcoma. J. C. Osmer, M.D., Ireland Army Hospital, Fort Knox, Ky.
177, B	1159465: Synovial chondrosarcoma. E. Ferrington, M.D., Veterans Administratoin Center, Jackson, Miss.
178, A	1220441: Synovial sarcoma. C. B. Reiner, M.D., Children's Hospital, Columbus, Ohio.
178, B	910828: Synovial sarcoma. R.

Contributors of AFIP Radiographs / 441

Figure	
	J. Wagner, M.D., Augustana Hospital, Chicago.
179	1050813: Adamantinoma. J. T. McClellan, M.D., St. Joseph Hospital, Lexington, Ky.
180	1122932: Adamantinoma. J. B. McAneny, M.D., Mercy Hospital, Johnstown, Pa.
181	1144688: Adamantinoma. F. L. Sturrock, M.D., Royal Colombian Hospital, New Westminster, Canada.
182, A, B	1209110: Chordoma. W. R. Pollard, M.D., William Beaumont General Hospital, El Paso, Tex.
182, C	950076: Chordoma. H. C. Dangle, M.D., St. John's Hospital, Springfield, Ill.
183, A	807795: Chordoma. O. H. Sauls, M.D., Veterans Administration Hospital, Indianapolis, Ind.
183, B	1165358: Chordoma. R. Terry, M.D., University of Rochester Medical Center, Rochester, N.Y.
184, A	1033960: Lipoma. R. Peterson, U.S.A. M.C., Fitzsimons General Hospital, Denver, Colo.
184, B, C	1058001: Lipoma. A. S. Katz, U.S.A.F. M.C., Headquarters 862nd Medical Group, Minot Air Force Base, N.D.
185	982228: Lipoma. W. J. Miller, M.D., Lafayette Home Hospital, Lafayette, Ind.
186	1068166: Myxolipoma. W. E. Harrison, Jr., M.D., Crippled Children's Service, Phoenix, Ariz.
187	1128364: Osteosarcoma. E. M. Wright, M.D., St. Mary's Hospital, Saginaw, Mich.
188	1180666: Metastatic cancer. J. McClellan, M.D., St. Joseph Hospital, Lexington, Ky.
189	1199710: Metastatic tumor. Chief of Radiology, Veterans Administration Hospital, Nashville, Tenn.

Index

An asterisk (*) indicates reference to an illustration.

A

ADAMANTINOMA(S)
  of femur, 418–19
  of fibula, 414–15
  in long bones—sites, 17
  in specific bones, 11
  of tibia, 416–17

AGE
  significance in diagnosis, 9
  and visibility of bone destruction, 34, 36*

ANGIOENDOTHELIAL TUMOR(S)
  of humerus, 390–91
  of ilium, 398

ANGIOMA: of lumbar spine, 399

ANGIOSARCOMA(S)
  of fibula, 394–95
  of humerus, 392–93

ANTRUM: ossifying fibroma of, 194–95
ARTERIOGRAPHY: evaluation, 358

ASTRAGALUS
  chondrosarcoma of, 226–27
  giant cell tumor of, 94–95
  osteoid osteoma of, 328–29

B

BAYES'S CONCEPT: definition, 4*
BAYES'S RULE OF INVERSE PROBABILITY, 66

BONE(S)
  cancellous—reduction of density in, 42, 131*
  flat—tumor locations in, 17
  long—Decision Tree for tumors in, 74*
  medullary—Decision Trees for tumors in, 73*, 75, 76*
  proliferation, *see* Proliferation
  shaft—Decision Tree for tumors in, 76*
  spongy
    destruction—visibility, 34, 35*
    Ewing's sarcoma in—with mottled proliferation, 50*, 348–49
    tumor matrix mineralization resembling, 29
    trabecular—metastasis to, rate factors, 52*
  tumor bone, *see* Calcification *and* Tumor Matrix Mineralization

BONE DESTRUCTION WITH TUMOR, 33 ff.
  combined patterns, 42
  and cortical penetration, 44
  geographic, 38, 39–41*, 42 ff., 49*
  and growth rate estimation, 44, 59
  kinds and significance, 38 ff.
  moth-eaten, 39*, 42, 43*
    vs. permeative, 366
    width, and growth rate, 42
  vs. normal aging loss, 34
  permeative, 42, 43*
    vs. moth-eaten, 366
  punched-out lesion of multiple myeloma, 42
  in spongy bone—visibility, 34, 35*
  terminology, 38
  visibility, 33 ff.

BUTTRESS: of periosteal proliferation, 48*, 53

C

CALCANEUS: tumor location in, 18
CALCIFICATION IN TUMORS
  see also Tumor Matrix Mineralization
  in cartilaginous tumors, 27 ff.
  evaluation, 26 ff.
  in necrotic fat with tumors, 32
  in necrotic tissue, 32, 348

CARPAL(S): tumor in—Decision Tree, 79*

CHONDROBLASTOMA(S)
  of femur, 240–43, 246–47
  flocculent calcification in, 32
  of humerus, 236–39
  hyperostoses with, 53, 54*
  in long bones—sites, 15
  rate factors, 49*
  size, 24
  of tibia, 236–39, 244–45

CHONDROMA
  benign, of thumb, 254–55
  flocculent calcification in, 32
  of humerus, 250–51
  periosteal
    of clavicle, 252–53
    of toes, 246–49
  synovial, of finger, 248–49
  of tibia, 250–51

CHONDROSARCOMA
  age and, 9
  of astragalus, 226–27
  bone and cartilage in, 30, 32
  of clavicle, 208–209
  consistency and contour, 40
  of femur, 216–17, 230–31
    arising in a benign lesion, 222–23
    arising in calcified enchondroma, 212–13
  of humerus, arising in calcified enchondroma, 220–21
  of ilium, 206–207
  ossified edge of, 32
  of pelvis, 214–15, 224–25, 232–35
  of pubis, 218–19
  rate factors, 49*
  of ribs, 218–19, 228–29
  synovial, of fingers, 408–409
  of tibia, 228–29
  velvety spiculation of, 57, 58*
CHORDOMA(S)
  of sacrum, 422–23
  of spine, 420–23
CLAVICLE
  bone cyst of, 136–37
  giant cell tumor of, 96–97
  periosteal chondroma of, 252–53
  reticulum cell sarcoma of, 364–65
  tumors in—Decision Tree, 74*
CLEAVAGE PLANE: with extraosseous mass, 32, 33*
CODMAN'S TRIANGLE, 48*, 55
  and growth rate, 61
COMPUTER DIAGNOSIS
  Hollerith cards for, 8
  image analysis, 4
  principles, 3 ff.
  probability
    and size of specific tumors, 24
  protocol, 7
    physical characteristics, 8
CONSISTENCY AND CONTOUR OF TUMOR: relationship, 40
CORTEX (OF BONE)
  displacement of bone through, 45*, 46
  expanded, of periosteal proliferation, 50*, 53
  penetration by tumor, 44 f.
    with geographic destruction, 44
  tumors centered in—Decision Tree, 72*
CORTICAL DEFECT, BENIGN
  in long bones—sites, 16
  size, 24
CYST(S), BONE
  aneurysmal, 80
  classification, 80
  of clavicle, 136–37
  consistency, 40
  of femur, 134–35, 138–39
  of fibula, 132–33
  of humerus, 122–23
    expanding, recurrent, 126–29
  of ilium, 124–25, 138–39
  of pelvis, 140–41
  of radius, 120–21, 142–43
  recurrent, 80, 126–29
  of tibia, 136–37
  of ulna, 122–23
CYSTOMA, 80

D

DECISION TREE, 67 ff.
  diagrams, 69 ff.
  and tumor location, 68
DESMOIDS, CORTICAL: of femur, 198–203
DISPLACEMENT PHENOMENON, 45*, 46

E

ENCHONDROMA
  chondrosarcoma (ossifying) arising in, in femur, 212–13
  in humerus, 220–21
  of dorsal spine, 254–55
  in tibia, fibrosarcoma in, 162–63
ENDOSTEAL ENVELOPE—BONE PROLIFERATION IN, see Proliferation of Bone
EPIPHYSIS: tumor centered in—Decision Tree, 76*
EWING'S SARCOMA
  age in differential diagnosis, 9
  bone proliferation with, 50*, 52, 57
  calcification in, 32
  of femur, 338–39, 356–57
  of fibula, 340–43
  general characteristics, 59
  hair-on-end spiculation of, 56*, 339*
  of humerus, 346–47, 350–51
  of metatarsal, 344–45
  of pelvis, 348–49
  of pubis, 356–57, 360
  rate factors, 48*, 50*
  of rib, 352–53
  of tibia, 340–41, 358–69
EXTRAOSSEOUS MASS
  cleavage plane, 32, 33*
  ossified edge, 32, 33

F

FAT NECROSIS: with calcification in tumors, 32

FEMUR
    adamantinoma of, 418–19
    bone cysts of, 134–35, 138–39
    bone destruction in, 35 f.*
    chondroblastomas of, 240–43, 246–47
    chondromyxoid fibroma of, 168–69
    chondrosarcomas of, 216–17, 230–31
        arising in benign lesion, 222–23
        arising in calcified enchondroma, 212–13
    cortical desmoids of, 198–203
    Ewing's sarcomas of, 338–39, 356–57, 361–63, 370–75
    fibrosarcomas of, 156–57, 164–65
    fibroxanthomas of, 186–89, 192–93
    giant cell tumors of, 84–93, 100–101
    lipoma of, 426–27
    myositis ossificans of, 296–99, 312–13
    myxolipoma of, 428–29
    osteoid osteoma of, 328–29, 332–33
    osteosarcomas of, 262–67, 270–71, 276–77
        with metastasis to opposite femur, 262–63
    parosteal sarcomas of, 278–89
    shaft—tumor in, Decision Tree, 76*
    solitary myeloma of, 388–89
    villonodular synovitis of, 404–405
FIBROMA(S)
    chondromyxoid
        consistency and contour, 40
        of femur, 168–69
        of fibula, 172–73, 178–79
        in long bones—sites, 16
        of os calcis, 182–83
        of pelvis, 170–71, 176–77
        of radius, 168–69
        rate factors, 48*
        of rib, 182–83
        size, 24
        of tibia, 176–77, 180–81
        of ulna, 174–75
    nonossifying
        in long bones—sites, 16
        size, 24
    ossifying
        of antrum, 194–95
        matrix mineralization of, 30
        periosteal, of radius, 190–91
FIBROSARCOMA(S)
    age and, 9
    amorphous periostosis of, 57
    bone destruction of, 40*
    classification, 81
    differentiation from giant cell tumor, 110
    displacement phenomenon with, 46

    of femur, 156–57, 164–65
    of fibula, 150–51, 158–59, 166–67
    of frontal bone, 146–47
    grading of growth rate, 64
    of os calcis, 148–49
    ossified edge of, 32
    of pubis, 160–61
    of scapula, 150–51
    of tibia, 152–55, 166–67
        arising in old enchondroma, 162–63
FIBROXANTHOMA(S)
    of femur, 186–89, 192–93
    in long bones—sites, 16
    of metatarsal, 190–91
    rate factors, 48*
    size, 24
    of tibia, 184–89
FIBULA
    adamantinoma of, 414–15
    angiosarcoma of, 394–95
    chondromyxoid fibromas of, 172–73, 178–79
    Ewing's sarcomas of, 340–43
    fibrosarcomas of, 150–51, 158–59, 166–67
    giant cell tumors of, 110–11
        cystic, 132–33
    hemangioma (ossifying) of, 396–97
    parosteal sarcoma of, 290–91
    tumor in—Decision Tree, 76*
FINGER(S)
    chondrosarcoma of, 210–11
    hemangioma (ossifying) of, 396–97
    myositis ossificans of, 304–11
    osteoid osteoma of, 334–35
    synovial chondroma of, 248–49
    synovial chondrosarcomas of, 408–409
FOOT (FEET)
    synovial sarcoma of, 410–11
    tumors in—Decision Trees, 74*, 71*
FRACTURE, PATHOLOGIC
    distinction from displacement, 46
    and tumor, 45
FRONTAL BONE
    fibrosarcoma of, 146–47
    fibrous osteoma of, 194–95

G

GIANT CELL TUMOR(S)
    anatomic relationship in bone, 18
    of astragalus, 94–95
    bone destruction of, 39*
    of cervical spine, 106–109
    classification, 81
    of clavicle, 96–97

GIANT CELL TUMOR(S) (*cont.*)
  consistency and contour, 40, 41*
  cystic
    of pelvis, 118–19
    of tibia, 130–31
  differentiation from fibrosarcoma, 110
  of femur, 84–93, 100–101
  of fibula, 110–11
  of humerus, 102–103
  in long bones—sites, 15
  of metacarpal, 112–13
  of metatarsal, 94–95
  of os calcis, 114–15
  of pelvis, 116–19
  of radius, 102–103
  rate factors, 50*
  of rib, 98–99
  of sacrum, 104–105
  of tibia, 130–31
GROWTH RATE
  IA, 61, 62*
  IB, 61, 62*
  IC, 61, 62*
  II, 61, 62*
  III, 61, 62*
  assessment of, 59 ff.
  and cortical penetration by tumor, 44
  grading, 59 ff.
    criteria, 59
  Paget's disease with tumor—effect on, 14
  and pathologic fracture, 45
  and patterns of bone destruction, 44
  tabulation of tumors, 68
  Truth Table, 60, 61

H

HANDS: tumors in—Decision Trees, 74*, 76*
HEMANGIOMAS (OSSIFYING)
  of fibula, 396–97
  of finger, 396–97
HIP: reticulum cell sarcoma of pelvis and, 370–71
HISTOLOGIC DIAGNOSIS OF TUMOR
  Decision Tree, 67 ff.
  prediction of, 65 ff.
  relation to site in bone, 18, 23*
HONEYCOMBING: of periosteal proliferation, 53, 55*
HUMERUS
  angioendothelial tumor of, 390–91
  angiosarcoma of, 392–93
  bone cysts of, 122–23
    expanding, with recurrence, 126–29
  chondroblastoma of, 236–39
  chondroma of, 250–51
  chondrosarcoma of, in calcified enchondroma, 220–21
  Ewing's sarcomas of, 346–47, 350–51
  giant cell tumor of, 102–103
  lipomas of, 424–25
  metastasis from prostatic carcinoma, 434–35
  osteosarcoma of, 268–69, 274–75
    with Paget's disease, 430–31
  reticulum cell sarcoma of, 376–77
  shaft—tumor in, Decision Tree, 76*
HYPEROSTOSIS: of periosteal proliferation, 53, 54*

I

ILIUM
  angioendothelial tumor of, 398
  bone cysts of, 124–25, 138–39
  chondrosarcoma of, 206–207
  reticulum cell sarcoma of, 380–81
ILLUSTRATED DICTIONARY OF TERMINOLOGY, 7, 8 ff.
IMAGE ANALYSIS, 4
ISCHIUM
  Ewing's sarcoma of, 360–61
  myositis ossificans of, 314–15

J

JOINT(S), TUMORS IN
  see also specific sites
  Decision Tree, 79*
  sites in, 16*
    axial position of center, 12*

K

KNEE
  synovial osteochondromatosis of, 406–407
  synovial osteosarcoma of, 406–407
  villonodular synovitis of, 402–403

L

LAMINATED NEW BONE, 48*, 54
LIPOMA(S)
  of femur, 426–27
  of humerus, 424–25
LOCATION OF TUMOR, 10 ff.
  axial position of center, 11 ff.
    axial—Decision Tree, 70*
  cortical penetration, 11
    estimated fraction of tumor outside bone, 13

and Decision Tree, 68
and histologic type—relation of, 11
in joint, 12*
significance in radiograph, 10 f.
in special bones, 18 ff.
in tubular bones, 15 ff.
LONG BONES, *see* Tubular Bones

M

MANDIBLE
   tumor in—Decision Tree, 77*
   tumor sites in, 18, 21*
MAXILLA: tumor in—Decision Tree, 78*
METACARPAL
   giant cell tumor of, 112–13
   osteoblastoma of, 324–25
METASTASES
   in humerus from prostatic carcinoma, 434–35
   from osteosarcoma of femur to opposite femur, 262–63
   in tibia from lung tumor, 432–33
   to trabecular bone—rate factors, 52*
METATARSAL
   Ewing's sarcoma of, 344–45
   fibroxanthoma of, 190–91
   giant cell tumor of, 94–95
MINERALIZATION, *see* Tumor Matrix Mineralization
MYELOMA
   amyloid calcification of, 32
   of skull, 386
   solitary
      of femur, 388–89
      of pelvis, 387
MYOSITIS OSSIFICANS
   of femur, 296–99, 312–13
   of fingers, 304–11
   of ischium, 314–15
   matrix mineralization of, 30, 31*
   vs. parosteal sarcoma, 82
   of radius, 300–301
   of ulna, 302–303
MYXOLIPOMA: of femur, 428–29

O

OCCIPUT: osteoblastoma of, 316–17
ONION-PEEL PATTERN, 54, 339*
OS CALCIS
   chondromyxoid fibroma of, 182–83
   fibrosarcoma of, 148–49
   giant cell tumor of, 114–15
   tumor in—Decision Tree, 77*
   tumor sites in, 18, 21*

OSSIFIED EDGE OF EXTRAOSSEOUS MASS, 32, 33*
OSTEOBLASTOMA(S)
   of cervical spine, 322–23
   contour, 41*
   of metacarpal, 324–25
   ossified edge of, 32
   of radius, 324–25
   of sacrum, 320–21
   of skull
      inner table, 318–19
      occiput, 316–17
   of tibia, 326–27
   tumor matrix, 30
   of vertebrae (cervical), 316–17
OSTEOCHONDROMA: in long bones—sites, 16
OSTEOCHONDROMATOSIS: synovial, of knee, 406–407
OSTEOMA(S)
   of astragalus, 328–29
   of femur, 332–33
   fibrous
      of frontal sinus, 194–95
      of skull, 196–97
   osteoid
      diffuse sclerosis of, 55*
      of femur, 328–29
      of finger, 334–35
      fleck of calcium in, 29*
      size, 24
      of tibia, 330–33
OSTEOSARCOMA(S)
   age and, 9
   bone and cartilage in, 30, 31*
   of femur, 262–67, 270–71, 276–77
      with metastasis to opposite femur, 262–63
   of humerus, 268–69, 274–75
   in Paget's disease, 430–31
   periosteal lamination of, 54*
   rate factors, 48*
   in specific bones, 11
   spiculation of, 56*
   synovial, of knee, 406–407
   of tibia, 258–61, 272–73

P

PAGET'S DISEASE
   with neoplastic bone—effect on growth rate, 14
   osteosarcoma of humerus in, 430–31
PAROSTEAL TUMORS
   Decision Tree, 71*
   grading of, 63

PELVIS
    bone cyst of, 140–41
    chondromyxoid fibroma of, 170–71, 176–77
    chondrosarcomas of, 214–15, 224–25, 232–35
    Ewing's sarcoma of, 348–49
    giant cell tumor of, 116–17
    reticulum cell sarcomas of, 368–71
    solitary myeloma of, 387
    tumor in—Decision Tree, 77
    tumor location in, 18, 19*
PERIOSTEAL ENVELOPE—BONE PROLIFERATION IN, see Proliferation of Bone
PERIOSTOSIS, see Proliferation of Bone, periosteal
PROBABILITY: and size of specific tumors, 24
PROBABILITY MATRIX, 65
    Bayes's rule of inverse probability, 66
PROLIFERATION OF BONE, 46 ff.
    in endosteal envelope, 47 ff.
        as diffuse sclerosis, 51, 55*
        as endostosis, 53, 54*
        as mottled density, 50*, 52
        as sclerotic rim, 51
        time factor in, 51
    in growth rate estimation, 59
    in periosteal envelope, 53 ff.
        amorphous response, 55*, 57
        buttress, 48*, 53
        coarse, 48*, 50*, 56*, 57 f.
        delicate, 48*, 50*, 54*, 56*, 57 f., 350
        expanded cortex, 50*, 53
        hyperostosis, 53, 54*
        lamination, 48*, 54
        onion-peel pattern, 54
        septation, 50*, 53
        spiculation, 56*, 57 ff.
        time factor in appearance, 53
        tumor encapsulation by, 57
    and qualitative factors, 46, 54–55*
    and rate factors, 46 ff.
    time of visualization, 47
PUBIS
    chondrosarcoma of, 218–19
    cystic giant cell tumor of, 118–19
    Ewing's sarcomas of, 356–57, 360
    fibrosarcoma of, 160–61
PUBLIC MODEL, 4*, 6 ff.

Q

QUALITATIVE FACTORS, 46, 54–55*

R

RADIUS
    bone cyst of, 120–21, 142–43
    chondromyxoid fibroma of, 168–69
    giant cell tumor of, 102–103
    myositis ossificans of, 300–301
    osteoblastoma of, 324–25
    periosteal fibroma of, 190–91
    shaft—tumor in, Decision Tree, 76*
RATE FACTORS: and bone proliferation, 46 ff.
RIB(S)
    chondromyxoid fibroma of, 182–83
    chondrosarcomas of, 218–19, 228–29
    Ewing's sarcoma of, 352–53
    giant cell tumor of, 98–99
    synovioma of vertebra and, 410–11
    tumors in—Decision Tree, 74*

S

SACRUM
    chordoma of, 422–23
    giant cell tumor of, 104–105
    osteoblastoma of, 320–321
    tumor in—Decision Tree, 79*
SARCOMA(S)
    see also Ewing's Sarcoma
    parosteal
        age and, 9
        cleavage plane of, 32, 33*
        of femur, 278–89
        of fibula, 290–91
        vs. myositis ossificans, 82
        of skull, 294–95
        spiculation of, 56
        of tibia, 288–89, 292–93
    pleomorphic—classification, 82
    reticulum cell
        age in differential diagnosis, 9
        amorphous periostosis of, 57
        calcification in, 32
        of clavicle, 364–65
        differentiation, 82
        of femur, 361–63, 370–75
        of hip and pelvis, 370–71
        of humerus, 376–77
        of ilium, 380–81
        of pelvis, 368–69
        —and hip, 370–71
        of tibia, 366–67, 378–79, 382–85
    synovial, of foot, 410–411
SCAPULA
    fibrosarcoma of, 150–51
    tumor in—Decision Tree, 77*
    tumor location in, 18, 19*

SCLEROSIS: diffuse, as tumor sign, 51, 55*
SEPTATION: of periosteal proliferation, 50*, 53
SESAMOID(S): tumor in—Decision Tree, 79*
SHAPE OF TUMOR: significance in diagnosis, 24*, 25
SINUSES, PARANASAL
  antrum—ossifying fibroma of, 194–95
  frontal
    fibrosarcoma of, 146–47
    fibrous osteoma of, 194–95
SIZE OF TUMOR
  and probability for specific tumors, 24
  significance in diagnosis, 23 ff.
SKULL
  see also Sinuses, paranasal
  fibrous osteoma of, 196–97
  inner table—osteoblastoma of, 318–19
  myeloma of, 386
  occipital osteoblastoma, 316–17
  parosteal sarcoma of, 294–95
  tumor in—Decision Tree, 78*, 79*
  tumor sites in, 22 f.
SOFT TISSUES
  calcification with tumors, 32
  tumors—grading of, 63
SPICULATION (PERIOSTEAL), 56*, 57 f.
SPINE
  see also Vertebral Body and Sacrum
  bone destruction in, 37*
  cervical
    chordomas of, 420–23
    giant cell tumors of, 106–109
    osteoblastoma of, 322–23
  chordomas of, 420–23
  dorsal, enchondroma of, 254–55
  lumbar
    angioendothelial tumor of, 398
    angioma of, 399
  tumor sites in, 20
STERNUM: tumor in—Decision Tree, 79*
SYNOVIOMA: of vertebra and rib, 410–11
SYNOVITIS, VILLONODULAR
  of femur, 404–405
  of knee, 402–403
  of toe, 402–403

T

TARSAL(S): tumor in—Decision Tree, 79*
TERMINOLOGY, 7, 8 ff.
  buttress, 48*, 53
  central position of center, 11, 12*
  clouds of tumor mineralization, 30, 31*
  coarse periosteal response, 57
  cortical position of tumor, 11, 12*
  delicate periosteal response, 57, 350
  eccentric position of tumor, 11, 12*
  expanded cortex, 50*, 53
  flecks of mineralization, 29*, 30
  flocculent mineralization, 28*, 29
  geographic bone destruction, 39, 39–41*, 42 f., 49*
    ill-defined edge, 38
    lobulated edge, 38, 41*
    nibbled (ME) edge, 38, 41*
    ragged or irregular edge, 38
    regular edge, 38, 40*
  ground-glass mineralization, 30
  hair-on-end spiculation, 56*, 57
  ill-defined bone destruction, 38
  lobulated bone destruction, 38, 41*
  lumps (tumor mineralization), 30, 31*
  ME (nibbled) bone destruction, 38, 41*
  moth-eaten bone destruction, 39*, 42, 43*
  mottled proliferation, 52
  nibbled (ME) bone destruction, 38, 41*
  parosteal position of tumor, 11, 12*
  permeated bone destruction, 42, 43*
  probability matrix, 65
  public model, 6
  qualitative factors, 46
  rate factors, 46
  reticulate contour or pattern, 40, 41*
  solid mineralization, 29, 30*
  sunburst spiculation, 56*, 57
  veillike mineralization, 30, 31*
  velvety spiculation, 57, 58*
THUMB: benign chondroma of, 254–55
TIBIA
  adamantinoma of, 416–17
  bone cyst of, 136–37
  bone destruction, 35*
  chondroblastomas of, 236–39, 244–45
  chondroma of, 250–51
  chondromyxoid fibromas of, 176–77, 180–81
  chondrosarcoma of, 228–29
  Ewing's sarcomas of, 340–41, 358–69
  fibrosarcomas of, 152–55, 166–67
    arising in old enchondroma, 162–63
  fibroxanthoma of, 184–89
  giant cell (cystic) tumor of, 130–31
  metastasis from lung tumor, 432
  osteoblastoma of, 326–27
  osteoid osteomas of, 330–33
  osteosarcoma of, 258–61, 272–73
  parosteal sarcomas of, 288–89, 292–93
  reticulum cell sarcomas of, 366–67, 378–79, 382–85
  shaft—tumor in, Decision Tree, 76*

TOE(S)
  osteoid osteoma of, 334–35
  periosteal chondromas of, 246–49
  villonodular synovitis of, 402–403
TROCHANTER: tumor in—Decision Tree, 76*
TRUTH TABLE, 60, 61
TUBULAR BONE(S)
  quadrants of circumference involved by tumor, 17
  tumor in—Decision Tree, 74*
  tumor location in, 15 ff.
TUMOR(S)
  see also Location, Shape, Size, etc., *and* specific types
  angioendothelial
    of humerus, 390–91
    of ilium, 398
  calcification in, evaluation, 26 ff.
  cartilaginous—calcification in, 27 ff.
  classification, 80 ff.
  in differential diagnosis (Decision Tree), 67
  displacement phenomenon, 45*, 46
  encapsulation by periosteal new bone, 57
  growth rates (tabulation), 68
  increased density
    see also Tumor Matrix Mineralization factors related to, 25
  parosteal, *see* Parosteal Tumors
  of soft tissues, *see* Soft Tissues
TUMOR MATRIX MINERALIZATION, 26 ff.
  see also Calcification
  in cartilaginous neoplasms, 27 ff.
  flocculent pattern, 28*, 29
    tumors typified by, 32
  in growth rate estimation, 59
  in neoplastic bone, 29 ff.
  patterns, 29 ff.
  resembling spongy bone, 29

U

ULNA
  bone cyst of, 122–23
  chondromyxoid fibroma of, 174–75
  myositis ossificans of, 302–303
  shaft—tumor in, Decision Tree, 76

V

VERTEBRAE; VERTEBRAL BODIES
  cervical—osteoblastoma in, 316–17
  in giant cell tumors
    of cervical spine, 106–109
    of sacrum, 104–105
  synovioma of, 410–11
  tumor sites in, 20, 21*